MW01659787

STUDENT HANDBOOK

MASSAGE THERAPIST

EDITION 2

ELSEVIER
SAUNDERS

CCi
CORINTHIAN
COLLEGES, INC.

ELSEVIER
SAUNDERS

3251 Riverport Lane
Maryland Heights, Missouri 63043

MASSAGE THERAPIST STUDENT HANDBOOK ISBN: 978-1-4377-2580-3
A Custom Publication for Corinthian Colleges

Chapters 1–4, 6–8, and 10–12 from Haroun L: Career Development for Health Professionals, ed 3, Philadelphia. Copyright © 2011, Saunders.

Chapters 5 and 9 from Palau SM and Meltzer M: Learning Strategies for Health Careers Students, Revised edition, St. Louis. Copyright © 2007, Saunders.

Appendix A from Fordney MT: Insurance Handbook for the Medical Office, ed 11, St. Louis. Copyright © 2010, Saunders.

Portions of Appendix B from Bonewit-West K: Clinical Procedures for Medical Assistants, ed 7, St. Louis. Copyright © 2008, Saunders.

Portions of Appendix B from Young AP and Proctor DP: Kinn's The Medical Assistant, ed 10, St. Louis. Copyright © 2007, Saunders.

Portions of Chapter 13–16, 19, and 20 from Fritz S: Mosby's Fundamentals of Therapeutic Massage, ed 4, St. Louis, Copyright © 2009, Mosby.

Portions of Chapter 13, 17, and 19 from Salvo SG: Massage Therapy: Principles and Practice, ed 3, St. Louis, Copyright © 2007, Saunders.

Portions of Chapter 18 from Fritz S and Grosenbach MJ: Mosby's Essential Sciences for Therapeutic Massage: Anatomy, Physiology, Biomechanics, and Pathology, ed 3, St. Louis, Copyright © 2009, Mosby.

Portions of Chapter 18 from Fritz S and Grosenbach MJ: Mosby's Essential Sciences for Therapeutic Massage: Anatomy, Physiology, Biomechanics, and Pathology, ed 2, St. Louis, Copyright © 2004, Mosby.

ISBN 978-1-4377-2580-3

Acquisitions Editor: Scott Weaver
Developmental Editor: Stephanie Roulias
Publishing Services Manager: Gayle May
Project Manager: Stephen Bancroft
Design Direction: Teresa McBryan

Printed in Canada

Last digit is the print number: 9 8 7 6 5 4 3 2 1

CREDITS

Editor and Project Manager

Jeffrey A. Simancek, BS, LMT, NCBTMB, Curriculum Manager, Massage Therapy & Fitness Training, Santa Ana, CA

Some material in this book is adapted from the following sources:

Chapters 1–4, 6–8, and 10–12 from *Career Development for Health Professionals*, 3rd edition, Lee Haroun, 2011, Saunders, Philadelphia.

Chapters 5 and 9 from *Learning Strategies for Health Careers Students*, Revised edition, Susan Marcus Palau and Marilyn Meltzer, 2007, Saunders, St. Louis.

Appendix A from *Insurance Handbook for the Medical Office*, 11th edition, Marilyn T. Fordney, 2010, Saunders, St. Louis.

Portions of Appendix B from *Clinical Procedures for Medical Assistants*, 7th edition, Kathy Bonewit-West, 2008, Saunders, St. Louis.

Portions of Appendix B from *Kinn's The Medical Assistant*, 10th edition, Alexandra P. Young and Deborah P. Proctor, 2007, Saunders, St. Louis.

Portions of Chapter 13–16, 19, and 20 from *Mosby's Fundamentals of Therapeutic Massage*, 4th edition, Sandy Fritz, 2009, Mosby, St. Louis.

Portions of Chapter 13, 17, and 19 from *Massage Therapy: Principles and Practice*, 3rd edition, Susan G. Salvo, 2007, Saunders, St. Louis.

Portions of Chapter 18 from *Mosby's Essential Sciences for Therapeutic Massage: Anatomy, Physiology, Biomechanics, and Pathology*, 3rd edition, Sandy Fritz and M. James Grosenbach, 2009, Mosby, St. Louis.

Portions of Chapter 18 from *Mosby's Essential Sciences for Therapeutic Massage: Anatomy, Physiology, Biomechanics, and Pathology*, 2nd edition, Sandy Fritz and M. James Grosenbach 2004, Mosby, St. Louis.

CONTENTS

About Corinthian Colleges, Inc. (CCi)

Corinthian Colleges, Inc. was founded in 1995 and completed an initial public offering in 1999. As of June 30, 2009, Corinthian Colleges, Inc. operated 89 schools in 24 states, operated 17 schools in the province of Ontario, Canada, and served the large and growing segment of the population seeking to acquire career-oriented education. Through hard work, dedication, and vision, Corinthian Colleges, Inc. is managed by an experienced executive team with considerable industry, operations, marketing, financial, and regulatory knowledge.

The mission of Corinthian Colleges, Inc. is to help students prepare for new careers or to advance in their chosen careers. With more than 86,088 students as of June 30, 2009, Corinthian Colleges, Inc. is one of the largest post-secondary educational companies in North America and Canada. Corinthian Colleges, Inc. offers short-term diploma programs and associate's, bachelor's, and master's degrees for occupations in demand. Corinthian Colleges, Inc. main program areas include healthcare, criminal justice, business, information technology, transportation technology and maintenance, and construction trades. In addition, Corinthian Colleges, Inc. offers online degree programs that include business, accounting, criminal justice, paralegal, and information technology.

GROWTH STRATEGY

Our growth strategy consists of the following components:

Enhance Growth and Existing Campuses

Integrated and Centralized Marketing Program. We employ an integrated marketing program that utilizes an extensive direct response advertising campaign delivered through television, the Internet, newspaper, and direct mail. A professional marketing staff at our campus support center coordinates marketing efforts with advertising agencies and utilizes our in-bound call center and our lead-tracking capability.

Curriculum Expansion and Development. We develop, refine, and acquire curricula based on market research and recommendations from our faculty, advisory board members, and our curriculum development team. We believe considerable opportunities exist for curriculum adoption and we expect to continue to acquire and develop new curricula and selectively adopt existing curricula into both existing and new locations. In fiscal 2009, we successfully implemented 114 programs into existing U.S. schools and Canadian schools.

Facilities Enhancement and Expansion. We remodel, expand, and relocate our existing colleges to ensure we have sufficient capacity to meet our expected enrollment demand, as well as to improve the location and appearance of our facilities. We believe modern attractive education environments enhance our students' learning experience. During fiscal 2009, we remodeled, relocated, or expanded 10 colleges. As of June 30, 2009, the total square footage of all our properties was approximately 4.6 million square feet.

Expand Online Education

As of June 30, 2009 we offer 326 online courses through 33 campuses. We serve approximately 15,157 online students.

OPERATING STRATEGY

Key elements of Corinthian Colleges, Inc. operating strategy include the following components:

Emphasize Student Outcomes. Corinthian Colleges, Inc. believes that positive student outcomes are a critical component of our long-term success. Accordingly, Corinthian Colleges, Inc. devotes substantial resources to maintaining and improving the retention and placement rates. Corinthian Colleges, Inc. has implemented a variety of student service programs, including orientation and tutoring, academic advising, ride-sharing, and referral programs, all of which are designed to improve student retention to assist our students in achieving their career goals. Utilization of a curriculum development team comprised of campus representatives, corporate program directors, and textbook publishers, which is assisted by the advisory board comprised of local business professionals, to help ensure that our curricula provide our students with the skills required by employers. Corinthian Colleges, Inc. has also maintain dedicated career services personnel at the schools that undertake extensive placement efforts, including identifying prospective employers, helping students prepare resumes, conducting practice interviews, establishing externship programs, and tracking students' placement success on a monthly basis.

Create a Supportive Learning Environment. Corinthian Colleges, Inc. views the students as customers and seeks to provide a supportive learning environment where student satisfaction is achieved. The wide variety of campuses offer flexible schedule of classes, providing our students with the opportunity to attend classes throughout the day, as well as nights and weekends. Schools operate year-round, permitting students to complete their course of study quickly. The campuses maintain reasonable class sizes and focus the efforts of our faculty on teaching students rather than research. Personal interaction between students and faculty is encouraged, and we offer several support programs, such as on-campus advising and tutoring, which are designed to help students successfully complete their courses of study. Corinthian Colleges, Inc. also maintains a toll-free student hotline to address and help resolve student concerns.

CCI BRANDS

Corinthian Colleges changes lives by providing students the skills they need to pursue the careers they want. This is done through two distinct school brands. Each brand was developed to offer essential skills and training to students in a variety of practical fields.

Everest

Everest campuses offer diploma and/or degree programs in the health care, business, and computer technology career field. There are over 106 Everest campuses located across the United States and Canada. Popular programs include medical assisting, accounting, business administration, dental assisting, massage therapy, medical insurance billing and coding, paralegal, and pharmacy technician.

Everest includes the following:

Everest College
Everest College of Business, Technology and Health Care (Canada)
Everest Institute
Everest University
Everest University Online, a division of Everest University
Everest College Online, a division of Everest College Phoenix

WyoTech

WyoTech is dedicated to college-level, career-oriented education in the automotive, diesel, motorcycle, watercraft, HVAC, electrician, and plumbing fields. The WyoTech campuses are located in: Blairsville, Pennsylvania; Daytona, Florida; Fremont, California; Laramie, Wyoming; Long Beach, California; and Sacramento, California.

Unlike traditional post-secondary institutions, we provide an education that is focused on the job-oriented needs of nontraditional students in a learning environment that fosters on-the-job success. We also go one step further by helping our graduates find the right jobs and, in the process, helping employers find the skilled workers they need.

Heald College

Established in 1863, Heald College is the nation's oldest business college in the Western United States, with such notable alumni as A.P. Giannini, founder of Bank of America; Trader "Vic" Bergeron, famous restaurateur, and Hiram Johnson, former California governor.

Heald has 11 campuses which are regionally accredited by the Accrediting Commission for Community and Junior Colleges of the Western Association of Schools and Colleges (WASC), an institutional accrediting body recognized by the Council for Higher Education Accreditation and the U.S. Department of Education. For more than 145 years, Heald has been an innovative leader in providing career-oriented education to students who have made the decision to begin their careers. This proud tradition continues at Healds' eleven campuses in California, Oregon, and Hawaii offering programs in fields of Healthcare, Business, Legal, and Technology.

Operational Structure

Operations at all Corinthian locations are coordinated through the executive vice president of operations, divisional presidents, regional vice presidents of operations, and regional vice presidents of admissions.

At the campus level, an academic dean or education director as well as admissions, placement, and finance directors assist a college president; the staff at corporate headquarters oversees the student body, individual campuses, and regional and divisional territories.

Integration Process. Acquired and new branch campuses have been successfully integrated into our operational structure since the original founding of the company. Prior to purchasing or opening a new campus, we develop intensive infrastructure and marketing plans to ensure a smooth transition, as well as optimize capital expenditures and marketing and acquisition investments.

On-line Education

Online education, or education delivered via the Internet, has become an increasingly important component of the higher education market. The online programs are designed to prepare students for successful employment in the workplace. The courses emphasize real-world training that is tailored to meet the needs of potential employers. Corinthian Colleges offer online learning to two categories of students: those attending online classes exclusively and those attending a blend of traditional classroom and online courses. The majority of our students participating in online learning are now registered in exclusively online programs.

Corinthian Colleges, Inc. began enrolling exclusively online students through our Florida Metropolitan University (FMU) colleges in fiscal 2002. In the fourth quarter of fiscal 2005, we started to offer exclusively online degrees through our regionally accredited Everest College in Phoenix, Arizona. Online degree programs are offered in business, criminal justice, accounting, higher education management, criminal investigations, applied management, homeland security, computer information science, and medical insurance billing and coding. In total, 18 accredited degrees are available exclusively online at the master's, bachelor's, and associate's levels.

During fiscal 2009, Corinthian Colleges, Inc. experienced a significant increase in the number of students taking our online courses. Our online learning participation increased by approximately 25% to 181,909 course registrations in fiscal 2009. As of June 30, 2009, Corinthian Colleges, Inc. offered 326 online courses through 33 campuses serving approximately 15,157 exclusively online students.

MISSION STATEMENT

We create, acquire, and operate educational units that deliver quality instruction at a fair price, while maintaining full regulatory compliance and ensuring an appropriate financial return to investors.

CHAPTER 1

Your Career Starts Now

YOUR FIRST STEP ON THE ROAD TO SUCCESS

"Today is the first day of the rest of your life."

Congratulations! By choosing to study for a career in health care, you have taken the first step toward achieving a productive and satisfying future. You have made a significant commitment to yourself and your community. By enrolling in an educational program, you have demonstrated your ability to set your sights on the future, make important decisions, and follow through with action. You have proven you have the strong personal foundation on which you can build the skills and habits needed to ensure your success in school and in your career.

The purpose of this book is to help you succeed in this building process by sharing the knowledge and techniques that have helped other students achieve their goals. It is written with the hope that you will apply what you learn here to maximize your investment in education, secure the job that you want after graduation, and find satisfaction in your career as a competent and caring health care professional.

CONNECTING SCHOOL AND CAREER

The process of becoming a health care professional began the day you started classes. In addition to providing you with opportunities to learn important technical skills, this process involves acquiring the attitudes, personal characteristics, and habits of a successful professional. What you think and do while in school will determine, to a great extent, the quality of the professional you will become. Students who demonstrate good work habits in school generally carry those same habits into the workplace. The opposite is true, too. Students who practice poor conduct in school tend to struggle on the job. You are faced with a great opportunity to determine your future. Your career has indeed started now.

The organizational and study skills presented in this handbook are designed to help you succeed in school. But they can also be applied to your professional and personal life. In fact, the term "study skills" is misleading, because these skills are not isolated sets of activities restricted to school situations. "Study skills" have many applications on the job. Let's look at four skills that will be discussed more fully in future chapters. Each one can be applied to your studies, your job search, and your future work in health care.

1. **Time management.** For busy people, time is one of the most precious possessions. Juggling class attendance and study time with family responsibilities, work, and personal time involves **prioritizing** and careful planning. Your success in school depends heavily on how well you organize your time.

   An effective job search typically requires you to devote time each day to identifying leads, making appointments, attending interviews, and completing follow-up activities. You must allocate adequate amounts of time for these efforts and organize your time to avoid delays that could cost you employment opportunities.

   Once you are on the job, effective use of time is critical in health care work. Many health care professionals are responsible not only for their own time, but also for planning other people's time. Medical assistants, for example, are often in charge of the physician's daily appointment scheduling, a task that can affect the profitability of the practice. Insurance coders and billers must submit claims on time to avoid rejections and financial losses. Nurses who have patient care responsibilities must plan a schedule that permits them to complete these during their shifts.
2. **Oral communication.** Strong communication skills are essential to success. Expressing yourself clearly is important for giving presentations, as well as for asking and answering questions in class. It is also necessary for establishing and maintaining satisfactory relationships with your instructors and classmates.

   A critical part of the job search process is the interview, in which you combine your ability to think clearly and use verbal skills effectively. Feeling confident about expressing yourself will enable you to present your qualifications in a convincing way.

All jobs today require good communication skills. This is especially true in health care because many positions involve constant interaction with others, including patients, co-workers, supervisors, and the general public. Physical and occupational therapy assistants are examples of the many health professionals who provide extensive patient education. The effectiveness of their explanations of exercises and self-care techniques influences the rehabilitation progress of their clients.

3. **Taking notes.** You may think of note-taking as being limited to use in lectures, but this skill is used extensively outside the classroom. During the job search, it will be important to accurately record information about job openings, as well as interview appointment dates and times and directions to facilities. After interviews, you may want to make notes about the job requirements, additional information you need to send to the prospective employer, and other important facts.

   When you become employed, you will be expected to absorb a lot of new information about your facility's rules and procedures, the location of supplies and equipment, people's names, and many other details. You can use your note-taking skills to create a personal reference notebook, a resource that will increase your efficiency on the job. Note-taking is also an important health care job skill. Many professionals are responsible for interviewing patients and taking notes on special forms called *patient histories*. Another specialized form of medical note-taking is called *charting*. Charting means making notes on patient medical records, in either written or electronic form. The notes include information about symptoms, treatments, and medications prescribed. These medical records not only affect patient care, but they also are legal documents. They must be clear, accurate, and complete.

4. **Taking tests.** You may think you have escaped the dreaded test once you leave school, but testing is not limited to the classroom. The truth is that life is full of tests. Job interviews are a form of test designed to assess your ability to present yourself and your qualifications. To legally work in many health care occupations, such as licensed practical nurse, radiologic technologist, and physical therapist, you must pass a professional exam. Other occupations, such as medical assistant, have voluntary tests to obtain certification that improves your chances of getting a job. In fact, many employers hire only certified medical assistants.

   Once on the job, you are in a sense, being tested every day. Although you may not think of your everyday tasks as tests, they are applications of what you have learned, and your ability to perform them correctly will be noted by your patients, co-workers, and supervisor. The annual employee performance evaluation may be considered a type of test in which your supervisor writes a report about your work and then meets with you to discuss it. Learning to perform "when it counts" is a valuable skill and represents the ultimate ability to take and successfully pass a test. The mother of an infant wants to know that the health care professional giving the injection has "passed the test" and is qualified to safely perform this task.

   From these examples you can see that skills traditionally labeled as personal or school skills have valuable applications during the job search and on the job. Throughout this book you will continue to see how "school skills" are also valuable job skills.

MAXIMIZING YOUR EDUCATION

You are making a significant investment of time, effort, and money in your education. You can simply get by, doing only what is required to pass your classes, or you can fully benefit from this investment. A worthy personal goal is to do everything possible to become the best health care professional possible. Both you and your school have responsibilities to ensure that this happens.

Your Rights as a Student

"Making mistakes is inevitable. Not learning from them is inexcusable."

1. **Make mistakes.** You may think this sounds a little strange. After all, aren't you supposed to do the best you can, earning the highest grades possible? Yes, but many students see grades as ends in themselves, rather than as signs of having mastered the skills they will need in the future. Good grades do not guarantee mastery, nor do you receive grades for all the skills that will determine your future success.

   Many students want to know "what's on the test" so they can focus their efforts on learning only what they will be tested on. But think about it—can you possibly be tested on everything you will need to know and do to perform your job? If you were, all class time would have to be devoted to testing, leaving little or no time for learning! Studying only what you need to pass tests and earn grades may make you a "good student," but a good student is not necessarily a good health care professional.

   Compare your educational experience with learning to ride a bike. First, you use training wheels, go slowly, and tip over once in a while. Eventually you become a proficient cyclist, ready for the big race. School offers you a rehearsal for professional life, providing you with opportunities to learn from mistakes that would be unacceptable if you were to make them on the job. If you do not score 100% on an exam, it has still served you by allowing you to make mistakes and learn from them so you avoid making them on the job when the consequences are more serious. A health care worker may have made mistakes when she practiced working with a classmate, but she learned from them and is now able to use correct techniques to help her patients.

2. **Ask questions.** You are attending school to benefit from the knowledge and experience of your instructors. Take advantage of this opportunity by being an active participant in your classes. Don't be an invisible student. Even if the textbooks and lectures are excellent, you may still need to ask for explanations, examples, and additional resources. If there is anything you don't understand, ask questions. Students aren't expected to understand everything the first time they hear or read it—maybe not even the second time. Consider this: there would be no need for you to attend school at all if you already knew the information presented in your program.

   Many adults are afraid of "looking stupid" and hesitate to admit they don't understand or are confused. However, failure to ask questions not only decreases the chances of maximizing your education, it prevents you from learning a critical health care skill—asking questions. Consider the serious consequences for professionals who are not sure of drug dosages or steps in a procedure but are afraid to ask their supervisors for direction. In these situations, risking the well-being of patients is indeed stupid, whereas asking questions demonstrates intelligence. Start learning now to be comfortable asking questions. If it is too difficult for you to speak up in class the first few times you have questions, start out by speaking with your instructor at the break, after class, or during office hours.

   Of course, you should not use questions to substitute for reading your textbook or studying assigned material before each class meeting. This results in the misuse of class time and is unfair to students who are prepared. A related on-the-job example is employees who arrive late and unprepared for meetings, thus wasting their co-workers' time. Develop habits that show consideration for others and will contribute now to the efficiency of the classroom and later to that of the workplace.

3. **Take advantage of school resources.** Every school wants every student who enrolls to graduate, and considerable resources are spent on services to support this effort. Find out now what services are available to you, the hours they can be accessed, and whether appointments are necessary. Two of the most important services that all students should become familiar with are the library (or resource center) and career services (sometimes called *job placement*).

   If you are having personal problems or academic difficulties, ask whether your school provides counseling and/or tutoring. Some schools refer their students to outside agencies that offer assistance for difficulties such as dealing with domestic abuse and finding reliable child care. Asking for help when you need it can make the difference between dropping out and graduating and becoming successfully employed.

   The school catalog is an often overlooked information resource that can help you succeed in school. Many students never take the time to read it and as a result are unaware of available resources. Even worse, they risk unknowingly breaking rules or missing important deadlines. Spend a few minutes becoming an informed student by reading the catalog and other printed information. On the job, you will likely be expected to read organizational handbooks and procedure manuals. Getting in the habit of reading informational literature is a good job skill.

Your Responsibilities as a Student

1. **Attend all scheduled learning activities.** Health care educational programs feature a variety of learning opportunities including lectures, lab sessions, guest speakers, field trips, and hands-on experiences in health care facilities. Your instructor may also recommend additional activities outside of those organized by the school, such as watching a television documentary, attending a professional meeting, or visiting a medical supply company. These activities are designed to help you understand and master all the knowledge and skills necessary for your future work, as well as to provide exposure to your future work environment. You cannot afford to miss them. They are opportunities to develop the competencies essential for working in health care. Learning to perform essential tasks, such as the administration of injections, requires you to spend time and put forth effort under the guidance of your instructors. Now is the time for learning and making mistakes, not when you are faced with your first patient. Someday you will be performing tasks that affect the well-being of others, so it is essential that you fully participate in every learning activity offered in your program.

   Employers routinely request information about a student's attendance record. Good attendance is considered a valuable job skill because health care services are driven by time requirements. The success of a private physician's practice depends heavily on efficient patient scheduling and service. Hospitals have daily responsibilities for performing hundreds of treatments, procedures, and surgeries that must be completed in a timely way. In both settings, effective care can be provided only if the staff is available to do the work. Patients who need help should not have to wait because someone didn't show up. Start now to develop the habit of consistent and punctual attendance.

2. **Apply your best efforts to learning.** As a student, you have the right to ask questions and make mistakes. At the same time, it is your responsibility to complete all reading, writing, and lab assignments and to participate actively in class. Instructors cannot cover everything you are expected to know. Learning will require effort on your part. The study techniques and suggestions for learning presented in the following chapters are intended to help you succeed as a student.

   In performing your work as a health care professional, you will encounter new situations in which you will apply what you learned in school. To be successful in those situations, you must now focus on your studies, work hard, and be persistent. Your willingness to do the "shoulds" when you would rather be doing the "wants" will be a major determinant of your success. You will not always feel like studying after a day that may include classes, a few hours on the job, and family responsibilities. Being a college student is not always easy. Keeping your long-term career goals clearly in mind will help you find the self-discipline to stick with it.

3. **Ask for help when you need it.** Instructors and administrators want to see their students succeed. Educators are interested in helping students complete their programs and graduate. At the same time, you must take responsibility for requesting assistance. Ignoring problems will not solve them; they usually only get worse. Don't wait until you are hopelessly lost in a class and cannot possibly be ready for the upcoming final exam before asking for help. Take charge of your learning and at the first sign of trouble, ask about tutoring, study groups, computer labs, and any other resources available through the school.

   If you experience problems of a personal or financial nature, refer to the list of school resources you prepared in Prescription for Success 1-2. Remember that asking for help when you need it is a sign of strength, not weakness, and it is one of the main actions that distinguish a graduate from a dropout.

   The flip side of asking for help is being willing to give it. Offer your assistance to others in the school community. Volunteer to hand out papers for the instructor. Give a student who lives in your area a ride to school. Tutor a classmate who is struggling with a subject you find easy. (This doesn't mean sharing your work; it means helping the other person understand and learn.) You have chosen a profession that is based on giving service, and this is a habit you can start practicing now in all areas of your life. Students who give of themselves are the type of people who become indispensable employees.

PLANNING FOR CAREER SUCCESS

The time to start thinking about your first job in health care is now, as you are starting your educational program. In the following pages, we look at how you can use job search tools, such as a resume, to help guide you to a successful career.

PERSONAL REFLECTION

What are some other ways you can take responsibility for your own learning so that you succeed in your health care program?

____

____

____

____

____

And the Product Is... You!

Marketing is a multi-step process that begins with an idea for a new product and ends with the sale of that product. Mastering this process is essential for the survival of any business. Successful marketing is similar to successfully starting a new career. You—the combination of your skills, characteristics, and talents—are the product. To make sure you have the skills and qualities needed by employers, you must prepare appropriately for the workplace and learn to present yourself effectively during the job search.

The marketing process can be organized into a five-part plan called the "Five Ps of Marketing," as follows:

1. Planning
2. Production
3. Packaging
4. Presentation
5. Promotion

You can use the 5 Ps to develop your own personal marketing plan now, as you begin your health care studies, to help ensure future career success. We will discuss the first P, planning, in this chapter and the remaining four Ps in Chapter 11.

PLANNING: THE FIRST "P" OF MARKETING

"Give yourself a running start."

Studying the needs of customers is called *market research*, and its purpose is to find out what customers want. Your customers will include your future employers and patients. Waiting until the end of your educational program to think about getting a job is like creating a product without doing market research. Designing and manufacturing a product that no one wants or needs doesn't make sense. Just like a business, you are investing time, effort, and money in the development of yourself as a product.

What Do Employers Want?

In recent years, employers in all industries have expressed concerns that entry-level workers are not adequately prepared for the modern workplace. Employers are looking for job candidates who not only are qualified technically, but who also bring essential supporting skills such as the ability to communicate effectively, work cooperatively with others, accept responsibility, and solve problems. These skills are especially critical in the health care industry because it is service-based and depends heavily on the quality of its personnel. This is even truer today as health care facilities strive to provide higher quality care and control costs.

National Health Care Skill Standards. A project of special interest to future health care professionals is the National Health Care Skill Standards, a list of entry-level worker competencies. Box 1-1 contains examples that apply to all health care occupations. You can see that they are not limited to technical skills, such as taking blood pressure, but include the ability to communicate, maintain good attendance, and demonstrate responsibility. Some employers report that these so-called "soft skills" are as important as technical skills in the provision of good health care.

Did you notice how many standards mention the ability to communicate well? The lack of effective communication skills among health care workers is reportedly the leading contributor to patient dissatisfaction and personnel problems in health care facilities. Your future success can be greatly enhanced by your ability to listen and to convey information effectively.

Professional Organizations. Many of the professional organizations that represent specific health care occupations have statements outlining the characteristics needed to work in their fields.

BOX 1-1 Examples of the National Healthcare Foundation Standards and Accountability Criteria

Health care workers will:

- Apply speaking and active listening skills
- Summarize basic professional standards of health care workers as they apply to hygiene, dress, language, confidentiality, and behavior
- Exemplify professional characteristics
- Engage in continuous self-assessment and career goal modification for personal and professional growth
- Apply ethical standards in health care
- Demonstrate respectful and empathetic interactions with diverse age, cultural, economic, ethnic, and religious groups
- Recognize methods for building positive team relationships
- Apply behaviors that promote health and wellness
- Recognize technology applications in health care[1]

What Do Patients Want?

"Patients do not care how much you know until they know how much you care."

Patients want to receive competent care delivered with consideration and respect. When seeking health care, people are often at their most vulnerable. They fear what might be discovered during a diagnostic test or that they will experience pain during a necessary treatment. The self-esteem of patients can be threatened by a feeling of powerlessness that often accompanies illness and injury.

Many patients want to participate in making decisions about their care. They have the right, both ethically and legally, to be fully informed about their condition, treatment options, and possible outcomes. Health care professionals must give clear explanations in everyday language and offer patients the opportunity to ask questions and receive honest answers. At the same time, patients want and have the legal right to confidentiality. As a health care professional, you must guard the privacy of your patients. Without the patient's permission, nothing can be discussed with anyone other than the health care team members directly involved with the patient's care, and all files and paperwork must be securely stored and electronic records protected.

Changes in American society and increasing costs of providing medical care have brought special challenges for patients and for health care professionals. In the past, many people had the same physician throughout their lives. Doctor and patient belonged to the same community, and a sense of trust developed over the years. Patients today may see a different physician each time they visit their health care facility. They may face a serious illness or life-threatening situation in the care of a stranger, adding to the stress of an already difficult situation. Studies have shown that patients who belong to a caring, supportive community recover more successfully than patients who don't. Providing a supportive health care community can improve patient outcomes. As a health care professional, you can demonstrate a caring attitude that helps develop a bond of trust with patients by being attentive, listening carefully, and practicing empathy.

Health care professionals today face the challenge of working with patients from many different ethnic backgrounds, some of whom have beliefs about health care practices that differ from those of traditional Western medicine. Patients also come from many different economic and social groups. They may have lifestyles or personal beliefs with which you disagree. All patients have the right to be respected and to receive appropriate, high-level care, regardless of your personal opinions about them. Every patient deserves your best efforts.

Patients seek help in solving their health problems, but your responsibilities in meeting their needs go beyond performing a painless blood draw, giving effective breathing treatments, or sending out accurate bills for payment. You must be willing to combine a caring attitude with technical competence by treating each patient as worthy of your full attention. Studies have found that even if a health professional excels in one area, poor communication skills or the appearance of not caring can cause patients to view that person negatively.[2]

The Patient Care Partnership. Health care organizations have formally recognized the rights of patients to receive proper care. The American Hospital Association has written a brochure for patients, entitled "The Patient Care Partnership: Understand Expectations, Rights and Responsibilities," which is used by many health care facilities nationwide. These include, among others, the rights of patients to do the following:

- Be treated with compassion and respect
- Receive information about the benefits and risks of treatments
- Have their privacy protected
- Participate in making decisions regarding their care, including the right to refuse treatment
- Have their health goals and values taken into account as much as possible

What Do You Want?

"If you don't know where you're going, chances are you'll end up somewhere else."

In addition to exploring the needs of your "customers" —your employers and patients—an important part of planning is to identify what *you* want. You must consider your own needs and desires as you create your professional self. The clearer you are about your career goals and expectations, the greater the chance you have of achieving them.

Beginning now to think about your specific career goals and workplace priorities will keep you alert to appropriate employment possibilities as you go through your educational program. Take every opportunity during your studies to observe, ask questions, and read about your field. Then compare your findings with your own interests. Many fields in health care today feature newly created positions and expanded responsibilities for traditional jobs. A wide variety of choices is available for new graduates. Being aware of these opportunities improves your chances of finding employment that matches your interests and preferences.

Developing a Philosophy of Work. Most of us spend a significant number of our waking hours on the job. How we spend that time determines, to a great degree, the quality of our lives. It makes sense, then, to think about what work means to you. Exploring your personal beliefs will help you increase the amount of satisfaction you get from your career. The following list contains a variety of reasons why people work[3]:

- Survive financially
- Define self
- Gain self-respect
- Demonstrate competence
- Gain power
- Help others
- Learn
- Experience variety
- Contribute to the community
- Experience enjoyment
- Fill time

People are generally happiest and most productive when their work provides them with more than material rewards. Some people are motivated by continual challenges, others value consistency, and still others are content with either condition as long as their work allows them to help others.

Health care is a complex, ever-changing field that offers both opportunities and challenges for those who choose to work in it. Here are some of the major sources of satisfaction you can expect.

1. **Meaningful work.** Good health is a basic need for both human survival and happiness. Working in a field that promotes health gives you the opportunity to make meaningful contributions to the well-being of others. Whether you provide direct patient care or perform supporting activities, your work directly affects patients, and the quality of your work can truly make a difference in their lives. A career in health care has purpose and value.
2. **Opportunity to serve.** People seek the services of health care professionals when they need help. They come with the hope that you can help them solve their problems, and they entrust themselves to your care. You have opportunities to enter both the physical and emotional space of others, sharing close personal contact. People who are ill or injured are often afraid and anxious. You are in a position to influence their recovery.
3. **Career stability.** The need for health care will always exist, even if job titles change over time. The reorganization taking place in today's health care delivery systems is causing continual shifts in the need for specific occupational positions. A decrease in the number of job openings for one position is often bal-

anced by an increase in another. You may need to redefine your job in the future, but you will always have a solid knowledge base on which you can add the experience or training needed to qualify for new positions.

4. **Interesting work environment.** The world of health care is changing at a rapid rate, both scientifically and organizationally. Advances in our understanding of how the body works, along with discoveries about the causes and treatments of diseases, are reported almost daily. Computers have increased our capacity to collect and organize information and are sophisticated tools that are constantly being upgraded. Medical scientists are making discoveries at an astounding rate. You will witness advances in knowledge that extend and improve the quality of human life. The health care environment is never boring. There will be a steady stream of interesting information to learn, apply, and use.
5. **Opportunities for advancement.** The health care field provides many opportunities for upward mobility if you are willing to continue learning and adding to your skills. Many jobs offer opportunities for on-the-job learning that enable you to increase your value to your patients and employer, as well as your eligibility for promotion. In addition, many occupational specialties in health care present the chance for **career laddering.** Career ladders contain jobs within one occupational area that require different levels of knowledge and skills. The higher-level positions almost always require further education and additional certifications or licenses, which are official approvals for working in a specific occupation.

Work Preferences. It is also a good idea to begin thinking about the kinds of tasks you like to do and the working conditions you prefer. A wide variety of work settings exists for health care professionals. Being clear about your own preferences will help you choose and prepare for the most appropriate types of positions in your career area.

Alignment with Employers

Although it is important to try to meet your personal needs when seeking employment, you must also have realistic expectations. An essential activity in career planning is to compare your work preferences with the needs of potential employers to see how well they match. Students sometimes have unrealistic goals for the positions they hope to fill immediately after graduation. Recent graduates are qualified for entry-level positions. You can avoid frustration and disappointment if you understand the workplace and adjust your expectations. This way, you can maximize the benefits of your first work experiences in health care.

Formal training is only the beginning of your journey to developing competence as a health care professional. Your skills will continue to grow and be refined as you accumulate hands-on practice and everyday experience in the field. When starting a new career, it may be wise—even necessary—to trade your "perfect job" requirements for opportunities that lead to long-term career success. Consider looking for a first-time job in which you can do the following:

1. Gain self-confidence
2. Work with a variety of people
3. Acquire additional knowledge
4. Increase your skill base
5. Explore specialties within your field of interest
6. Network with other professionals
7. Demonstrate your abilities

Your first employer is giving you the gift of his or her confidence in your abilities. You will be entrusted with serious responsibilities that may include patient welfare, accuracy and confidentiality of important records, and other matters that influence the reputation and success of the facility. You will have a chance to prove your value by learning as much as possible, finding ways to help your employer and co-workers, and contributing to the overall success of the organization. Entry-level jobs, performed well, can be the first important step leading to positions that meet all your hopes for a fulfilling career.

Alignment with Your Profession

Health care professions vary in the type of work performed. You need to be aware of the daily tasks and working conditions of the occupation you have chosen. For example, respiratory therapy and radiology require the technical aptitude to work with complex equipment. Occupational therapy requires the ability to apply oral communication skills to teach patients and their families. Health information technology and insurance coding require accuracy and attention to detail when creating, filling out, and organizing medical records and forms.

You may need to consider tradeoffs to obtain a balance that offers maximum career satisfaction. For example, a recent nursing graduate who wants the excitement of a hospital emergency room and the convenience of a 9:00 AM to 5:00 PM weekday schedule may have a conflict. To avoid a mismatch between your expectations and the real world, learn as much as possible about the specific requirements of your future profession so you can rethink and reprioritize your requirements, if necessary.

Adjusting your short-term expectations doesn't mean giving up your long-term goals. In fact, purposeful planning now can help you arrive where you want to be in the future. If you discover that the specific type of job you want requires previous work experience, you can set short-term goals to serve as stepping stones to acquire that experience. Find out now what skills are emphasized in your target position and look for opportunities to learn as many of them as possible during your studies, clinical experience, and first job. For example, Rosa wants to work as a back-office medical assistant with a plastic surgeon, helping the physician with outpatient procedures. Her research shows there are only a few plastic surgeons in her area and they prefer to hire assistants with previous work experience. Rosa decides to look for a job with a general practitioner or pediatrician who does minor surgery in the office. Her short-term goals are to gain experience with sterile technique, standard precautions, surgical assisting, and patient care. While in school, she asks her instructor to recommend books and articles about plastic surgery and to allow her to spend extra practice time in the lab so she can reach a high level of competence with sterile technique, surgical instruments, wound care, and related topics.

Employees who are willing to meet the expectations of their employers are often rewarded with additional (and interesting) responsibilities and promotions. Some employers even create new positions so they can use the talents of their employees. For new health care professionals who are well prepared and who contribute enthusiastically to the success of their employers, entry-level jobs can serve as launch pads for career success. You, too, may benefit by having new and interesting responsibilities added to your job description, receiving a promotion, or having a job created that brings you satisfaction. Serving the needs of others can provide you with opportunities to meet your own needs.

To Learn More

About.com: Health Careers
http://healthcareers.about.com
This web page contains links to articles about choosing and succeeding in a health care career.

American Hospital Association: *The Patient Care Partnership*
www.aha.org/aha/issues/Communicating-With-Patients/pt-care-partnership.html.
This brochure contains an explanation of the rights of hospitalized patients.

Covey SR: *The 7 habits of highly effective people*, New York, 2004, Free Press.
This popular book lists seven principles that help individuals live effective lives. Students may find it helpful to learn about the seven habits, which are as follows:

- Habit 1: Be Proactive: Principles of Personal Choice
- Habit 2: Begin with the End in Mind: Principles of Personal Vision
- Habit 3: Put First Things First: Principles of Integrity and Execution
- Habit 4: Think Win/Win: Principles of Mutual Benefit
- Habit 5: Seek First to Understand, Then to Be Understood: Principles of Mutual Understanding
- Habit 6: Synergize: Principles of Creative Cooperation
- Habit 7: Sharpen the Saw: Principles of Balanced Self-Renewal

Explore Health Careers
www.explorehealthcareers.org
This noncommercial site contains general information about working in health care, as well as articles about specific careers.

Health Care Career Professional Organizations
All health careers have organizations that set standards and provide support and information for both students and working professionals. Many organizations are listed, along with contact information, in Appendix A.

National Consortium on Health Science and Technology and Technology Education
www.nchste.org
This website contains the foundation standards developed for health care students in all types of career programs. Reviewing these standards will give you an idea of what employers expect of their employees.

U.S. Department of Labor: *Occupational Outlook Handbook*
www.bls.gov/oco
This is a source of detailed information about hundreds of careers, including typical job descriptions, educational requirements, and average salaries. It is updated every 2 years.

REFERENCES

1. National Consortium on Health Science and Technology Education. "National Healthcare Foundation Standards and Accountability Criteria." www.nchste.org/cms/wp-content/uploads/2008/03/foundation_standards_ac_rev_01_08. (Accessed 2/13/09)
2. Anderson R, Barbara A, Feldman S: "What patients want: a content analysis of key qualities that influence patient satisfaction." www.drscore.com/press/papers/whatpatientswant.pdf (Accessed 2/9/09)
3. Binghang M, Stryker S: *Career choices and changes*, Washington, UT, 2005, Academic Innovations.

PRESCRIPTION FOR SUCCESS 1-1 RESOURCE TREASURE HUNT

When you need help, school services can seem like treasures. But to take advantage of everything your school has to offer, you must know about it. Take a tour of your school and record your findings for future reference. If your school does not offer all these services, find out if they are available elsewhere in the community.

Resource	Services Provided	How to Access and When Available
Advising or Counseling	______________	______________
Academic	______________	______________
Personal	______________	______________
Career Services	______________	______________
Job search assistance	______________	______________
School job fairs	______________	______________
Part-time jobs	______________	______________
Resume preparation	______________	______________
Interviewing skills	______________	______________
Employer contacts	______________	______________
Classes or workshops	______________	______________
Financial Aid	______________	______________
Information Sources and Referrals	______________	______________
Child care	______________	______________
Financial help	______________	______________
Transportation	______________	______________
Other	______________	______________
Learning Assistance	______________	______________
Learning center	______________	______________
Study skills	______________	______________
Instructors	______________	______________
Tutors	______________	______________
Other students	______________	______________
Study groups	______________	______________
Refresher and basic skills classes	______________	______________

PRESCRIPTION FOR SUCCESS 1-1 | RESOURCE TREASURE HUNT—cont'd

Resource	Services Provided	How to Access and When Available
Library	____________	____________
Books	____________	____________
Periodicals	____________	____________
Internet Access	____________	____________
Journals	____________	____________
Reference assistance	____________	____________
Other	____________	____________
Professional Organizations (student chapters)	____________	____________
School Organizations	____________	____________
Special interest groups	____________	____________
Social clubs	____________	____________
Service clubs	____________	____________
Special Needs and Referrals	____________	____________
Alcohol abuse	____________	____________
Drug dependency	____________	____________
Family planning	____________	____________
Domestic abuse	____________	____________
Other	____________	____________
Volunteer Opportunities	____________	____________

PRESCRIPTION FOR SUCCESS 1-2 | OVERCOMING OBSTACLES

1. List any obstacles that might interfere with your school attendance (e.g., problems with child care).

____

____

2. What can you do now to overcome these obstacles (e.g., find backup for child care)?

____

____

PRESCRIPTION FOR SUCCESS 1-3 | SELF-ASSESSMENT

How would you rate yourself on each of these general employment competencies? Fill out the following self-assessment guide as a first step in creating an action plan to fully develop the competencies most needed in the modern workplace. Check the column that best describes you.

	Sometimes	Seldom	Often
1. **Creative thinking:** I generate new ideas and come up with original approaches to everyday problems and situations.	______	______	______
2. **Decision making:** I gather information, identify alternatives, consider consequences, select an alternative, and evaluate the effectiveness of the results.	______	______	______
3. **Problem solving:** I recognize problems that need attention, identify possible solutions, create a plan, and carry out the plan.	______	______	______
4. **Continuous learning:** I am interested in knowing everything I can that will help me succeed in my work and life, and I try to keep up with advances that will help me to do so.	______	______	______
5. **Reasoning:** I understand the relationships among ideas and am able to apply them when learning and problem solving.	______	______	______
6. **Responsibility:** I am dependable and complete any tasks I am given or for which I volunteer.	______	______	______
7. **Self-worth:** I believe in myself and my ability to succeed.	______	______	______
8. **Empathy:** I make an effort to understand the experiences and feelings of others and to see situations from their points of view.	______	______	______
9. **Self-management:** I set personal goals, monitor my progress, and use self-discipline to ensure that I achieve them.	______	______	______
10. **Integrity:** I guide my actions by a set of principles that defines right and wrong.	______	______	______
11. **Honesty:** I tell the truth to myself and to others.	______	______	______

- Review the ratings you gave yourself, and list any areas you believe need further development.

____

____

____

- What can you start doing now to improve in these areas?

____

____

____

Success Tip: Review your completed assessment and self-development plan periodically to see how you are progressing.

PRESCRIPTION FOR SUCCESS 1-4 | THE IDEAL CANDIDATE

Imagine yourself running a clinic in a low-income neighborhood. You need to hire a health professional. You have found a candidate who appears to have the necessary technical skills and experience.

1. What are five other characteristics you would want the candidate to have?

____

____

2. Why did you choose these five characteristics?

____

____

Now answer the following questions for yourself:

3. Explain how understanding the needs of employers can help you to better prepare for your future career.

____

____

4. Which of your own personal qualities do you believe will be most valuable to future employers?

____

____

PRESCRIPTION FOR SUCCESS 1-5 | CHECK OUT YOUR PROFESSIONAL ORGANIZATION

Find the website of the professional organization for your chosen occupation. Read through the material and look for answers to the following questions:

1. What kinds of personal characteristics are needed to succeed in this occupation?

____

____

2. Are there characteristics mentioned that also appear in the SCANS and National Health Care Standards examples? If so, list them here.

____

____

3. On the basis of what you read, in your own words describe an ideal person for this occupation.

____

____

PRESCRIPTION FOR SUCCESS 1-6 | AND THE PATIENT IS...YOU

Imagine you have just arrived at an urgent care facility with a suspected broken arm. You were out for an enjoyable Sunday afternoon, skating with friends, when you hit a hole in the pavement and fell. Your arm is very painful, and you are worried about your ability to work if you end up in a cast.

1. Describe how you would feel if you found yourself in this situation.

2. How would you hope to be treated by the health care professionals at the urgent care center?

3. What would be most important to you?

4. What would be least important to you?

5. Did you learn anything from this exercise that might influence your approach to working with future patients?

PRESCRIPTION FOR SUCCESS 1-7 | MY PHILOSOPHY OF WORK

1. What meaning does work have for you?

2. What needs do you want to be filled by your work?

3. Why did you choose a career in health care?

4. What do you hope to accomplish?

5. What do you hope to contribute?

PRESCRIPTION FOR SUCCESS 1-8 WHAT DO I WANT?

Think about the characteristics you would prefer in your place of employment.

1. Type of facility
   Examples: large, small, urban (in the city), rural, inpatient (such as a hospital), outpatient (such as a clinic), home care

   ____

   ____

2. Type of population served
   Examples: economic status, age range, gender, ethnic groups

   ____

   ____

3. Work schedule
   Examples: steady employment with one employer; per diem (daily, contracted to different facilities); flexible, changing hours; fixed hours; frequent overtime; days only; evenings and weekends

   ____

   ____

4. Specialty
   Examples: emergency care, orthopedics (bones and muscles), hand therapy

   ____

   ____

5. Type of supervision
   Examples: closely monitored, work more independently

   ____

   ____

6. Work pace
   Examples: fast, moderate (There is no slow-paced work in health care!)

   ____

   ____

7. Amount of interaction with others (All health care professionals are part of a team, although some work more independently than others.)

   ____

   ____

8. Range of duties performed
   Examples: wide variety of tasks, concentrate on a few, somewhere in between

   ____

   ____

CHAPTER 2

Strategies for Students with Special Situations

ADULT STUDENTS

PORTRAIT OF THE ADULT STUDENT

Just what is an adult student or a mature student? There are a variety of definitions, depending on the source. Generally, students are considered to be mature if they have one or more of the following characteristics:

- Have been out of high school for at least 5 years
- Are over the age of 25
- Work either full- or part-time
- Have children or other dependents

COME JOIN THE CROWD

"Through education, you hope to give a new direction to life."

—Linda Simon

If you've been out of school for a number of years, you may be quite nervous about the idea of returning to school. Something you should know is that returning to school after a few—or even many—years is becoming much more common these days. In fact, the crowd of older students is getting larger. Some sources report that up to 50% of all college students are over the age of 25. The world is changing rapidly, and education is increasingly important for securing good jobs and moving up in careers. This is especially true for health care careers.

Continuing your education will ultimately add to the quality of your life—and to the lives of those around you. But you may be experiencing a number of fears and wondering if you have made the right decision. It is not unusual for adults to have a variety of concerns about their ability to succeed as students. Table 2-1 lists common fears, along with suggestions for overcoming each one.

One proven way to deal with fears is to share and discuss them with others, especially those who are in the same situation. It can be comforting to know that other students have the same concerns. You will find that you are not the only one feeling the way you do and that your fears are not irrational. Talking with someone else, however, should not simply be an "ain't it awful, this is tough" gab session. Rather, use it as an opportunity to help each other focus on the positive, exchange ideas for managing difficulties, and share resources. Examples of such resources include the following:

- Trading childcare
- Carpooling
- Teaching each other, such as computer skills
- Sharing class notes when one of you is absent

According to Al Siebert, an expert in helping adult learners, "Creating a personal support group and issue-specific learning teams is the most effective thing you can do to help assure your success in college."[1] This makes sense because research has shown that social support—relationships with other people—has powerful positive influences. For example, people with good social support have been shown to have reduced stress, improved resistance to disease, and improved recovery from illness.

Once you have graduated, consider maintaining your support group as you navigate the job search and the first few months on the job. You will likely encounter new challenges, and sharing these experiences can help smooth the road during these times.

Another suggestion for overcoming fears is to grit your teeth and face them head on. Ask yourself if the fear is based on reality. Then think about ways you can deal with it: ask for help; take a class; use the suggestions in this book. Do your best to get through what needs to be done and then reflect on your success. Over time, with each new triumph, your fears will decrease.

ADVANTAGES OF BEING A MATURE STUDENT

It is quite possible that you have a number of advantages over more traditional students—those who are entering college directly from high school or who have been out for only a couple of years. Perhaps you left school to get married and raise a family, join the military, or go to

TABLE 2-1 Common Fears of Adult Students

Fear	Suggestions for Overcoming
My brain is rusty and I won't be able to learn quickly.	Think of it this way: your brain may not have been in school, but if you have been working and/or raising a family, your brain has had plenty of workouts! You have simply been using it in different ways, but they all involve thinking and learning.
I won't be able to compete with younger students.	You actually have certain advantages over younger students. These are described in the next section of this chapter.
My academic abilities are not that great. I didn't do well in math/science/English, etc.	This book can help you review basic skills and overcome special fears such as math anxiety. See Chapters 6 through 9. Take advantage of any resources available at your school such as the learning center and tutors.
I don't have a computer or Internet access.	Computers have become quite affordable. If purchasing one is not an option, check with your school and the public library. Most have computers that students and the public can use.
I don't know how to use computers like the kids do.	Technology does have a way of moving on, and it's not uncommon to feel left behind. (The manual for the car I bought last year was 506 pages long!) If possible, take a computer class. Your school may have them. If not, they are often available for free or at a small charge at public libraries, adult schools, and community centers. There are also many good books and websites for beginners.
I might not be able to do it all—work, study, and raise a family.	This is a problem faced by many students. See the suggestions in this chapter as well as the sections in Chapter 3 on time management and personal organization.
My family will feel neglected.	There are actions you can take to help prevent you family from feeling this way. This chapter contains many specific ideas.
People in my life will try to sabotage my efforts.	People who truly care about you will support your efforts to improve your life. It may be that they feel threatened or left out. This chapter contains suggestions you can try to gain their support.
The thought of taking tests worries me.	Taking tests is a skill discussed in detail in Chapter 8.
Instructors might not like older students.	Actually, many instructors believe that older students are more motivated and committed.

Adapted from: Siebert A, Karr MK: *The adult learner's guide to survival and success,* ed 6, Portland, 2008, Practical Psychology Press.

TABLE 2-2 Skills Acquired through Life Experience

Skill	Application in School
Meeting deadlines	Turning in assignments on time
Handling several activities at the same time	Coordinating studying, caring for children, and completing household tasks
Interacting and working with others	Developing working relationships with instructors; getting along with other students
Solving problems	Determining the best ways to learn; balancing adult responsibilities so you can study; completing assignments that require solving problems
Adapting to new situations	Adjusting to being in school; adapting to the role of student
Having patience and knowing that situations will improve over time	Staying with your studies even if the going gets tough

work. If so, you have almost certainly accumulated a wealth of experience that will help you as a student. In fact, it is likely that as an older adult you have acquired many skills you can apply at school. Examples of these are listed in Table 2-2. In fact, many educators believe that lessons learned from life are the most valuable.

Certain life experiences are especially helpful for health care students. If you are a parent, for example, you have undoubtedly taken your children to the doctor. You understand how important it is to have faith in those who are caring for your loved ones. You yourself may have had health problems. These experiences can motivate you to do your best in school to become a truly qualified health care professional.

Okay, now you're feeling more confident about being a mature student. At the same time, adult students who find themselves with instructors and classmates younger than themselves should take care not to assume a know-it-all attitude. Adults who are used to being in charge at home—and perhaps even on the job—can find it difficult to become a student and follow the directions of others. You may believe that you have more practical experience than the instructor and many of the other students. At times like this, it is especially important to focus on your goal of becoming a competent health care professional. Recognize the need to learn from individuals who, although younger, have health care experience and knowledge. On the other hand, don't hesitate to share your experiences when these are appropriate for the topics being presented in class. Offer your comments courteously, and take care not to dominate the discussion.

PERSONAL REFLECTION

1. Which of the life skills listed in Table 2-2 do you believe will most help you in your role as a student?

___

___

___

2. Can you think of others that you can apply to help you succeed in school?

___

___

___

MEETING NEW CHALLENGES

"Believe in yourself and take things one day at a time.
—Al Siebert

The greatest challenge faced by most adult students is the matter of time—having enough of it! Adults have multiple responsibilities that may include running a household, caring for children, and holding down a job. They may even include helping elderly parents and holding volunteer positions in the community. Balancing these demands can be stressful, even overwhelming. At times your responsibilities may seem like acceptable excuses for being late to class, or even absent. You may feel that your instructors are not caring or understanding if they don't accept your excuses. But you must remember that the goal of health care education is to prepare you for a career. You will have important responsibilities, and your employer and your patients will count on you to know what you are doing. Being prepared to serve requires being in class regularly. If instructors were to let students slide through school because they have good excuses and good intentions, the instructors would be doing a disservice to their students and to the future employers and, most important, the future patients of these students.

Time Management—Advanced Techniques

This section is called "Advanced Techniques" because good time management is especially important for adult students. The fact is there are only 24 hours in a day. When you combine typical adult responsibilities with attending class and studying, no day will seem long enough to take care of everything that needs to be done. Adding the role of student may require some major adjustments and new strategies.

As discussed in Chapter 3 in the section on time management, prioritizing is the key to effective use of time. Recall that prioritizing means determining which tasks are most important and then making sure that they are completed. Start by determining which activities are critical to your success as a student, and focus on these. If you are a parent and/or a spouse, maintaining these relationships will also be high on your list of priorities. For example, when time is short, spending an hour with a child may be more important than dusting and vacuuming the house or performing volunteer activities. The fact is you may have to temporarily put off some of your customary activities. Attending school—and putting in the necessary time to study—is a big commitment and will almost certainly require some sacrifices. You may have less time for social and volunteer activities and household chores. See which of these can be put off, without endangering the health of you or your family, until after you graduate.

In addition to the ideas presented in Chapter 3, adult students may benefit from the following suggestions:

- Let family members and friends know your schedule. Consider putting up a large calendar where everyone can see it. Mark the dates when assignments are due and you have tests so everyone knows when you will be especially busy. Include events that are important to others as well, such as a child's music recital.
- Work with your family to delegate tasks. Organize a family meeting to discuss your need for study time and to assign age-appropriate chores. Have follow-up meetings to evaluate how things are going and make any needed adjustments to schedules and tasks.
- Schedule dedicated fun time with your family. Plan activities together that everyone enjoys. Aim for days that follow a major exam or project due date.
- Treat your studies as you would a job. After all, you wouldn't just leave your job to visit with a friend or stay on the phone for an hour catching up on the latest news.
- Plan to study each day, even if some days it is for only a short period. Don't wait until you have long periods of uninterrupted time—this luxury may happen rarely, if at all! (I have learned that 20 minutes here and there eventually results in a book.)
- Add 15 minutes to each day, either by getting up earlier or staying up later. This will actually add 91 hours a year to your waking—and hopefully productive—hours.[2]

Managing with Children in the House

Being a parent presents special challenges for adult students, especially if you are a single parent. In spite of comments throughout this book about committing yourself to your studies, the truth is that your children are your top priority. If they are young, finding appropriate childcare is critical. Even with a good provider, you should develop a backup plan to cover emergencies. For example, preschools can close during severe weather, individual caretakers can become ill, or your child can get sick and be required to stay home.

Your children's school and the adults who care for them should be able to reach you in an emergency. Be sure they have your school's phone number. If your instructors require that you turn off cell phones during class (not an unreasonable request), ask the administration about their policy for taking emergency calls and notifying students in class.

Handling childcare issues now is excellent preparation for later when you are employed. Although employers understand true emergencies, they cannot tolerate employees who regularly miss work because of child-related issues. Health care providers must make patient care and achieving work goals their highest priorities.

Your children may be upset by changes in your schedule, absences from home, and limitations in the time you have to spend with them. It can help if they know where you are spending your time and what you are doing. Ask your school for permission to show your children the classrooms, labs, and other areas. Explain how you are learning new things to help others and to help them have a better future. Explain to your children why you are in school. Show them a picture of a health care professional, and tell them about your future job. Make it a habit to tell them about your day in school, something interesting that happened, and what you learned.

Make time for each child to do activities you enjoy doing together, talk about their concerns, and let them know how much they mean to you. Focus on them during this time so they feel included and loved. Neighbors of mine have a busy family with two working parents and four school-age children. They eat dinner together whenever possible, and during the meal each person is allotted 2 minutes (they set a timer) to give a presentation about their day. The message is that each person, even the 6-year-old, has something of value to contribute.

When your children help around the house, show appreciation. Even if the beds aren't made perfectly or dinner isn't as nutritious as you would like, let them know that you are grateful for their efforts. Al Siebert offers the following ideas[1]:

- Say "thank you."
- Buy or fix their favorite food.
- Give hugs and kisses.
- Give treats or little gifts.
- Leave nice notes for them; send cards.
- Tell them about something interesting at school.
- Speak highly of them to others.
- Let them feel that your success is their success.

Finding quiet time to study can be challenging when children are present. Here are a few suggestions:

- If your children are old enough, work on homework together.
- Have young children "help" you by drawing, coloring pictures, filling in sticker books, or performing other "desk work."
- Try turning your study time into a positive experience for the kids by saving their favorite videos, toys, and other activities for the times when you are busy.
- Set up a special place for children to play quietly while you study. Childproof a room in the house where older children can play while you study.
- Set a timer for quiet periods. If children know there is an end to the quiet time, they may be more willing to oblige.
- Let children help you study, such as by showing you flashcards or asking you questions. Exchange babysitting services with friends and family members, arranging to help them out when your study load is lightest.

Working with your children in these ways can be a win-win situation. Not only will you accomplish more, but you serve as a positive role model for your children. They will see your behavior as a disciplined, goal-oriented person who enjoys learning and self-improvement.

Explore combining resources with other students. For example, see about organizing a study group with classmates who have children. Contribute to a babysitting fund, and hire someone to watch all the children while you study together. Or you might exchange childcare with one other student, trading off watching the children for an afternoon. For older children, investigate activities such as day camps, sports teams, and craft classes. Organizations such as churches and community centers offer these at reasonable prices. There may also be opportunities for single parents who are continuing their education.

Finally, if it becomes necessary, try studying before and after classes in the school library. You may accomplish more there in shorter periods of time than if you are at home with constant interruptions.

Maintaining Personal Relationships

Adults have many relationships with others. These may include aging parents, a spouse or significant other, friends, and co-workers. Becoming a student can put a strain on these relationships because you will have less time to devote to them. In addition, your new status as a student may cause others to feel frustrated, jealous, or even threatened.

Include people who are important to you when making your educational plans. Let them know what you are doing and why—how pursuing a career in health care is going to contribute to the quality of your life, the quality of your family, and even to the welfare of the community. Assure them that you will schedule time with them, and let them know how you are doing. Consider throwing a going-back-to-school party. Invite friends and family and tell them about your plans, what you'll be studying, and the great future you anticipate working in health care. Let them know how important this is to you and ask for their support.

When adult students are interviewed, married women report more difficulties in their role as "caretaker of family needs" when they assume the role of student.[1] It can be hard for a spouse or significant other to accept your new status as a student. They may worry you will leave them behind or not have time for them, or they may be jealous of your opportunity. Here are some things you can try if you find yourself with an unhappy spouse[1]:

1. Ask your spouse what is really bothering him or her. It will be easier to deal with if you are both clear on the nature of the problem.
2. Focus on the future. Emphasize that attending school is temporary.
3. Discuss how your studies can benefit your relationship.
4. Schedule time together to do something you both enjoy.

Being pulled in many directions can be stressful for everyone, and it is important to make a special effort to include family members in your decisions. If behavior problems develop, such as being upset and refusing to talk, allow some time for adjustments. If the reactions of others are extreme, it may be necessary to seek help such as family counseling. If this is financially difficult, check with your school about free or low-cost services in your community.

When you do spend time with others, try to minimize complaining. That is, don't go on and on about how difficult you are finding a subject, how a certain instructor gives difficult tests, how stressed you feel, and so on. These issues should be addressed with people at your school who can help you with these problems. It's best to focus on the positive when visiting with friends. The same advice applies at home. If there is already some stress over your attending school, the last thing you need to do is cast a dark cloud over everything when you are home. Describing how tired you are, how difficult your classes are, how unfair your instructors are will take away from the time you do have to spend with loved ones.

Personal relationships can cause problems as you begin your studies. At the same time, strong support systems can increase your chances for success. This is not surprising because studies have shown that social support is associated with good mental health and the ability to handle stress. There is even some evidence that social support positively influences physical health. For example, the survival rates of individuals who have heart attacks are higher in those with the greatest emotional support.[3,4]

Your personal support system may extend beyond your immediate family and can include anyone who encourages you and supports your goals: your health care provider, spiritual advisor, and members of your place of worship and other groups to which you belong.

There are three basic types of social support, and you can benefit from each:

1. **Emotional:** provided by people who make you feel loved and cared for and increase your sense of self-worth
2. **Instrumental:** provided by those who help you with specific tasks such as childcare, household tasks, and transportation
3. **Informational:** provided by instructors and others who give you information you need in order to succeed as a student[5]

Don't hesitate to ask for support: explanations from your instructor, encouragement from your spouse. Show appreciation and let people know how important their help is to you. And don't forget to give back—even if you are busy, you can offer to provide these same kinds of support to others. In fact, giving of yourself is a valuable characteristic of the health care professional.

Combining Work and School

Working takes time, but according to government surveys, many working students believe that employment helps them with their coursework; more than half think it helps them prepare for a career.[6] If possible, work as few hours as is financially possible. Working full-time while attending school is doable, but it is very difficult for most people.

Either way, try to enlist the support of your employer. Discuss your educational plans and see if there are ways you can tie school assignments to your work. Take care not to use work time inappropriately. At the same time, if you are seeking a new job, see if you can find a position that would permit studying while working, such as receptionist or security guard. (This would be with the employer's permission and without performing poorly.)

Overcoming Academic Weaknesses

You may have had difficulties during your previous educational experiences. This is very common for students of all ages who are pursuing career training. You may be a practical person who learns best through hands-on activities. If so, a health care career is a good choice

Q&A With a Health Care Professional

Kim Fruge

Kim is a manager and caregiver in a care home for older and disabled adults. She shares her experience going back to school as an adult student with a family and full-time job.

Q When did you return to school to study medical assisting?

A Six years ago. I was married with grown children—they were 20 and 21 at the time—and had worked many years in retail. When I decided to make a change, I was a scan supervisor. That means I was supervising the coding and pricing of items in a large grocery store.

Q Why did you decide to change careers and return to school?

A I never really liked working in retail, but it was something I could do without any education beyond high school. I had always wanted to work in something where I could work directly with people, helping them in some way. I loved raising my kids and we always had their friends around the house. So I checked around and found out I could earn my certificate in medical assisting in a reasonable amount of time.

Q How did your family react when you decided to return to school?

A When I first decided to go back to school, my family thought I was crazy! They didn't think I would do it. But after I started talking about it and what I would achieve, they were 100% behind me. Then, after I started, they thought I would give up. But when they saw how well I was doing and the grades I was getting, they started encouraging me and trying to help me in any way they could. They helped me to study and to research. My son was still living at home. Actually, both my son and daughter helped me with homework and quizzed me. My daughter helped me with math.

When accomplishments were done, they were very happy for me and patted me on the back. My son's friends were so nice—they would call me, help me study. Then my children's friends came to my graduation. They were so proud of me and what I had done because I graduated with a 3.8. And that was after 20 years of not being in school!

Q Did you find returning to school difficult?

A Oh, yes. I was still working 40 hours a week at the store, from 4 am to noon or sometimes 2 pm. I'd go home for a quick nap and then go to class. My classes met Monday through Friday for 5 hours a night, so my schedule was intense. Including my externship, this all lasted about a year.

After not being in school for all those years, trying to learn how to study again was really hard until I found a way to make it easier for myself. I discovered flashcards and that really helped me. I made my own flashcards for whatever we were studying. I learned about these when we used them for medical terminology. Then I started making them for facts and questions in all my subjects. I don't think I could have made it through without those flashcards.

I did get discouraged sometimes—with pharmacology, for example. I had trouble learning to convert ratios so I could calculate medications. Math was always my worst, worst subject. I didn't think I would have to worry about math studying medical assisting, but I was wrong about that!

Q What helped you most when you had problems with math?

A Actually, my husband, Jimmy, was great about helping. He could explain things in words I understood. Also, my instructors were wonderful. I always stayed after class and got as much help as possible. I always asked lots of questions. I would get help from Jimmy at home and then ask my teachers. Talking with my teachers really helped. I'm a hands-on learner, so once I saw it on paper, I could do it. So ask for help when you need it!

Q What other advice do you have for adults who are returning to school?

A Set your goals and work to achieve them. Study hard. Do lots of research. Make sure you have the time to spend on school. You have to make this a priority. Always tell yourself what the outcome will be—what you will achieve by doing this. Do lots of research on things you don't understand. I spent lots of my time in the library trying to understand certain things. I did extra practice, too. I did lots more blood draws than were required to make sure I got it.

Q How did you handle time management?

A Very carefully! I stayed on a schedule that worked best for me and my family. I spent all my spare time studying, getting ahead on courses—doing extra homework ahead of time as much as possible because I always liked to be ahead of where we were, always doing extra credit to learn and better understand.

Q How did you handle the pressure of balancing so many activities?

A I look deep breaths and told myself, "I am smart enough to do this." I said that to myself at least once a week. I had pressure to make sure I got all my classwork done. And at work the pressure was making sure I met all my deadlines. As scan coordinator, I had to be sure the prices were all up to date.

Q How did you balance your job and school?

A The other employees and my boss were really great. I got their support when I started school. For example, when I did my externship from 8 to 5, I worked at the store on the weekends. They were all really good about accommodating me and my scheduling needs.

because much of the work is hands-on. At the same time, health care requires a knowledge of what you are doing. Therefore academic skills are needed for the reading, writing, and studying necessary to learn important background information.

If your academic and study skills are not what they should be, the first step is to acknowledge this. There is nothing to be embarrassed about. In fact, it is a sign of strong character to recognize our weaknesses and seek the means to make improvements. It is very important to seek help as soon as you realize you need it. Many health care programs move along quickly. You may have only 1 month or a few weeks in a class. You cannot wait until just before the final exams to seek help. There are a couple of good reasons for this. First, it may simply be too late to catch up. Second, even if you are able to pass the class, have you really learned what you should? Have you mastered the information and skills you need to perform your future health care duties?

If you believe that your academic skills are not strong, plan to spend a little time each day working on them. For example, spend 15 or 20 minutes working on math skills or spelling. Over time, you are likely to acquire the skills needed to master your classes.

There are many ways to strengthen your study and academic skills, including the following:

1. Read the information and try the suggestions presented in this book. They include everything from understanding what you read to overcoming math anxiety to writing a well-organized paper. See Chapters 6 through 9.
2. Investigate learning resources at your school: learning center, review courses, tutors, writing lab.
3. Look for helpful classes open to the public in your area: computer literacy, basic skills, using the Internet.
4. Organize a study group with other students.
5. Most important, don't hesitate to ask your instructors for help. They have chosen to teach because they want to share what they learned working in the health care field. They want successful graduates—in other words, they want their students to succeed!

Many adults have trouble admitting when they don't know something or when they need help. But think of it this way: you are paying for your instructors to help you learn. That is their job, and seeking this help is one way to ensure that you are getting what you pay for, just as you would with any service. One difference with education, of course, is that you must do your part, too, by reading assignments, attending class, and doing the homework.

Achieving academic success is important. At the same time, a common cause of stress among adult students is striving for perfection. You may feel that because you are older, you should do as well as or perhaps even better than younger students. You may believe that others expect more of you. However, just as age doesn't mean your brain is rusty, neither does age equate with intelligence and ability. If your previous experiences in school were not all positive, don't stress yourself out thinking you must earn an A in every class. Your goals should focus on learning and preparing yourself for your health care career.

If you are paying for your education yourself, you may see grades as a reflection of the value you are receiving for your money. Again, focus on your goals and purpose in attending school. Your future performance on the job, not your transcript, is the product you are paying for. Doing it all perfectly—studying, working, parenting—is not possible for anyone, so decide what is most important and work to achieve balance.

ENGLISH-AS-A-SECOND-LANGUAGE STUDENTS

ENGLISH FOR THE NON-NATIVE SPEAKER

English may be your second—or even third or fourth—language. This may be because you grew up in a family that spoke another language. Or you may have moved to the United States from another country. In either case, you probably speak English pretty well—perhaps very well. However, you may have concerns such as the following:

- I'm not always sure which verb tense to use. In fact, I could use some help with many parts of grammar.
- English spelling is difficult. How can I remember words that have so many letters that aren't even pronounced?
- I have an accent and am self-conscious about speaking.
- I'm worried about doing writing assignments in school or having to write on the job.

These are natural concerns when English is not your first language, and they, along with other language difficulties, will be discussed in this chapter. First, let's look at some of the advantages of knowing more than one language. You may have heard the term "global economy," which is evidence of just how interconnected the countries of the world have become. You also know that the people of the United States come from a variety of countries and cultures. Large numbers of people living in the United States do not speak English well. Some do not speak it at all. Knowing at least two languages can be a real advantage in this environment. This is especially true in health care. Think about how frightening it can be for patients who are being treated by someone with whom they can't easily communicate. If you speak a language that is spoken by many people in your area, this is a valuable and helpful skill. You have something extra to offer your future employers.

If you speak a Romance language, such as Spanish, you may be surprised to find that some medical terms you will be learning are similar to everyday words in your language. (Even if the spelling is different, the sounds are similar.)

IMPROVING YOUR ENGLISH

"Surround yourself with English; practice it, study it, and you will learn it."

—Kathy Ochoa Flores

To be successful at improving your English, it is important to be motivated. This means that you *want* to improve your English communication skills. Working on language skills takes time and effort, as well as taking risks, so it really helps to be clear about why you want to improve.

The best way to improve any skill, and this includes communicating, is to practice. Although this is the best way, it is not always easiest. For example, you may speak a language other than English with the people with whom you spend most of your time. Perhaps your parents don't speak English. You may be more comfortable with friends who speak your language and understand your cultural background. But if you are serious about improving your English, you will need to seek opportunities to use it. Here are some suggestions:

- Make friends with classmates who speak only English. Invite them to have coffee and use the time to practice speaking English. This is a good way to learn slang and informal conversational English.
- Organize or join a study group in which the majority of the members speak English. Use this time to work on vocabulary related to your studies.
- Speak up in class if you have questions. If this is too difficult at first, ask to speak with your instructors outside of class.
- Talk with everyone you can, such as people you do business with: clerks in stores, the librarian, the receptionist at the doctor's office.

It can be scary speaking English with people you don't know, especially if you are self-conscious about your speaking ability. It is especially hard for adults who worry about looking dumb. But this is the best way to learn. The first chapter said that students have the right to make mistakes. This is also true for people who are learning to speak English well—they have the right to make mistakes. In fact, you must give yourself permission to make mistakes. Think about it this way: if you only repeat what you already know and don't try new things, you won't learn anything new. English instructors believe that their best students are the ones who are willing to take risks. They are not afraid to make mistakes and don't worry about using perfect grammar, vocabulary, and pronunciation. When they make mistakes, they are not discouraged. Instead, they learn from their errors. Good students visit with other people (not during class when the instructor is speaking, of course!), ask and answer questions, and interact as much as possible or as much as they can. If your instructors have you work in groups, this is an excellent way to practice. Health care involves working with others, and interacting with your classmates is excellent practice for this on-the-job skill. If you sit quietly in class every day, you will lose many (good) opportunities to learn and practice.

You might try practicing at home. If you have family members who are interested, try teaching them new English words and phrases. Teaching others is an excellent way to learn and reinforce what you know.

Language teachers agree that to learn or master another language, you need to spend some time—even if it is only 20 minutes—studying or practicing every day. They believe this is more effective than working on it once a week for several hours. Teachers also recommend that you set reasonable goals and try to make your language studies fun.

The following sections cover topics that can be difficult for learners of English. They are *not* intended to provide an English course. Rather, the purpose is to provide encouragement, suggestions about how to improve your English, and examples of common problems in areas such as pronunciation, spelling, and grammar. For more in-depth study, you might take an intermediate or advanced English class, explore the websites listed at the end of this chapter, or spend time practicing with native English speakers. The important thing is to find what works best for you and then "go for it."

Increasing Your Vocabulary

The English language has more words than any of us—even teachers and textbook writers—will ever know. Depending on how you count them (for example, are "talk" and "talking" one word or two?), there are more than 250,000 words in English! And new ones are added every day. To just get along in English, you should know about 2000 frequently used words. To succeed in college, that number grows to 10,000 to 15,000 words.[7]

Here are a few suggestions for increasing your vocabulary:

1. Set a goal of learning a certain number of new vocabulary words each week. While you are studying health care, you might want to concentrate on terms related to your future career.
2. In a notebook or on your computer, list new words as you encounter them. Write the word, its definition, and a sentence using the word. Write something personal to make the word your own.[7] Use the new words, in both oral and written forms, as often as possible.
3. If you are a visual learner, make posters of your new vocabulary and post where you will see them every day. Use pictures and drawings when appropriate.
4. If you are an auditory learner, record your new words along with a sentence for each one. Listen to the recording over the following weeks.
5. Study word lists such as vocabulary, key terms, and the glossaries in your textbooks.
6. Find other basic English word lists, such as those on the websites listed at the end of this chapter.

Idiomatic Expressions. Idiomatic expressions exist in many languages and can present difficulties to language learners. This is because they consist of words that when used together have meanings that are different from the dictionary definitions of the individual words. Because these expressions are commonly used in English, consider adding these to your vocabulary learning goals. A good list is available at www.usingenglish.com/reference/idioms.

Improving Your Pronunciation

Pronunciation can be a problem, especially if you learned English as an adult. Once our habits are established and the muscles in our tongue and mouth become accustomed to making the sounds of our first language, it becomes more difficult to form "foreign" sounds. A problem for some people is distinguishing between similar sounds. For example, I knew a gentleman from Peru who could not hear the difference between the words "duck" and "dock." If you can't hear the difference, it is nearly impossible to pronounce them differently.

If you can be understood easily, you may not need to worry too much about having an accent. Some people find accents interesting, even charming. If you are working on developing an "American accent," it is a good idea to model your speech after television newscasters. This is because they speak what is considered standard or neutral American English rather than one of the many regional ways of speaking found throughout the United States.

Perhaps even more important than the pronunciation of individual words is how they are combined into sentences and on which words and syllables (parts of words) the stress (emphasis) is placed. Using a rhythm that is different from the way Americans speak makes speech difficult to understand. Therefore listening carefully to native speakers and practicing entire sentences are important parts of pronunciation practice.

Combining Sounds. A common custom in spoken English is to link words together when there is a vowel sound between them. An example is the sentence "I want an apple." If each word is pronounced carefully and separately, this results in a "foreign" accent. Spoken by a native speaker, this sentence sounds like "I wannanappul." The words are run together, and the letter "t" disappears. Another example is "Would you like an apple?" which becomes "Would juh likeanappul?" Consider the following examples:

1. "An elephant" sounds like "a-nelephant" or "uh-nelephant"
2. "An orange" sounds like "a-norange or "uh-norange"

You may not realize it, but many languages do this. French is especially full of linked sounds in which whole parts of words seem to disappear. When spoken quickly and naturally, Spanish does the same thing. We grow accustomed to understanding our own language. It's just more difficult when we don't know a language well.

Here are a few more examples of English pronunciation challenges:

- The common use of the sound "uh" for vowels: mother—m*uh*ther; the—th*uh*; complicated—complicat*uh*d.
- The letter "t" pronounced as a "d" when the word requires a faster sound: little—liddle; anatomy—anaduhmy; thirty—therdy. (Note, however, that "thirteen" retains the "t" sound. This is because the word parts before and after the "t" in "thirteen" are longer than in "thirty.")
- Many words are pronounced differently than they are spelled: have to—haffto; bright—brite.
- Some words are spelled the same but pronounced differently to convey different meanings: "read" is pronounced "reed" when meaning the present tense and "red" when meaning the past tense.
- Combinations of consonants. In many languages, there are vowels between consonants that give kind of a running start to the tongue. For example, the word just used—"start"—begins with two consonants, s and t. When first learning English, speakers of some languages may say "e-start"—they need that extra first vowel to get the word going.

As you can see, English pronunciation is not easy to learn by studying the language's written form. So just how do you learn to speak this language well? The answer is *by listening and practicing*. The best way is to spend time communicating with native English speakers who don't slow or simplify their speech. They also must be willing to correct your mistakes. Their being too nice to say anything will not help you to learn. Practicing this way may sound challenging, but trying to learn English speech from rules is much more difficult. There is just no way to list and memorize all the different combinations of words and sounds. And it certainly is a lot more fun to work with someone else.

Improving Your Reading Comprehension

Reading has the advantage of time—you can take your time and read a sentence over and over. You can also stop and look up new words in the dictionary. At the same time, this can create a problem. This is because you may be tempted to look up every word you don't know and end up spending hours reading. English-language professor Kathy Flores recommends that students read an entire assignment first without stopping.[7] Your purpose during this first reading is to look for the main ideas. This can be difficult to do if you are constantly stopping to look up words. Here are some suggestions for completing this first reading[8]:

1. Ignore words that seem unimportant.
2. Use the context to guess the meaning.

3. Scan for specific information.
4. Skim for general information.
5. Read in units or chunks of words.

When reading textbook assignments, review any key terms given at the beginning of a chapter. This will highlight the vocabulary that the author considers to be most important for understanding the chapter. Second, read the learning objectives. These will help you identify what is most important and what you should be looking for as you read.

Once you have finished the first reading, write a list of the main ideas as you understood them. Then read the chapter again, this time listing and looking up the words you don't know. Later you can practice the words by writing sentences and using your preferred learning method, such as using flashcards. This is especially important if these are key words for the subject you are studying.

Improving Your Spelling

Spelling is difficult for both native and non-native English speakers (including me!). In Chapter 7 there is a section on spelling written for native speakers of English. The spelling of English words is difficult for several reasons:

1. One letter can be pronounced in different ways, depending on the word. This is different from languages such as Spanish, in which the letters do not vary much in sound. Note the variations for the letter "o" in the following words:
   - once
   - only
   - woman
   - women (These last two words can be really confusing! The words are almost identical, but in the plural form the "o" sound changes to "i"!)

   (If you are unsure of the differences in sound, ask a native speaker to read them aloud.)
2. Different combinations of letters can be pronounced in the same way, such as in l*ie* and rel*ie*ve. The letters "ough" have a variety of pronunciations, none of them including the letter g:
   - t*ough*—pronounced "tuhf"
   - thr*ough*—pronounced "throo"
   - d*ough*—pronounced "doe"
   - b*ough*t—pronounced "bawt"
3. Different spellings can be pronounced the same way. Consider the following examples with the sound "ee":
   - m*e*
   - m*ee*t
   - m*ea*t
   - ch*ie*f
   - p*eo*ple

TABLE 2-3	**Examples of Words with Silent Syllables**	
Word	**Syllables in Written Form**	**Syllables in Spoken Form**
aspirin	as-pi-rin	as-prin
different	dif-fer-ent	diff-rent
temperature	tem-per-a-ture	tem-pra-ture
comfortable	com-fort-a-ble	comf-table
vegetable	veg-e-ta-ble	veg-table

   Following are a few more with the sound "oo":
   - f*oo*d
   - r*u*de
   - cr*ew*
   - gr*ou*p
   - thr*ough*
   - bl*ue*
   - sh*oe*
4. In some words, not all the syllables are pronounced. For example, some words with three syllables have only two sounds when spoken, and some with three syllables have two sounds. See Table 2-3 for some examples.

These examples demonstrate why you simply have to memorize the spelling of many words. In fact, according to one source, to become a moderately competent speller of English, you have to memorize at least 3700 words that have unpredictable spellings.[9] This is almost four times the number of unpredictable spellings of any European language. You may wonder why English has such a variety of vocabulary and spellings. It is largely because English has a number of different of roots: Anglo-Saxon, Latin, and Greek.

Other languages have contributed vocabulary to English, including Danish and Norman French. This is why we have so many different and overlapping spelling patterns. It also explains why English has such a large vocabulary: different words meaning the same thing were adopted from various languages.

There are some major spelling rules, and these are listed in Chapter 7 (more proof that even native English speakers need this help!). These rules can be helpful. However, as one author puts it, they are like weather reports. We can use them but cannot depend on them to be correct 100% of the time.[10]

STUDENTS WITH LEARNING DISABILITIES

THE CHALLENGE OF LEARNING DISABILITIES

When people hear the term "learning disability," many of them picture a child struggling to learn to read or

BOX 2-1 Challenges Associated with Learning Disabilities

- Rarely completing projects you start
- Rarely meeting deadlines
- Being unable to manage time realistically
- Constantly feeling the need to move around or fidget
- Being unable to handle sequential or serial information
- Being unable to stay focused for more than very short periods of time
- Getting distracted very easily
- Seeing letters and numbers in the wrong order
- Having letters go blurry or jumping around when you are reading
- Experiencing great difficulty remembering oral instructions
- Having trouble judging distance and determining direction, such as left and right
- Always feeling disorganized and out of control
- Being unable to write legibly or neatly, even when you try
- Easily forgetting material that is presented visually
- Experiencing great difficulty in communicating thoughts orally or in writing
- Constantly losing your possessions

perhaps a youngster who can't sit still in the classroom. The fact is that there are a variety of conditions that interfere with learning, and many of these present problems for adults as well as children. There are no typical profiles of a "learning disabled student" of any age. Rather, there is a variety of learning disabilities, and some individuals may experience different combinations of challenges that interfere with their learning or even with carrying out their daily activities. (See Box 2-1 for examples of common challenges.)

You may have been diagnosed with a learning disability as a child or teenager. Or you may have simply wondered why you had, or are having, certain difficulties in school or even in learning on the job. Learning disabilities are not always obvious, even to the person who has them, and for this reason they are sometimes referred to as "hidden" or "invisible" disabilities. Actually, it doesn't really matter if you "have" a learning disability. What matters is that if you have noticed you have more difficulty than most people with certain tasks and this often gets in the way of your learning and living productively, there are positive actions you can take. As an adult, you have self-awareness and can monitor your own behavior and work to make changes.

First, however, there are some things you should know about learning disabilities:

- They are *not* related to intelligence. In fact, some research indicates that individuals with attention deficit disorder tend to have above-average IQs.
- They are based on biologic factors, mostly involved with certain specific brain functions. They are not a person's fault or caused by a person's unwillingness to try to do better.

BOX 2-2 Contradictions in Performance

- You can think logically but cannot write your thoughts in a paragraph.
- You are alert and skilled but have trouble following directions.
- You understand mathematical theories but get confused performing calculations.
- You practice for hours, but your handwriting is illegible.
- You have creative ideas but cannot explain them clearly to others.
- You write beautiful stories and essays, but your spelling is very poor.
- Having a learning disability does *not* mean you can't learn. It simply means you learn in different ways from the crowd.
- There are many strategies you can use to overcome the challenges of learning disabilities.

- They are not always obvious and can result in puzzling contradictions. (See Box 2-2 for examples.)
- They do not prevent people from having successful and high-level careers.
- Some people with learning disabilities are creative and able to come up with innovative ideas.
- Being learning disabled has *nothing* to do with a lack of effort or laziness.

You are encouraged to try the strategies presented in this chapter. They are organized by academic and life skills, such as reading and time management, and presented in Tables 2-4 through 2-14. Select strategies that correspond to difficulties you are having and that look appropriate for you. Not all of them will work for every student. For example, let's look at the following suggestion: "Take notes as you read your textbook to increase your concentration." Now, if one of your problems is difficulty with your handwriting, this might not be good advice. In that case, you could place your book next to your computer and take notes on your word processing program. But if you are very slow at keyboarding or very easily distracted, this might not work for you. So perhaps underlining key words in your text and making short notes in the margins might work best. Repeating the important points out loud may also work. Consider your own situation to determine what might work best for you.

If the suggestions don't work and you find yourself struggling with your studies, speak with your instructors and perhaps an administrator at your college. Don't wait until you experience feelings of desperation or panic. There is no need to miss achieving your academic and career goals when help is available.

GENERAL SUGGESTIONS

This section contains suggestions for individuals with all types of learning disabilities. The first involves your

Text continued on p. 35

TABLE 2-4 Communication

Difficulties	Suggested Strategies
You find it difficult to follow what people are saying.	Keep your eyes on the speaker to avoid getting distracted. Ask the speaker to speak more slowly or to repeat things, when necessary. If the person is the instructor, request a meeting outside of class. Ask if lecture outlines are available to help you follow along. Develop active listening skills (see Chapter 6).
You think you know what you want to say, but it doesn't come out right.	Practice speaking alone in front of a mirror. Use notes when engaging in an important conversation. Before speaking, take a few moments to think and be clear in your own mind about what you want or need to say.
You tend to ramble on and get lost in details when you are speaking.	Think about the purpose of your conversation: what do you want to get across? Practice being self-aware and observing your own behavior. When you catch yourself, use humor and say: "Oops, I'm rambling on again. The important thing is. . . ." If appropriate, explain to your listener(s) that communication is difficult for you and that you may experience some problems.
You miss nonverbal signals that people give you during conversations.	Read about nonverbal communication. Practice observing others. Work with a friend who is willing to observe you and help you identify nonverbal language.

TABLE 2-5 Focusing

Difficulties	Suggested Strategies
You are easily distracted by extraneous noise.	When studying, wear headphone or earplugs or use a white noise machine. Sit close to the instructor during lectures (if seats are assigned, request permission to sit up front). Avoid sitting near students who talk during class. Choose quiet places to study, such as the library. Turn off your phone when you are studying.
You are easily distracted by visual stimuli.	Choose a seat where there are minimal distractions, such as away from a window or an interesting wall display. Work in an uncluttered area. Minimize the number of items on your desk that might draw your attention.
You are distracted by your own ideas that come up but are not needed at the moment. You are just bombarded with competing thoughts and ideas.	Keep a brainstorming log to note the ideas for consideration later. (I have 27 pages of writing ideas that popped into my head while I was working on something else.) Try doing meditation, a practice that has been shown to increase focus and attention.
It is very difficult to stay with a task for any length of time—even a few minutes.	Try doing meditation, a practice that has been shown to increase focus and attention. Train yourself to keep on task by deciding how many minutes you will focus, even if it is just 5 or 10 to start. Write down the time, and keep bringing yourself back to your task until the stop time. Try focusing on what you will gain by completing the task at hand.
You find it difficult to both start and complete projects.	Think about your goal. Why is this project important to you? Build in rewards to encourage yourself to get things done. Break projects into small chunks with interim deadlines. Trying to do too much can be overwhelming and result in doing nothing.

TABLE 2-6 Hyperactivity

Difficulties	Suggested Strategies
You cannot sit still or refrain from fidgeting for any length of time.	Engage in regular physical exercise. Choose something you enjoy doing. When appropriate, move around when you study. Try relaxation exercises, yoga, or guided imagery to help you relax and slow yourself down (see Chapter 3 for a relaxation exercise). When you are attending gatherings where you must sit for extended periods of time, engage your hands in an activity such as taking notes.
You have trouble settling down at night and sleeping.	Thirty minutes before bedtime, turn off the television and computer to reduce the sensory stimulation. Instead, engage in a quiet, relaxing activity. Develop a "going to bed" ritual that signals your body to slow down.

TABLE 2-7 Memory

Difficulties	Suggested Strategies
You cannot remember information given to you orally, especially things like multi-step instructions.	Ask the speaker to speak slowly, if necessary. Take notes. Ask if the instructions are available in written form. Ask the speaker to repeat anything you do not understand (it is very difficult for anyone to remember something they don't understand). Check your understanding of what people have said: "Let me make sure I've got this right...," then repeat what you heard or read from your notes. See the suggestions for improving your memory in Chapter 3.
You cannot remember what you have read or studied in class.	See the suggestions for reading in Chapter 6. Take notes of the main points as you read to increase your concentration. Writing also helps reinforce memory traces in the brain. Try the following to reinforce the material. Suppose you are studying diabetes. • *Visualize* how you might use what you are learning, such as in patient education. • *Associate* it with anyone you know who has diabetes. • *Think* about the causes and the increase in cases in the United States. • *Create* a mental picture of the pancreas. • *Discuss* what you are learning with others. • *Explain* what you are learning to others, such as the effects of untreated diabetes. • *Read* other sources, such as information on the Web or brochures about diabetes. • *Review* the material periodically.
You cannot remember new vocabulary.	Create a word list that you review daily. Use some of the techniques above to visualize, associate, and so on to "plant" the word in your memory. Try creating mnemonics such as the following: • Create a silly or interesting mental picture. Example: picture a *crane* lifting a large skull to remember *cranium*, the medical term for skull. • Link the new word to one with a similar sound and meaning. Example: *-stasis* is the medical word element for stoppage. It sounds like *stay*. If something stops, it stays in place.

TABLE 2-8 Note-Taking

Difficulties	Suggested Strategies
You cannot listen and write at the same time.	Request permission in advance to record class lectures. (Take care, however, to listen in class.) It is best if you use a recorder that has variable speed control so you can speed up or slow down the speech as needed. Request permission to copy notes from another student. Ask your instructors if they can give you outlines of their lectures. Try to copy down any information written on the board or screen.
You can listen and take notes, but what you write down doesn't make much sense.	See the sections on note-taking in Chapter 6.

TABLE 2-9 Numbers

Difficulties	Suggested Strategies
You have trouble copying strings of numbers in the correct order.	Break strings of numbers into groups of two or three digits. Write each small group, and check as you proceed. Cover part of the number as you read, especially if there are series of zeroes. When copying two numbers, cover the one that you are not copying.
You find it difficult to read tables that contain lots of numbers.	Draw an extra thick line under every third row. Highlight the sections in different colors.
You have difficulty performing math calculations.	Go over the review material in Chapter 9. Request permission to use a calculator when doing your work. If you have trouble reading numbers and following your calculations, try a talking calculator. It may be easier for you to catch errors if you hear them.
It is hard for you to measure accurately.	Take a deep breath and work calmly and slowly. Write down measurements as you go along so you don't forget them. Double check your work. If in doubt, have someone else check your work.

TABLE 2-10 Organization

Difficulties	Suggested Strategies
You lose things all the time.	Designate a place for everything, especially items such as keys and eyeglasses. Store items close to where you use them. Set up specific places for important items such as bills to be paid and assignments you are working on. Keep your desk and work areas as free of clutter as possible so important items don't get buried. Keep items such as your cell phone attached to your purse or belt so they can't get away from you.
Your desk is covered with piles of papers, folders, and notes, with many of their contents a mystery to you.	Work on clearing a small area at a time. Discard papers you no longer need. Create a simple filing system. Use colored file folders for different projects. (If you have trouble sequencing letters, and keeping files in order, make an alphabet arc. This is a semicircle with the letters of the alphabet written from left to right along the curved portion. Alternate idea: purchase a home filing system that comes with files, labels, and instructions for organizing papers and forms. Set up two accordion files: one with a section for each day of the week, and the other with a section for each month of the year. Place items that need attention in the corresponding file section. Be sure to check these files regularly. Alternate method: set up three trays labeled "This Week," "This Month," "This Term (or Semester)." Sort tasks accordingly; check the file labeled "This Week" daily and the other two weekly.
You frequently miss deadlines or appointments.	Keep a calendar or planner, either paper or electronic. Today's PDAs (personal digital assistants) include everything from calendars to wireless phones. Be disciplined about recording everything you need to do and checking your calendar frequently. Maintain a daily and weekly to-do list, either on paper or electronically. If on paper, use a small notebook, not little slips of paper that are easily lost.
You often find you don't have what you need for class, work, or household duties such as paying bills.	Create a list of things you must have each day and post it where you will see it, perhaps next to the front door. Each evening, set out what you will need for the next day. Do the same for your children to prevent the morning rush.
You feel so overwhelmed by everything that needs to be done that you often become "paralyzed" and don't do anything.	Get an "organization buddy" who can help you get things into perspective, make a plan, and keep you motivated. Your buddy can be a family member, a friend, or even an organization professional. It just needs to be someone who is organized, patient, and sympathetic to your situation. Work on gradually clearing clutter that can cause an overload of stimuli, visual stress, and distraction. Think about what really needs to be done and what can be put off until later. Consider the consequences of your choices. Divide large projects that seem impossible to complete into small pieces; estimate the time needed to complete each; designate deadlines for each piece and for the final project.

TABLE 2-11 Reading

Difficulties	Suggested Strategies
You can't seem to remember anything you read.	Study the section on reading in Chapter 6 and try the methods suggested. The previewing and reviewing steps are especially helpful for students with retention problems. Use the following strategies, which are also listed in Table 2-7 (Memory). This time, let's suppose you are studying the process of digestion: • *Visualize* the path of a donut as it goes through the digestion system, naming each part of the anatomy it passes through. • *Associate* the digestive process with the energy you use going about your day. • *Think* about the functions of the various digestive organs. • *Create* a mental picture of the digestive organs. Imagine each one in a bright color. • *Discuss* what you are learning, such as the causes of indigestion, with others. • *Read* other sources, such as illustrated material on the Web. • *Review* the material periodically.
You have trouble keeping your place when reading.	Move your finger along text as you read. Place a ruler or piece of paper under the line. Use an eye-level reading ruler, a special ruler made of opaque and transparent plastic in a variety of colors. Its serves to underline and highlight text in a colored tint, thus helping with both tracking and reducing the glare. Use a reading window, a slotted piece of plastic that shows one line at a time to reduce distraction from surrounding text.
You have problems distinguishing letters and their order: 1. See letters in the wrong order 2. Confuse reversible letters, such as *b* and *d, m* and *w* 3. Confuse words that look similar, such as *were* and *where* 4. Mis-sequence letters in long words, such as *conversation* and *conservation*	Pay attention to the context and meaning of sentences. If a word doesn't fit, examine it carefully to see if you have misread it. Practice seeing words as separate groups of letters (syllables) instead of as long strings of letters. Examples: presentation = pre-sen-ta-tion, terminology = ter-mi-nol-o-gy Learn common prefixes and suffixes. A prefix is a letter or a group of letters attached to the beginning of a word that partly indicates its meaning. Examples: • *anti-* means against: anti viral → antiviral • *mis-* means wrong or bad: mis diagnose → misdiagnose • *trans-* means across: trans plant → transplant A suffix is a letter or a group of letters attached to the end of a word to form a new word or to alter the grammatical function of the original word. Examples: • *-less* means without: pain less → painless • *-ment* means action or process: treat ment → treatment • *-ed* indicates past tense: inject → injected
You have difficulty reading print on white backgrounds because it seems to glare. Letters are blurred and jump around on the page.	Copy written materials, such as class handouts, onto light colored paper (investigate to see which color works best for you). Use a colored overlay on your computer monitor screen, or change the background color on your screen, if possible. Investigate the use of colored overlays for placing on text or colored eyeglasses.

TABLE 2-12 Taking Tests

Difficulties	Suggested Strategies
You misunderstand instructions and what the questions are asking.	Ask the instructor to privately explain the questions. State what you think a question is asking and ask for feedback to let you know if you understood it correctly. *Note:* If you believe you will need this extra help, advise the instructor *before* the day of the test.
You read and write so slowly that you don't have enough time to finish all the questions.	Request extra time to complete tests. *Note:* If you believe you will need this accommodation, submit your request *before* the day of the test.
You are too distracted by noises in the environment to focus on the test.	Request permission to take the text in a quiet environment *Note:* If you believe you will need this accommodation, submit your request *before* the day of the test.

Note: See also the section on test anxiety and test-taking strategies in Chapter 8.

TABLE 2-13 Time Management

Difficulties	Suggested Strategies
You never come close to estimating the amount of time it will take to complete any given project or activity.	Keep a time diary for a couple of weeks. Write down start and stop times for your daily activities. Then analyze to see how long things really take. You may be astonished to discover that something you thought takes 15 minutes actually takes closer to an hour. Estimate how long it will take to complete an activity, then start by adding 50% to the time. You can adjust over time as you learn to set realistic goals.
You try to do too much during the time available and often end up feeling exhausted or burned out.	See the suggestion above for keeping a time diary. Try planning fewer activities than you normally would, and see how much you actually accomplish. Prioritize your tasks, and always do the most important ones first. Pace yourself. When doing something that requires concentration, work in blocks of 20 to 30 minutes at a time. Use a planner or calendar to mark final deadlines. Set interim deadlines for completing parts of the project, studying for a test, and so on.
You easily lose track of time. A 10-minute break becomes a 2-hour session of lost time.	Set timers or alarms when you go on a break, answer the phone, or look at your e-mail. Vibrating timers are available if more appropriate. Practice being aware of where you are, what you are doing, and the time.
You are rarely on time for appointments, classes, or social occasions.	Start recording how much time it actually takes you to get to places you commonly visit, such as school. Then try adding 5 minutes to your travel time. Resist doing "one last little thing" as you head for the door.

See also the section on time management in Chapter 3.

TABLE 2-14 Writing

Difficulties	Suggested Strategies
You have serious problems with spelling.	Review the spelling rules and strategies presented in Chapter 7. Use the spell-check feature on your word processor. Carry a handheld spell-checker. Consider purchasing a medical terminology spell-checker. Investigate abbreviation-expander software. You can enter codes for often-used words so you don't have to continually reenter—and possible misspell—them. Check into proofreading software to supplement what came with your word processing program. This is available in medical report versions.
You make mistakes copying written material.	Work slowly and carefully. Copy onto colored, nonglare paper. Use paper with a slot cut into it or a reading window to cover the lines you are not copying.
You have difficulty organizing your thoughts and presenting them logically on paper.	Use a computer to do writing assignments so you can easily correct mistakes and move text around. When students aren't worried about the mechanics of writing, they can focus on the content and meaning. Ask your instructor to review your first draft to help you get on the right track. Have someone critique and proofread your written work. See also the suggestions about writing in Chapter 7. Request extra time to complete long writing assignments. *Note:* If you believe you will need this accommodation, submit your request *before* the assignment is due.
You find that the white paper you are writing on seems to glare.	Request permission in advance to submit your work on colored paper (experiment with colors to see which works best for you).

physical health and fitness. Because learning disabilities are biologically based, it makes sense that maintaining good health habits is important. Physical exercise, which has been found to help prevent diseases of all kinds, is also helpful in relieving some of the problems that accompany learning disabilities. Some students report that they are more able to concentrate and learn if they engage in just a little exercise each day.

On the other hand, it is important to get adequate rest. This may seem like a contradiction for a busy adult student, but if you have a learning disability, it is quite important. This is because it takes effort to concentrate and learn, especially when you are overcoming learning difficulties. If you become overly tired, your learning efforts become counterproductive. The brain simply cannot function as it should when it is deprived of sleep and rest breaks. It is recommended that students break up their studying into chunks of 20 minutes or so, taking short breaks between sessions. The emphasis here is on "short" because you may need only a few minutes to rest your eyes and your mind. Because you may have to spend more time studying than students without learning disabilities, good time management and teaching yourself not to waste time are especially important skills. For example, if you leave things until the last minute, you will find yourself rushed. This creates anxiety, even feelings of panic, and these feelings can prevent you from getting anything done at all.

There is a variety of groups and services you might find helpful. These include the following:

- Services for learning disabled students that may be available at your college or in your community
- Support groups that consist of students with learning disabilities, in which they share their experiences and ideas for overcoming challenges
- Study groups with a variety of students
- Learning centers and tutors who help with specific academic skills and subjects

Lastly, what may be the most important advice of all: seek help from your instructors. Students with learning disabilities report that their greatest mistake was not getting help before they were struggling and feeling desperate. Your instructors want you to succeed. Give them the opportunity to help make that happen.

Tables 2-4 through 2-14 outline different learning challenges and offer strategies on how a student can work with these challenges.

ACCOMMODATIONS

Knowing yourself and your needs is the first step toward self-advocacy, which means seeking solutions to your learning difficulties, trying alternate ways of learning, and asking for appropriate and necessary help. You may need to explain the nature of learning disabilities to people who don't understand them.

Accommodations are often available for students whose learning challenges prevent them from learning in traditional ways and who cannot demonstrate what they actually know through typical testing methods. The laws that protect individuals with disabilities apply to some people who have learning disabilities, depending on the nature and severity of the condition. These laws are *not* intended to excuse students from having to fulfill the requirements of their certificate or degree programs. Their purpose is to help students find ways to acquire needed knowledge and skills and demonstrate that they have mastered them.

It is important that if you do seek extra help or time to complete a test, you do so only when absolutely necessary. Taking advantage of the situation is unethical and unfair to other students. You must also consider carefully the possible effects of your learning disability on your work in health care. Using this time during your training to find solutions you can apply to your working conditions will help ensure your future success.

LEARNING DISABILITIES DURING THE JOB SEARCH

Personal organization and good oral and written presentation are important aspects of a successful job search. You may want to seek assistance from qualified helpers to work with you as you look for a job. These might include the following:

- Career services personnel at your school
- Your organization buddy
- Your instructors
- Your mentor, if you have one (see Chapter 3)

If writing is a problem, have someone proofread your resume and any letters you send out. See if potential employers have applications you can fill out online; if not, ask if you can take the application home to fill out so you can check it over carefully. If you are called for an interview and communicating orally is difficult for you, ask for help from your school's career services personnel or an instructor. Perhaps they can spend some extra time helping you prepare.

A question many students have is if they should disclose their learning disability to a potential employer. The opinion of experts is that if your disability does not affect your job performance, then it is not necessary to mention it. If, however, you plan to request accommodations, you must disclose it to be eligible. (Do note that if you are not legally defined as "disabled," you may not be entitled to accommodations.)

Once on the job, there are things you can do to work more effectively, as follows:

- Ask your supervisor to help you prioritize tasks.
- Ask that oral directions be repeated or given to you in written form.
- Apply the strategies you used in school. For example, if you used an eye-level ruler to help with reading, keep one with you at work.
- Request permission to take notes at employee orientations, workshops, or important meetings.
- Copy material you must read onto colored paper.
- Keep a timer at your desk or work area—or a small one in your pocket—to limit phone calls and conversations with co-workers.

As discussed previously, the important thing is to identify your own weaknesses and work to find ways to overcome them. People with learning disabilities have successful careers and productive lives. Sometimes, it just takes a bit of extra effort.

To Learn More

Adult Students

Adult Student Center
adultstudentcenter.com
Explore this website for inspiring stories about adults who return to school. Also contains links to dozen of Web resources providing help with specific subjects, locating references, and acquiring study skills.

Doolin M: *The success manual for adult college students*, ed 3, 2006, Booklocker.com.

Hardin CJ: *100 Things every adult college student ought to know*, Williamsville, NY, 2000, Cambridge Stratford Study Skills Institute.

Siebert A, Karr MK: *The adult learner's guide to survival and success*, ed 6, Portland, Ore, 2008, Practical Psychology Press.
www.adultstudent.com
The Internet companion to the book provides help with study skills and includes success stories and suggestions from other students.

Simon L: *New beginnings: a reference guide for adult learners*, ed 3, Upper Saddle River, NJ, 2006, Pearson Prentice Hall.

Walstrom C, Williams BK, Dansby CK: *The practical student*, Clifton Park, NY, 1999, Wadsworth Cengage Learning.

- Apply the strategies you used in school. For example, if you used an eye-level ruler to help with reading, keep one with you at work.
- Request permission to take notes at employee orientations, workshops, or important meetings.
- Copy material you must read onto colored paper.
- Keep a timer at your desk or work area—or a small one in your pocket—to limit phone calls and conversations with co-workers.

As discussed previously, the important thing is to identify your own weaknesses and work to find ways to overcome them. People with learning disabilities have successful careers and productive lives. Sometimes, it just takes a bit of extra effort.

English-as-a-Second-Language Students

Activities for ESL Students
http://a4esl.org
The activities include grammar explanations, quizzes, and vocabulary practice.

Dave's ESL Café
www.eslcafe.com
The "café" contains links to many ESL sites, including grammar lessons and lists of idioms.

e Learn English Language
www.elearnenglishlanguage.com
This site contains short lessons, which include good examples, on dozens of topics.

English Club
www.EnglishClub.com
English Club provides grammar explanations with examples. Also included are quizzes with immediate access to correct answers. The site originates in England, so a few words, such as "favourite," have British rather American spelling. The grammar, however, is the same.

English Page
www.englishpage.com
Explore the online tutorials that teach English grammar and vocabulary. There are good practice exercises and links to dozens of other useful sites.

Flores K: *What every ESL student should know: a guide to college and university academic success*, Ann Arbor, 2008, University of Michigan Press.
Flores shares tips for learning English gathered from her years of teaching English to college students from around the world who come to the United States to study.

Hacker D: *A writer's reference*, ed 6, Boston, 2007, Bedford/St. Martin's.
This is an excellent, easy-to-use book that includes explanations and examples of grammar, sentence structure, punctuation, and organization of content. One entire section is devoted to special help for ESL students.

Hospital English
www.hospitalenglish.com
Vocabulary is grouped into families of health care words such as diseases, patient-interaction vocabulary, and body systems. The site includes audio for pronunciation help and quizzes to check understanding.

To Learn More—cont'd

Learn English Today
www.learn-english-today.com
This site has lessons on all aspects of English, including a good list of phrasal verbs.
Resources for English as a Second Language
www.UsingEnglish.com
This is a comprehensive site with lists of idioms, phrasal verbs, irregular verbs, grammar, and more. There are quizzes on all aspects of English, plus links to other useful websites.
Vocabulary University
www.vocabulary.com
This site contains links to groups of basic vocabulary, including one for health terms.
Purdue University Online Writing Lab
http://owl.english.purdue.edu/owl/resource/678/01/
A section of this excellent Writing Lab is designed for ESL students.

Students with Learning Disabilities

ADDitude Magazine
www.additudemag.com
The emphasis of this website is "living well with ADD and learning disabilities." It contains useful articles for adults with ADD, such as how to focus at a job interview.
Children and Adults with Attention Deficit Disorder (CHADD)
8181 Professional Place, Suite 201
Landover, MD 20785
800-233-5050
www.chadd.org
This organization provides helpful information and support as well as publishing *Attention!* magazine. The website contains questions to help adults identify the signs of ADHD.
Crossbow Education
www.crossboweducation.com/Eye_Level_Reading_Ruler.htm
Although this is a British website, it has good visual presentations of useful products to assist with dyslexia and reading problems, such as eye-level rulers and reading windows.
Dolber R: *College and career success for students with learning disabilities*, Chicago, 1992, VGM Career Horizons.
This book provides specific strategies for college students, including study techniques and personal organization tips.
Great Schools
www.greatschools.net/cgi-bin/showarticle/2479
This Web page contains an article on evaluating assistive devices.
www.greatschools.net/cgi-bin/showarticle/3080
This Web page provides information about abbreviation expanders and lists various types available.
International Dyslexia Association
www.interdys.org
This website contains fact sheets and other resources.
Learning Disabilities Association of America
www.ldanatl.org
Find comprehensive information that includes help for adults with learning disabilities in postsecondary education and in the workplace.
Learning Disabilities Research and Training Center
The University of Georgia
Roosevelt Warm Springs for Rehabilitation
http://people.rit.edu/easi/easisem/ldnoelbw.htm
This website contains many links to resources for learning disabled teens and adults.
Moody S: *Dyslexia: surviving and succeeding at college*, New York, 2007, Routledge.
This book provides practical information to help students succeed.
National Attention Disorder Association
1788 Second Street, Suite 200
Highland Park, IL 60035
847-432-5874
mail@add.org (e-mail address)
www.add.org
This organization is specifically for adults with attention deficit disorder. It prints newsletters and brochures, holds conferences, and maintains a helpful website.
National Center for Learning Disabilities
www.ncld.org
This organization provides useful information for adults as well as children with learning disabilities.
National Resource Center on AD/HD
www.help4adhd.org
Information and resources for all ages.
National Resource Center on AD/HD: *Succeeding in the Workplace*, 2003.
www.help4adhd.org/en/living/workplace/WWK16
This article discusses dealing with ADD in the workplace.
Sarkis SM: *10 Simple solutions to adult ADD: how to overcome chronic distraction and accomplish your goals*, Oakland, Calif, 2005, New Harbinger Publications.
This book provides tips for personal organization to help adults cope with attention deficit disorder.
Technology Matrix
www.techmatrix.org
This is a Web tool for finding and comparing products that address special learning needs.

REFERENCES

1. Siebert A, Karr MK: *The adult learner's guide to survival and success*, ed 6, Portland, Ore, 2008, Practical Psychology Press.
2. Ellis D: *Becoming a master student*, updated 8th ed., Boston, 1998, Houghton Mifflin.
3. Berkman LF, Leo-Summers S, Hoewitz RI: Emotional support and survival after myocardial infarction: a prospective, population-based study on the elderly, *Ann Intern Med* 117:1003-1009, 1992.
4. Williams RB, Barefoot JC, Califf RM, et al: Prognostic importance of social and economic resources among medically treated patients with angiographically documented coronary artery disease. *JAMA* 267:520-524, 1992.
5. Seeman T: Social support and social conflict. John D. and Catherine T. MacArthur Research Network on Socioeconomic Status and Health, 1998. Available at: www.macses.ucsf.edu/Research/Psychosocial/notebook/socsupp.html. Accessed January 12, 2009.
6. Special Analysis 2002: http://nces.ed.gov/programs/coe/2002/analyses/nontraditional/sa04.asp. Accessed 1/12/09.
7. Flores K: *What every ESL student should know: a guide to college and university academic success*, Ann Arbor, 2008, University of Michigan Press.
8. *Reading strategies.* John's ESL Community. Available at: www.johnsesl.com/templates/reading/strategies.php. Accessed 1/24/09.
9. Bell M: *Problems in learning to read and write.* Available at: www.englishspellingproblems.co.uk. Accessed 1/24/09.
10. Norquist R: *Top 4 spelling rules.* Available at: http://grammar.about.com/od/words/tp/spellrules.htm. Accessed 1/24/09.

PRESCRIPTION FOR SUCCESS 2-1 | WHAT ARE THE BENEFITS?

List all the ways that your attending school and pursuing a career in health care will help your family. Share the list with them and ask them to add ideas of their own.

Your Ideas

____

____

____

____

____

____

Ideas from Family

____

____

____

____

____

____

PRESCRIPTION FOR SUCCESS 2-2 | MY SUPPORT TEAM

List the names of everyone you know who supports your decision to go to school.

From these names, who can you rely on when you need help?

PRESCRIPTION FOR SUCCESS 2-3 | WHAT ARE MY CHALLENGES?

Look over the classes you will be taking and read any available descriptions. On the basis of these, list academic challenges that concern you.

What can you do now to improve your skills? Create a plan with resources and timelines.

PRESCRIPTION FOR SUCCESS 2-4 BREAKING IT UP

Handling your various roles won't seem so overwhelming if you break what you need to do into bite-sized pieces. Choose a project or task you are currently working to achieve. Break it into a series of independent steps.

What is the task?

Step 1:

Step 2:

Step 3:

Step 4:

Step 5:

PRESCRIPTION FOR SUCCESS 2-5 | MY PROBLEMS WITH ENGLISH

Write a short description of up to five problems you have with English.

1. ____________________

____

2. ____________________

____

3. ____________________

____

4. ____________________

____

5. ____________________

____

PRESCRIPTION FOR SUCCESS 2-6 | HELPING YOURSELF

1. List up to five difficulties listed in the tables you believe to be obstacles to your academic and/or personal success.
2. From your list, choose one you want to work on.
3. Choose at least one strategy to try for 1 week.
4. Evaluate the strategy: how did it work for you?

Difficulties:

1. ____________________
2. ____________________
3. ____________________
4. ____________________
5. ____________________

Choose one: ____________________

Choose a strategy and describe how you will use it: ____________________

____

____

Describe if the strategy worked for you. Why or why not was it helpful? ____________________

____

____

CHAPTER

3

Developing Your Personal Skills

SETTING UP YOUR MISSION CONTROL

Starting on a new career path is a lot like launching a spacecraft. Both students and astronauts are entering new worlds, and for their missions to be successful, careful planning and preparation are required. Final destinations must be clearly defined so progress can be continually monitored and adjusted as needed to stay on course.

A helpful activity when planning a career launch is writing a mission statement, a statement of your basic beliefs and what you want to accomplish in your life. Stephen Covey, the author of personal success books, suggests mission statements as a way to identify what is really important to you. Individual mission statements are based on personal values. Values are our beliefs about what is important in life. They are the result of the teachings of family, school, religion, and friends as well as our experiences in life. Values provide a foundation for making important life decisions, such as what we hope to contribute to the world, how we perform our work, and what we believe our obligations are to others and to ourselves.

A personal mission statement can help you choose an appropriate destination and then stay on track until you arrive. Many people, Covey points out, get sidetracked in life because they either lose sight of their basic values or fail to identify them clearly in the first place. Mission statements are usually written out, but there is no set format. You might want to write yours as a list, a series of paragraphs, or even a letter addressed to yourself. If you prefer, you can create a poster or collage, with each picture illustrating a value.

Mission statements can serve as powerful motivators when you feel adrift or discouraged. For example, if you are committed to the well-being of your future patients, this value, rather than the need to pass a test, should guide your studying. Suppose you have an anatomy test tomorrow morning. It is 10:00 pm and you have just finished a day filled with classes, work, and family responsibilities. Studying the skeleton becomes more meaningful when placed in the context of your dedication to helping future patients. You are not simply memorizing a collection of bones. You are learning about the source of Mrs. Jones's painful arthritis, and the more you know and understand about the bones and joints, the more you will be able to help her.

Keep in mind throughout your program that your future patients will be directly affected by both what and how you are studying now, so you should be guided by your highest values. Here's another example: your mission statement includes the statement, "Provide high-quality care to all patients." You have an important exam for which you feel unprepared, and you are offered an opportunity to cheat. Cheating may take care of what you believe to be your most urgent need—getting a passing grade. But the consequences of this action—not learning the material and compromising your integrity—do not align with what should be your major goal of competently serving the needs of future patients. A well–thought-out mission statement functions as the control center that keeps guiding you in the right direction toward achieving what is most important to you.

GOALS—SIGNPOSTS ON THE PATH TO SUCCESS

"The purpose of goals is to motivate, not to paralyze."
Maureen Pfeifer

Goals are based on your mission statement and serve as signposts, giving your life direction and measuring your progress on the road to success. You can use them to motivate yourself and mark your accomplishments. Effective goals have the following characteristics:

- They are based on your values and mission statement: The goals help you achieve what you believe to be important in life.
- They are reasonable: You may have to work hard, but you can accomplish them.
- They are measurable: You'll know when you have achieved them.

- They are clearly stated and written: Writing goals greatly increases your chance of reaching them.
- They are worth your time: They are related to your career success, personal growth, and so on.

Here are two examples of well-stated goals for a health care student:

1. Over the next 10 weeks, I will learn the definition, pronunciation, and spelling of 150 new medical terms.
2. Within the next month, I will attend one professional meeting and talk with at least two people I have not met before.

Making Goals Work for You

Many people fail to achieve what they want in life because they fail to set clear goals for themselves. The first step, then, to is to spend some time deciding what it is you want to accomplish. The next step is to put together an action plan in which you outline what you need to do to reach each goal. Include reasonable deadlines for completing these actions. This is also the time to identify and locate any resources you might need to carry out your action plan. Examples of resources include people, materials, classes, equipment, and money. Greg, a medical transcription student, is taking a medical terminology course.

Incorporate working on goals into your daily life. What can you do each day—even if it is something small—to move closer to achieving them? Long-term goals often get put aside in the scramble to meet everyday obligations, so it's a good idea to periodically review your goals to track your progress.

Long-Term Goals

Goals vary in the time and effort required to achieve them. Write your long-term goals first; then prepare short-term supporting goals. Link them together in a progressive series so each one supports the next. For example, Jaime's long-term career goal is to become successfully employed as an x-ray technician in a large city hospital. Here is his plan:

- **Long-term goal:** Employment as an x-ray technician
- **Supporting goals:** Graduate from an approved x-ray training program
  - Take a study skills course
  - Earn at least a B in all courses
  - Maintain perfect attendance for all classes
  - Complete all homework assignments on time
  - Receive a rating of at least "above average" on clinical experience
  - Pass the state licensing exam on the first try

As we discussed in Chapter 1, you may have to set short-term employment goals as a means of achieving your long-term ideal job goal. In Jaime's case, he discovers that the large urban hospital where he wants to work hires only technicians who have had at least 1 year of experience. Furthermore, they prefer technicians who are able to perform specialized x-rays not taught in most x-ray technology programs. So Jaime adjusts his goals as follows:

- **Long-term goal:** Employment in x-ray department at Grand Memorial Hospital
- **Short-term goals:** Receive a rating of "Excellent" on clinical experience
  - Improve communication skills
  - Work for at least 1 year in a facility that performs a variety of x-ray studies
  - Complete three specialized x-ray courses
  - Network with local professionals
  - Become active in the x-ray professional organization's local chapter

Jaime knows his clinical experience will provide valuable opportunities to demonstrate his hands-on competence as a technician. This will serve him well when he applies for his first job after graduation and will also supplement his work experience when he applies at Grand Memorial. His action steps to achieve his short-term goals include arranging reliable transportation (his old car is no longer dependable) so he can always arrive at his clinical site on time. By planning ahead, setting goals, and identifying appropriate action steps, Jaime has greatly increased his chances of achieving what he really wants.

Success Tips for Achieving Your Goals

- Visualize yourself achieving your goals.
- Use affirmations.
- Work on goals even when you don't feel like it. (Especially then!)
- Don't give up!

IT'S ALL IN THE ATTITUDE

"Man is not disturbed by the things that happened, but by the perception of things that happened."

Confucius

Your attitude, the way you mentally look at things, can be your strongest ally or your worst enemy. It is more powerful than physical strength, is more important than natural talents, and has helped people overcome seemingly impossible difficulties. Many survivors of concentration and prison camps, for example, attribute their survival to having a positive attitude. The best thing about attitude is that it does not depend on other people or circumstances. It is yours alone, one of the few things in life over which you have complete control.

We hear about positive and negative attitudes to describe how people interpret things. Is the weather partly sunny or partly cloudy? Is a difficult class an opportunity to grow intellectually or a nightmare? Dr. Philip Hwang, a popular professor at the University of San Diego, tells his students he prefers to interpret a popular offensive gesture as "half a peace sign." He chooses his reaction, and this is the key to the power of attitude: we all can choose how we react to any situation.

"Well," you may say, "that doesn't make sense. If someone insults me or I'm having a bad day, it's natural to get angry or feel frustrated." It does seem natural because we are in the habit of responding negatively to situations that are annoying or upsetting. But how does this benefit you? In most cases, nothing is gained except bad feelings. For example, if you develop a negative attitude about a class ("I'll never learn how the endocrine system works," or "She really can't expect us to perform 20 perfect venipunctures after 2 weeks!"), you are working against yourself. Your attitude, whether positive or negative, will not change the circumstances. Your negative attitude, however, can make it more difficult, or even impossible, for you to understand the endocrine system or master venipunctures. A negative attitude is distracting, drains your energy, and interferes with your ability to concentrate. Choosing to approach life with a positive attitude releases you from the control of circumstances and frees you to focus fully on the priorities and actions that are in line with your mission and goals.

TRIPPED UP BY YOUR THOUGHTS

"The only thing we have to fear is fear itself."

Franklin D. Roosevelt

What we expect is often what happens—we get or become what we think! In fact, negative expectations can be just as powerful as positive ones, sometimes even more powerful. This is because our mental images, whether positive or negative, create our reality. It is important to understand that doubts and worries can actually bring about the outcome you fear. For example, Melinda thinks her supervisor dislikes her, so she avoids him and reacts defensively whenever he makes suggestions about her work. As a result of Melinda's behavior, chances are good the supervisor will have a problem with her. Tripped up by her thoughts, Melinda ends up creating what she expects and fears.

The fact is, your attitude greatly influences your performance in school and your ability to secure and succeed in the job you want. Expect the best for yourself, and you are likely to get it.

MAKE TIME WORK FOR YOU

"Plan your work and work your plan."

Your success in life depends, to a great degree, on how you manage your time. Learning to use it to your advantage requires planning and self-discipline, but the payoffs are well worth the effort. One fact of life is true for everyone: there will never be enough time for everything you want to do. There are ways, however, to use your time more effectively. Two key strategies are prioritizing and practicing efficiency. Prioritizing means deciding what is most important and taking care of those tasks first. Your goals should determine your priorities. What do you most want to accomplish? Are you spending enough time and energy on activities that will help achieve your goals? For example, if your goal is to graduate from a medical lab technician program with honors, are you spending the necessary time attending class, studying, and developing the work habits required of a lab technician? Or are phone conversations with friends and television viewing taking up a lot of your time?

Efficiency means planning and making the best use of time—getting the most done with the least effort. Examples of inefficiency include running to the grocery store to pick up a forgotten item, spending time looking for misplaced homework, and stopping for gas when you're already late for class rather than filling up the tank the day before. It's easy to feel very busy and yet be inefficient. Pay attention to how you spend your time. A short break from studying to "rest your eyes" can stretch into an evening of lost hours in front of the television set.

Keeping a calendar is an important part of good time management. Many types of calendars and planners, such as PDAs (personal digital assistants) that include everything from calendars to phones, are becoming very popular.[1] They allow you to store lots of information, including your schedule, telephone numbers, and other reference information. Many now enable you to access the Internet. Paper planners also work very well, and some people even prefer them over the electronic variety. The important thing is to select the best kind for you—one you will use. It should be convenient to carry with you and should have room to list several items for each date.

Collect all sources of important school and class dates: schedules, catalogs, and class syllabi. Mark important items on your calendar, including dates of quizzes and tests; due dates for assignments, projects, and library books; school holidays (for both you and your children); and deadlines for turning in required paperwork, such as financial aid and professional exam applications, and for paying fees. Add important personal dates: birthdays of family members and friends, deadlines for bills and taxes, doctors' appointments, and back-to-school nights for your children. If you work, note dates you need to remember: company potluck party, performance review, project deadlines. Colored ink is a good way to mark events you don't want to miss, like the day your professional exam is given! Again, the important thing is to create a planning tool that works for you.

Success Tips for Managing Your Time

- **Consider your priorities and goals** when you plan your schedule and decide how to spend your time.
- **Write out a weekly schedule.** Take a few minutes every week to plan ahead. This allows you to coordinate your activities with family members, plan ahead for important days (to avoid trying to find just the right birthday present on the way to the party), combine errands to save time, and plan your study time to avoid last-minute cramming.
- **Schedule study time every day.** This is your top priority! Give yourself a chance to succeed. Arrange not to be disturbed, and let friends and family members know that when you are at your desk, the time is yours.
- **Schedule around your peak times.** We all have individual body rhythms, specific times of the day when we feel most alert and energetic. Some people do their best work late at night. Others accomplish the most between 5:00 am and 9:00 am. Class and work schedules cannot always accommodate your needs, but when you have a choice, do the most challenging tasks during your best hours.
- **Do the hardest thing first.** When you have a number of things to do or subjects to study, try tackling the most difficult (or boring or tedious) one first, when you are freshest. Completing unpleasant tasks gives you a surge of energy by removing a source of worry and distraction from your mind and rewarding you with a sense of accomplishment.
- **Be realistic about what you can accomplish and how much time tasks will take to complete.** For example, thinking you can complete a research paper in one weekend can be a serious mistake because you may run into difficulties and end up with no time to spare. You will learn more about your work speed as you progress through your program. At the beginning, it is best to plan more time than you think you will need. On the other hand, take care not to spend more time than necessary on one project or assignment, causing you to neglect all others.
- **Prevent feeling overwhelmed by breaking work into small segments.** (The thought of writing this book was overwhelming until I broke it down into chapters, topics, and pages.) Plan deadlines for each segment, and put them on your calendar.

Ask for help and cooperation from family members and friends.

- **Learn to say "no."** Your schedule cannot always accommodate the requests of other people. It's difficult, but sometimes necessary, to turn down demands on our time such as an invitation to a party or a request to help at the church rummage sale. An instructor who reviewed this book said the following response works very well: "I'm really sorry, but I won't be able to help. I wish you the best in finding someone who can."
- **Use down time to your advantage.** There are many pockets of time that usually go to waste, such as when waiting for an appointment or using public transportation. Use this time to study flash cards, write lists, review class notes, brainstorm topics for a research paper, review the steps involved in a lab procedure, or summarize the major points of a class lecture. (I did about half of the work toward my last college degree while sitting in airports and on airplanes!)

DEFEATING THE PROCRASTINATOR

To procrastinate is to put off doing what needs to be done. Procrastinating can cause late assignments, failed tests, poor recommendations, and increased stress. Yet many of us fall victim to this self-defeating habit. Although it's natural to delay what we perceive to be difficult, tedious, or overwhelming, there are steps you can take to break the habit.

The first step is to identify the reason for your procrastination. What is holding you back? Are you afraid of failing? Do you believe you lack the ability to do what needs to be done? Does the task seem so unpleasant you cannot motivate yourself to start it? Is the project so large you feel overwhelmed and are the victim of "overload paralysis"? Once you have identified the reason, examine it carefully. Is it true you don't have the ability? Can the job be broken down into manageable portions? Can you match completing the task to a meaningful long-term goal?

The next step is setting a time to start, even if you simply work on planning what you are going to do. Accomplishing even a small amount can inspire you to keep going. Look for ways to break large projects into manageable pieces and plan deadlines for each. Develop a controlled sense of urgency (not panic!) to encourage yourself to meet self-imposed deadlines.

If you find yourself stuck, identify sources of help, such as your instructor, your supervisor, or a friend. Perhaps you need additional materials or more information to get started. Try using affirmations such as, "I am capable of understanding how the nervous system functions. My presentation to the class will be interesting and well organized." Visualize yourself completing the work. Experience the feeling of satisfaction. Finally, focus on your future. Think about how completing the work will help you achieve your goals to graduate and get a good job.

PERSONAL ORGANIZATION: GETTING IT ALL TOGETHER

"A vital key to success is learning to work smarter, not harder."

The purpose of personal organization, like time management, is to make life easier. Organizational techniques build consistency and predictability into your daily routines, saving you time and energy. Surprise-filled adventures are great for vacation trips, but efficiency is a better way to ensure academic and career success. Hunting for your keys every morning and arriving late for class is a waste of your time and a sign of inconsideration for your instructor and classmates. On the job, lack of organization can reduce patient satisfaction. No one wants to wait while the massage therapist scurries about to gather clean sheets or the relaxation tape she wanted to play.

Organization, however, should never be an end in itself. It doesn't mean keeping a perfectly tidy house, with clothes arranged according to color and season. It does mean surveying your needs and developing ways to avoid unnecessary rushing, repetition, and waste.

Success Tips for Getting Organized

- **Write lists.** Most people today, especially students, have too many things on their minds to remember grocery lists, all the day's errands, who they promised to call, which lab supplies to take to class, and so on. Scraps of paper are easy to lose. Commercial organizers and planners, both paper and electronic, give you a place to record phone numbers, addresses of stores, recommendations from friends, ideas you think of throughout the day, and so on.
- **Carry a big bag.** A typical student's day may include classes, work, shopping, and errands such as returning a video. Start each day—either in the morning or the night before—by checking your calendar and to-do list to see what you need to take with you. If you go directly to class from work, pack your books, binder, uniform, and other necessary supplies. Take along a healthy snack to avoid having to raid the vending machines. Always carry your planner or calendar.
- **Stock up.** Running out of milk, shampoo, or diapers can lead to a frustrating waste of time and energy. Even worse is discovering at 11:30 pm, while finishing a major assignment due in the morning, that your printer cartridge is empty and you don't have another. (Cartridges seem to be well aware of deadlines and choose to dry up accordingly!) Keep important backup supplies on hand. A handy way to monitor these is to keep a shopping list on the refrigerator and instruct everyone in the household to list items as they run low. You can note needed study supplies on the same list.
- **Give things a home.** Keeping what you need where you can find it can save countless hours of search time. It will also prevent redoing lost assignments or paying late fees on misplaced bills. If your study area is a dual-use area such as the kitchen table, try keeping your books and supplies in one place on a shelf or in a large box where everything can stay together. This way you can set up an "instant desk" when it is time to study. Organize your class notes and handouts by subject in a binder. Color-coded files work well for keeping ongoing projects and notes from previous classes in order.
- **Keep things in repair.** Life is easier if you can depend on the car and other necessities. If money is tight, focus on keeping the essentials in working order and look for ways to economize elsewhere.
- **Cluster errands.** Modern life requires trips to the grocery store, the mall, the children's school, the post office—you name it, we go there! Save time and money by doing as much as possible on each trip. Look for shopping centers that have many services to avoid running all over town.
- **Take advantage of technology.** If you are connected to the Internet, take advantage of opportunities to shop, pay bills, and perform other tasks online. If you don't a have a PDA, investigate the use of one.
- **Handle it once.** If you find that mail, bills, announcements, and other paperwork accumulate in ever-growing piles, try processing each item as it comes in. Sort the mail quickly each day and do something with each piece: discard the junk, pay the bills (or file them together for payment once or twice a month), answer letters with a short note, read messages and announcements, and place magazines in a basket to be looked over when you have time. Handle other papers that come into the house—permission slips for the kids, announcements from work—the same way.
- **Get it over with.** Certain unpleasantries, like parking tickets and dental work, come into everyone's life. It's easy to spend time worrying about them. A good strategy is to get them over with as quickly as possible: pay the ticket or make an appointment with the dentist. Seek help if you need it, and do your best to take care of what needs to be done. Procrastinating and worrying can drain your energy and interfere with your concentration.
- **Plan backups.** Prearrange ways to handle emergencies: a ride to school if the car breaks down, child care to cover for a sick babysitter, a study buddy who will lend you notes if you miss a class. Backups are like insurance policies—you hope you won't need them, but if you do, they're good to have. And whenever possible, plan backups for your backups!

If getting organized seems like a waste of time, too much work, or just "not your style," consider the alternative: using even more time and energy in unproductive ways that result in frustration and inconvenience. You can start now to help yourself get it together at the same time you develop organizational skills that are valuable in all health care occupations.

WHAT IS THIS THING CALLED STRESS?

We hear a lot about stress these days. One friend says, "I'm so stressed over this exam." Another exclaims, "I just can't take any more of this stress." Stress refers to our physical and emotional reactions to life's events. These reactions can either help us or hurt us, depending on the circumstances. "Good stress" motivates us when we are called on to perform outside our usual comfort zone. For example, if you witness a car accident and stop to help the victims, your body probably experiences certain reactions: your heart rate speeds up, your blood pressure rises, and the blood vessels in your muscles and the pupils of your eyes dilate. These changes increase your energy, strength, and mental alertness so you can best deal with the situation.

You can draw on these natural reactions to help you in important, although less dramatic, situations such as taking a professional licensing exam, giving a speech in class, or planning your wedding. This is making use of good stress to maximize your performance. The excitement experienced when you pass the exam and start a new career or get married and begin a new life with the person you love is also a form of good stress.

Pressure and unresolved worries experienced over long periods of time can create "bad stress." When the physical responses to stress are repeated over and over, with no resolution or action taken, they can actually decrease your ability to cope with life's ups and downs. In a sense, your body wears itself out as it continually prepares you to handle situations that are never resolved. Signs of long-term stress include insomnia, headaches, digestive problems, muscle tension, fatigue, frequent illness, irritability, depression, poor concentration, excessive eating and drinking, and use of illegal substances. It's easy to see that these don't work in your favor and are likely to increase your stress level. It's possible to get caught in a vicious cycle of ever-increasing stress that leads to feelings of hopelessness. Your mental images become dictated by worry and fear and may bring about, as previously discussed, the very thing you fear.

Sources of Stress

The first step in dealing with long-term stress is to identify its source. The following list contains some of the common sources of stress (stressors) for students:

- Financial difficulties
- Family problems: unsupportive partner, abuse, children's behavior, overdemanding parents
- Poor organizational skills
- Inability to manage time; having too much to do
- Lack of self-confidence and poor self-esteem
- Feeling unsure about study skills and ability to learn
- Loneliness
- Health problems, pregnancy
- Believing that instructors are unfair or don't like them
- Poor relationships with peers
- Believing the assignments and tests are too difficult or not relevant
- Difficulty following school rules and requirements

The second step in handling stress is to examine the source to see whether it's based on fact or fiction. For example, if you worry about failing your courses because you are not "smart enough," this may be based on a false belief about yourself. It is very likely you are intellectually competent. But believing you aren't can create stress that discourages you from even trying. After all, what's the point of making a significant effort if you're going to fail anyway? (The self-fulfilling prophecy at work!) A better approach is to seek guidance from your instructor or student services.

Finally, look for a practical solution. What are your options? Can you distance yourself from the stressor (for example, a negative friend who constantly asks why you are returning to school at your age)? Can you get help to resolve the problem (free financial counseling for budget and credit problems, tutoring in a difficult subject)? Can you empower yourself (math refresher course, speed-reading tapes)? The important thing is to face the stressor and look for ways to take control. Convert bad stress into good stress by using it as a signal that you may have issues that can prevent you from achieving your goals and attaining the success you want and deserve. Then take action to deal with the issues.

Success Tips for Handling Stress

The very nature of being a student and working in health care brings a certain amount of ongoing stress that cannot be avoided entirely. Many of the practices that promote good health are excellent for relieving stress: exercise, adequate sleep, eating properly, and avoiding excess caffeine. Here are some other things you can try:

- **Practice mentally.** If your stress is caused by an upcoming event such as a job interview, you can anticipate and mentally practice the event. Athletes use this technique to prepare for the big game. They "see" themselves performing the perfect tennis serve or making the foul shot. Employ your stress to motivate you to prepare in advance.
- **Use time-management and personal organization strategies.** Try the techniques suggested in this chapter to help you take control of your life. Work on eliminating the conditions that have you feeling like you're racing downhill with no brakes.
- **Seek the support of others.** People do better when they have the support of others. Studies have shown that students who have just one other person who really cares whether they graduate are more likely to finish school than those who have no one. Seek the help of trusted friends, family members, classmates, or school personnel.

- **Perform relaxation exercises.** Meditation, yoga, deep breathing, and muscle relaxation can relieve physical discomfort and promote emotional well-being.
- **Engage in physical exercise.** Even a short walk can be a very effective stress reducer. Find something you enjoy doing and make a little time for it on a regular basis.
- **Adjust your attitude.** Focus on your goals, acknowledge all progress, and concentrate on the benefits you will receive.
- **Keep your sense of humor.** Look at the humorous side of life and its events. Laugh therapy has been found to strengthen the immune system and positively affect health.
- **Use school and community resources.** Refer to the chart you prepared in Prescription for Success 1-2. Helpful information may be available from student services, your religious organization, or the local community center.
- **Make use of this book.** Chapters 3 through 9 contain many suggestions for developing effective study and life skills. Try them out and use the ones that work best for you.

PERSONAL REFLECTION

1. Do you believe you may be experiencing long-term stress?

____

____

____

2. If yes, what are the signs?

____

____

____

3. Can you identify the cause or causes?

____

____

____

4. List at least three strategies you will try for dealing with stress:

____

____

____

LEARNING FOR LIFE

Learning means much more than getting by in school and remembering information long enough to pass tests. It means storing information mentally and mastering hands-on skills that you can retrieve and use when you need them on the job. Furthermore, it means being able to apply what you have learned to solve problems and make informed decisions. For example, if you are learning about the circulatory system, you are not simply memorizing the parts of the heart and the path of blood through the body. You are acquiring information to help real patients who have heart problems. If you are studying a form of therapy, your study of the muscular system will have practical applications. Your purpose for learning is far more important than simply studying to earn a grade. Your future patients and clients will depend on your knowledge, and they deserve your best efforts to learn now.

How Do You Learn Best?

If you ever have trouble following your instructors' lectures or find that your class notes are a confusing jumble, you are not alone. It is possible that you learn better when instruction is presented visually or through hands-on experience. Research has demonstrated that people learn in different ways, called learning styles, and that by identifying your own preferred learning styles you can be more successful in your studies. The three learning styles most commonly discussed are grouped by the senses used when acquiring and processing new information: auditory, visual, and kinesthetic (hands-on). Table 3-1 contains a description of each of these styles.

There are other learning preferences, in addition to the styles related to our senses. Table 3-2 describes six other approaches to learning.

None of us learns in just one way. And it is important to understand that there is not a "best way" to learn. Just as we have different personalities, we have different combinations of learning styles. The purpose of discovering your preferred learning styles is to help you study more effectively. Sandra, a nursing student, has found the following methods to work best for her:

1. Receive new information from a class lecture (auditory)
2. Review by studying notes alone (individual)
3. Concentrate first on memorizing the important facts (inductive)

Developing Learning Strategies

Identifying your preferred ways of learning does not mean you will avoid the others. This would be impossible in a health care program that includes both theoretical and practical knowledge and skills. And individual

TABLE 3-1 Three Major Learning Styles

Learning Style	How Student Learns Best	Examples of Effective Learning Activities
Auditory	Through *hearing.* Remembers information from lectures and discussions better than material read in textbook. Prefers music over art and listening over reading. Understands written material better when it is read aloud. May spell better out loud than when writing. Misses visual cues. Prefers doing oral rather than written reports.	Lectures, CDs, tapes, music, rhymes, speaking
Visual	Through *seeing.* Remembers information presented in written or graphic form better than in lectures and discussions. Often needs people to repeat what they have said. Takes notes when oral instructions are given. Prefers art to music and reading to listening. Understands better when the speaker's face is seen. Prefers doing written rather than oral reports.	Reading, pictures, diagrams, charts, graphs, maps, videos, films, chalkboard, overhead projections
Kinesthetic (hands-on)	Through *doing.* Remembers information acquired through activities. Reads better when moving lips and saying words silently or moving finger along the page. Enjoys moving around while studying. Likes to touch things, point, use fingers when counting or calculating. Prefers doing a demonstration rather than an oral or written report.	Lab activities, skills practice, experiments, games, movement, building models

TABLE 3-2 More Approaches to Learning

Deductive Versus Inductive	
Deductive	**Inductive**
Deductive learners prefer to learn facts before forming generalizations (the big picture). They prefer to first memorize dates, study individual events, and know the details. When learning about the circulatory system, for example, they would rather study the various parts of the system before learning how they all work together to circulate the blood.	Inductive learners want to see and understand the big picture which they use as a framework for learning the details. When learning about cells, for example, they would want to know the purpose and function of the cell before learning the individual components.
Linear Versus Global	
Linear	**Global**
Linear thinkers learn best when material is organized in a logical sequence. They like to do things in order, building on material previously learned.	Global thinkers like to work with all the facts, regardless of the order. They are interested in forming relationships within the material.
Individual Versus Interactive	
Individual	**Interactive**
Individual-type learners prefer to work on learning tasks alone. They like to figure out all aspects of assignments and projects on their own.	Interactive-type learners like to work with another student or in groups. They want to share their ideas and hear the ideas of others.

instructors use a variety of approaches to teaching. Some will match your learning styles; others won't. For example, when teaching students how to take a blood pressure reading, the instructor might introduce the topic with a lecture (auditory), give a reading assignment (visual), demonstrate and describe the procedure (auditory and visual), assign a worksheet (individual), and have partners practice on one another (kinesthetic and interactive). In her lecture, she might list the individual steps first (inductive) or explain the purpose and significance of blood pressure before explaining how to take it (deductive). The good news is that you can learn in a variety of ways and benefit from your strongest methods while developing your weakest.

DOWN MEMORY LANE

Memorizing is not the same as learning, but it is an important component of the learning process. Although you may be able to rely on your short-term memory to complete assignments and pass tests, it is the material stored in long-term memory that will serve you throughout your studies, when taking your professional exam, and afterward on the job. There are many ways to improve your memory and better retain the material you study.

The way to start is by making sure you understand the new material. Experiments have shown it is much more difficult to remember nonsense syllables or lists of unrelated numbers than material that has meaning. In other words, it is very difficult to remember what you don't understand in the first place. So ask questions in class, look up words you don't know, and read difficult passages several times.

Repeat, repeat, repeat. The very best way to retain new material is repetition over an extended period of time. In fact, the length of time information is remembered is often in direct proportion to the length of time over which it is learned. Review new material as soon as possible after you first encounter it and continue to review it on a regular basis, at least weekly.

Use strategies based on your learning styles. If you are an auditory learner, listen to or say new math formulas over and over. Visual learners can post the formulas on the bathroom mirror. And kinesthetic learners can try writing each new formula 10 times. Use your imagination. Studying does not necessarily mean working quietly at a desk. Create rhymes or funny images. Make up movements associated with each item you have to remember. One method, called "pegging," has you place imaginary pegs on walls around the house. On each one, "hang" a fact or idea you must remember. As you walk through the house each day, review the material on each peg.

Look for ways to relate new information to your own experience by connecting it to something you already know. When you study something new, start by making a list of what you know—or would like to know—about the topic.

Success Tips for Improving Your Memory

- **Relax.** Your ability to store and remember things does not work well when your body is tense and your mind is distracted with worry. Try doing a relaxation exercise before starting a study session.
- **Remove distractions.** Studying for mastery requires concentration. Find a place where interruptions are limited and where you can use your chosen techniques. (For example, auditory learners who plan to use singing and tapping should probably not study in the school library!)
- **Break up your study sessions.** Most people can't concentrate fully for very long periods of time. The great thing about reviewing over time, rather than at the last minute, is that you can take time for short breaks.
- **Overlearn.** Continue to review and repeat material you already know. This helps to firmly lock it into long-term memory.
- ***Quiz yourself.*** Make up your own quizzes. Review one day and take the quiz several days later to evaluate your retention.

THE PERILS OF CRAMMING

Cramming is a well-known student activity consisting of frantic last-minute efforts, sometimes fortified with coffee and junk food, to finish assignments or prepare for tests. The major problem with cramming is that it serves only the immediate goal of meeting a school deadline. True learning rarely occurs. The conditions required for learning, such as the opportunity for repetition over time, are absent. Most of what is crammed is forgotten within a few days—or hours! Work in health care demands a higher level of competence than you are likely to achieve as a result of cramming. Do your future patients deserve your best efforts to learn, or are the bits you may remember after a night of cramming good enough? This is an important consideration for students who claim that cramming works well for them because they can study only at the last minute when the deadline is close. This is true only if passing the test is their only goal.

Another problem with cramming is it leaves you with few options. If you are writing a paper the night before it is due and you discover that the information you have is inadequate (and the Internet is not available), you have no time to consult other sources. If you are studying for a test and realize there are several points you don't understand, it's too late to ask the instructor to explain them.

Finally, cramming adds more stress to an already busy life in which you may be balancing various responsibilities. If it costs you a night's sleep, it can deplete your energy, and it can interfere with your ability to concentrate. You end up creating a nonproductive cycle consisting of a continual game of catch up and the danger of creating ongoing stress.

The reality is that things happen, you get behind, and you run out of time. Almost every student occasionally finds it necessary to cram. Here are some tips to make the best of a bad situation2:

1. Don't beat yourself up and waste energy feeling guilty. You'll only distract your attention from what you have to do. Just make a mental note to change your study habits to avoid the need for future cramming.
2. Do a very quick visualization in which you see yourself accomplishing what you need to do in the time you have available.
3. Minimize all distractions. For example, see if you can find someone to watch the children.
4. Focus on the most important material. What is most likely to be emphasized on the test? What are the main requirements of the assignment?
5. Use the learning and memory techniques described in this section. Draw on your learning style to help you learn the necessary material.
6. Try to stay calm. Physical tension distracts from mental effort. Breathe deeply, stretch, and do a quick relaxation exercise.

MENTORS MAKE A DIFFERENCE

"People seldom improve when they have no other model but themselves to copy."

Oliver Goldsmith

A mentor is an advisor you choose for yourself, someone who has the experience and background to give you sound advice about your studies and career. This is a person you respect and see as a positive role model. Your chances of succeeding are greatly increased when someone you respect cares about your progress. This has been proven in both school and business settings. Where can you find such a person? It can be an instructor, school staff member, administrator, or someone who works in health care. You might find a graduate of your school who is working successfully. It is important to choose someone with whom you feel comfortable.

Once you have identified a person you would like to have as your mentor, ask for an appointment. Let him or her know you want to talk about mentoring. At the meeting, explain that you are pursuing a career in health care and would like this person to serve as your mentor and give you guidance. Ask how much time he or she has to meet with you. You should meet or talk with your mentor periodically to ask questions, stay motivated, and learn more about becoming a health care professional. Mentors who work in health care can give you information about the current state of your targeted occupation, suggest what you should emphasize in your studies, and introduce you to other health care professionals. If the first person you approach does not have the time or is not interested, don't be discouraged. Continue your search—it will be worth the effort!

PERSONAL REFLECTION

What would you look for in choosing a mentor?

____

____

Who do you know who might be a good mentor?

____

____

____

What can you do to find a mentor who works in health care?

____

____

____

LEARNING PRACTICAL SKILLS

Most jobs in health care involve a lot of hands-on activity, and the level of your performance is critical to your success on the job. Future health care professionals must master a variety of skills. Depending on your specific occupation, these skills range from filling out forms accurately to performing a urinalysis to taking an x-ray film. Learning to apply the theory you learn in class to practical situations is one of the most important components of your education.

It is important that students take learning practical skills as seriously as studying for their theory courses. This is because hands-on practice builds a bridge between school and the world of work. There is a big difference between knowing about a procedure and being able to actually do it well. Actually performing a blood draw, for example, is much different from hearing about it. Practice sessions provide you with opportunities to take risks in a safe, monitored environment where you can learn from your experience—and from your mistakes.

At the same time, it is important to learn the theory and background information that support the procedures you will practice in the lab. For example, giving injections requires an understanding of the principles of infection control. Insurance coding requires knowledge of basic human anatomy terminology and medical diagnoses.

LEARNING IN THE LAB

Depending on your program of study, practice may include performing procedures, engaging in role play, working on the computer, and completing pencil-and-paper activities. You may solve problems, work with "patients," conduct tests, or do calculations.

Being Prepared for Lab Sessions

Advance preparation will help you benefit fully from lab sessions. Lab time is often limited, and the instructor will expect you to get started on the assigned activities without delay. The first step in being prepared is to read your textbook. Don't depend on your instructor's explanations or on being able to "figure it out." Reading gives you time to think through the steps and, as we discussed in Chapter 6, gives you a framework for lectures and demonstrations. Many health care textbooks present procedures in recipe or how-to format. Read through each step. Note all hints and cautions that contain important safety information for you and the patient.

In addition to reading your textbook, study the illustrations. Are the health care professionals wearing gloves? How are they positioned in relation to the patients and equipment? What do the equipment and instruments look like? How are they held? In which direction should movements be made? For example, in disinfecting a surgical site on the skin, it is important that cleansing be done in a circular motion, moving from the center toward the outside edges, to not contaminate areas already cleaned. The effectiveness of a procedure is often based on details such as these.

If your instructor demonstrates a procedure in class, focus on the steps or actions involved. Take notes only if doing so doesn't prevent you from watching and listening. If action is involved, mirror the instructor as closely as possible. For example, when watching a demonstration of the proper way to hold a syringe, use your highlighter or pen to copy the motion. Developing the ability to observe carefully is, in itself, a valuable health care skill.

Don't hesitate to ask questions about any point you don't understand. Get as complete an understanding as possible before going to the lab, to minimize mistakes and avoid wasting practice time.

Last—but very important!—pay special attention to learning safety rules. Many textbooks, as well as labs, use warning diagrams. Your future job may require you to operate expensive and potentially dangerous equipment and to handle chemical and biological hazards. The human immunodeficiency virus (HIV) and the hepatitis B virus can be spread by mishandling blood and certain body fluids. Laws regulate the proper disposal of contaminated items. All health care professionals must learn and follow the standard or universal precautions developed by the U.S. Centers for Disease Control and Prevention. The time to start applying these precautions is in your lab classes.

Success Tips for Learning in the Lab

- Take along any study materials, reference books, supplies, or protective equipment needed to participate in the scheduled activities. Set them out the evening before if you have an early start the day of the lab.
- Work with "real patients." Treat the students you work with in lab as you would if you were on the job. Demonstrate courtesy and concern. (Remember, "Your career starts now.") If you are entering patient data on the computer or practicing patient scheduling, work as if the exercises involved real people who are depending on your ability to maintain accurate and efficient records and schedules.
- Aim for accuracy. All health care tasks depend on accuracy to ensure safe, high-level patient care. You will also be expected to follow various laws and regulations, both in the lab and on the job. In many procedures, "almost correct" is not good enough. Only perfection is acceptable. For example, a sterile field is a germ-free area prepared to prevent infection during procedures such as minor surgeries. It is either sterile or it is not. Brushing an ungloved hand against an object in the sterile field may seem like a small error, but the field is no longer sterile. Work carefully in the lab. Never skip a step because this is "just practice" and these are not "real surgeries" or "real medications." When establishing your work habits, it is important that everything you do be done as realistically as possible.
- Respect your instructor's time, but do ask questions as needed. If the instructor is busy observing or assisting other students, write down your questions so you won't forget them.
- Understand that there may be more than one correct way to perform a task. Your instructors, as well as future supervisors, may each have different ways of performing a procedure. The important thing is that your technique follows accepted practice and is safe for both you and your patients.
- Keep up with your lab assignments. Many health care classes feature "check-off" sheets that the instructor uses to observe student performance of each required procedure. Each step is listed separately. This is because health care procedures must be done in a certain way (called a *protocol*), with many of the steps essential for the success of the procedure. When the procedure is completed satisfactorily, it is checked off on the sheet. Strive to complete these sheets in a timely way as you progress through each course.

Lab Follow-Up

It is important to follow up and review what you learned in lab sessions, just as it is for note taking and reading. You can do a number of things to help move what you learn in lab to your long-term memory.

1. Join or organize a study group to practice procedures and quiz one another on the rationale, safety concerns, and supporting theories.
2. Write out the steps of each procedure from memory. Include any safety concerns or rationale.
3. Make flash cards to help you remember important facts—rules and regulations, normal values (blood cell counts, body temperature, purpose of various lab tests, and so on).
4. Make charts, using color and illustrations to highlight important points about each procedure.
5. Recite the steps out loud, or record them and review by listening.
6. Rehearse the steps for each procedure in your mind. Act them out. Develop mental checklists of the steps. Some students find it helpful to use mnemonics (techniques to help the memory). For example, RICE is a popular way to remember the immediate first aid treatment for sprains:
   R = rest
   I = ice
   C = compression
   E = elevation

To Learn More

Chapman E: *Life is an attitude!* Menlo Park, Calif, 1992, Crisp Publications.

Elwood Chapman has been an "attitude guru" since the 1950s. This is the latest in his bestselling books on how to control your outlook on life by beating negativity, eliminating doubts, and setting positive goals. The book is short and very easy to read.

Covey S, Merrill AR, Merrill RR: *First things first,* New York, 1995, Simon and Schuster. (Also available on a CD.)

This book connects your mission statement and goals with time management. Rather than describing ways to get more done, it explains how to do what you decide is the most important. Covey teaches a method of categorizing tasks to help you focus on what is really important, not just on what is urgent. As he puts it, "Doing more things faster is no substitute for doing the right things." Important items are identified by focusing on a few key priorities and roles that will vary from person to person, then identifying small goals for each role each week, in order to maintain a balanced life.

Felder RM, Soloman BA: Learning styles and strategies. Available at: www.ncsu.edu/unity/lockers/users/f/felder/public/ILSdir/styles.htm.

This article, written by a professor and an advisor at North Carolina State University, categorizes and describes a variety of learning styles along with strategies for effective learning.

Hansen K: *The value of a mentor.* Available at: www.quintcareers.com/mentor_value.html.

This article includes tips on finding and benefitting from a mentor as you pursue your career goals.

Lakein A: *How to get control of your time and your life,* New York, 1989, Penguin Group (USA).

Although first published 30 years ago, this book is still a classic. Many consider it to be *the* authoritative source on which all other time-management books are based. Lakein explains the importance of prioritizing tasks and learning to work smarter, not harder.

Mind Tools. Available at: http://mindtools.com.

This website contains hundreds of helpful articles about important life and career skills, including time management, memory improvement, and stress management.

REFERENCES

1. *Saunders Health professional's planner,* Philadelphia, 2002, Saunders.
2. Ellis D: *Becoming a master student,* ed 12, Boston, 2009, Houghton Mifflin.

PRESCRIPTION FOR SUCCESS 3-1 NAME THAT GOAL

1. Write a goal and two action steps to help you achieve your goal.

   My goal: ______________________________

   Deadline: ______________________________

   Action step 1: ______________________________

   Deadline for action step: ______________________________

   Resources I will need: ______________________________

   Action step 2: ______________________________

   Deadline for action step: ______________________________

   Resources I will need: ______________________________

2. Explain how your goal relates to your mission statement and supports your values.

   ____

   ____

   ____

3. Create a visualization to help you achieve your goal. Briefly describe it here.

   ____

   ____

   ____

4. Write two affirmations to help you achieve your goal.

   a. ______________________________

   b. ______________________________

PRESCRIPTION FOR SUCCESS 3-2 | IT'S ALL HOW YOU LOOK AT IT

Scenario 1

Your medical terminology class is more difficult than you expected. You must memorize long lists of words and word parts and take quizzes twice a week. To make matters worse, the instructor is quite strict and does not seem very sympathetic. For each of the following options, indicate whether it reflects a positive or negative attitude. Then describe the probable outcome of each attitude.

Attitude or Action	Positive?	Negative?	Probable Result of Having This Attitude
Be angry with the instructor and his "ridiculous" expectations.	______	______	______
Focus on the fact that learning terminology relates to your goals of becoming a health care professional.	______	______	______
Complain to your classmates about the unfairness of the situation.	______	______	______

Organize a study group with your classmates.

______ ______ ______

Meet with the instructor privately and ask for study suggestions.

______ ______ ______

Look for ways to apply your learning style (discussed later in this chapter) to learning the terms.

______ ______ ______

Skip class whenever possible because it doesn't really do any good to attend.

______ ______ ______

Create and say affirmations stating you are mastering the vocabulary.

______ ______ ______

Don't waste your time studying because you won't remember the words anyway.

______ ______ ______

Think about how you will use medical terminology on the job.

______ ______ ______

PRESCRIPTION FOR SUCCESS 3-2 | IT'S ALL HOW YOU LOOK AT IT—cont'd

Scenario 2

You are working as a health professional. Overall, you like your job and enjoy helping patients. However, one of your clients is a teenager who is recovering from a cycling accident. You find her very difficult to work with. She is rude and seems to resent your efforts to help her. List six ways of handling this situation, and label each as being either a positive (effective) or negative (ineffective) reaction.

1. ______________________________

2. ______________________________

3. ______________________________

4. ______________________________

5. ______________________________

6. ______________________________

PRESCRIPTION FOR SUCCESS 3-3 | DEFEATING THE PROCRASTINATOR

Note: Students who never procrastinate may skip this exercise.

1. What have you been putting off doing?

   ____

   ____

2. Why do you think you have been procrastinating on this task?

   ____

   ____

3. Which of the techniques listed in this chapter do you think would help you most?

   ____

   ____

4. Develop a plan to get started, including the date you will begin.

   ____

   ____

PRESCRIPTION FOR SUCCESS 3-4 LEARNING STYLES INVENTORY

Check the boxes for the statements with which you agree or that best describe you. When you finish the three checklists, total your score for each. The checklist with the highest number of points is likely to be your strongest or preferred learning style.

Auditory Checklist

- ☐ I follow oral instructions better than written ones.
- ☐ I enjoy listening to music more than looking at art.
- ☐ I would rather listen to a lecture than read the material in a textbook.
- ☐ I prefer to listen to the news on the radio rather than read the newspaper.
- ☐ I spell better out loud than when writing words out.
- ☐ When I read, I sometimes confuse words that look like other words.
- ☐ I remember things the instructor says better than what I read.
- ☐ I don't copy well from the board.
- ☐ I enjoy jokes told orally more than cartoons.
- ☐ I like games with action and noise more than quiet board games.
- ☐ I understand material better when I read it aloud.
- ☐ Sometimes I make errors in math because I don't see the sign or I read the numbers or directions incorrectly.
- ☐ I am often the last one to notice something new that requires observation—for example, if a room is painted or a wall display is changed.
- ☐ Reading a map is difficult for me.
- ☐ I like to use my finger as a pointer when I read. Sometimes when reading I get lost or skip lines.
- ☐ I often sing, hum, or whistle to myself.
- ☐ I frequently tell jokes, tell stories, and make verbal analogies to demonstrate a point.
- ☐ Matching tests are difficult for me, even when I know the answers.
- ☐ I often talk to myself when I'm alone.
- ☐ I sometimes need to have diagrams, graphs, or printed directions explained orally.
- ☐ *Score (total of all checked items)*

Visual Checklist

- ☐ I often have to ask people to repeat what they have just said.
- ☐ The best way for me to remember something is to picture it in my head.
- ☐ I typically prefer information to be presented visually on the board, PowerPoint slides, etc.
- ☐ I often find myself "tuned out" in class when the instructor is talking.
- ☐ Sometimes I know what I want to say, but I just can't think of the exact word.
- ☐ I am good at drawing graphs, charts, and other visual displays.
- ☐ I take notes during lectures so I can look at them later to review what was said.
- ☐ I can usually follow written instructions.
- ☐ I can understand maps and use them to find my way.
- ☐ I have difficulty understanding instructors or speakers when their backs are turned and I can't see their faces.
- ☐ Other people sometimes accuse me of not listening to them.
- ☐ I'd rather show someone how to do something than explain it in words.
- ☐ I prefer board games to games that require listening.
- ☐ I have trouble remembering things that are announced unless I see them written or write them down myself.
- ☐ Sometimes I confuse words when I am speaking, especially words that sound similar.
- ☐ When trying to recall the order of letters in the alphabet, I have to go over most of it from the beginning. For example, recalling whether "j" comes before or after "g."
- ☐ I would choose art over music activities.
- ☐ I do better when the instructor demonstrates how to do something instead of just explaining it in words.
- ☐ I often forget things I've been told, such as phone messages, unless I write them down.
- ☐ I often draw pictures or doodle on the edges of my notes, on scrap paper, etc.
- ☐ *Score (total of all checked items)*

Kinesthetic Checklist

- ☐ I read better when I say the words quietly to myself.
- ☐ I often draw pictures or designs when taking notes in class to help me concentrate and remember the lecture.
- ☐ When I shop I frequently touch the items displayed for sale; when I walk through a room, I tend to touch the furniture.
- ☐ I often count on my fingers.
- ☐ I like to smoke, eat, drink, or chew gum while I study.
- ☐ I am comfortable being touched by others. I often hug others or touch them when I'm speaking to them.
- ☐ I learn best by doing an activity, rather than reading or hearing about it.
- ☐ I enjoy hobbies that involve making things.
- ☐ I like to be able to move around as I learn. For example, moving about in the classroom helps me concentrate on the lesson.
- ☐ I would rather do a demonstration than give an oral or written report.
- ☐ I fidget a lot, such as tapping my pen or jiggling my leg.
- ☐ I usually prefer to stand while working.
- ☐ I use my hands more than the average person to communicate what I'm trying to say.
- ☐ I'm pretty coordinated and good at sports.
- ☐ I'm always on the move.
- ☐ I tend to talk and eat faster than most people.
- ☐ I would rather participate in an activity, such as a ballgame, than watch it.
- ☐ It's hard for me to sit still for long periods of time.
- ☐ I work well with my hands to make or repair things.
- ☐ I enjoy labs more than lecture classes.
- ☐ *Score (total of all checked items)*

CHAPTER

4

Developing Your People Skills

THE IMPORTANCE OF PEOPLE SKILLS

The last few chapters focused on you as an individual and the personal attitudes, habits, and skills that influence your academic and career success. In this chapter, we shift our focus to other people and how you relate to them. You can expect to work closely with many kinds of people in your career, and your ability to create and maintain mutually beneficial relationships will be an important factor in your career success.

The quality and consistency of patient care are affected by how well health care professionals communicate among themselves as well as with patients and their families. Poor communication with patients contributes to the growing number of malpractice lawsuits. When patients feel they are listened to and understood, they are less likely to sue. This is true even if their treatment outcomes are negative.

At the same time, one of the most frequent complaints from employers today is that their employees lack good people skills. They don't know how to work well with others. More people fail on the job because of poor interpersonal skills than because they lack the necessary technical qualifications.

Good interpersonal skills are also important for academic success. Throughout your studies, you will have opportunities to learn from both your instructors and your fellow students. Your ability to communicate effectively will influence how much and how well you learn. Activities such as working on teams, practicing hands-on skills with other students, and joining study groups are ways you can start now to practice working with others. Most of life's activities take place in relation to other people, and improving the quality of these relationships can improve the overall quality of your life.

RESPECTING OTHERS

"Be kind. Remember, everyone you meet is fighting a hard battle."

Plato

By choosing a career in health care, you have accepted the responsibility to serve others. Your duties may range from performing an uncomfortable medical procedure to explaining a complicated bill for a hospital stay. It will be your obligation to serve all patients or clients with an equal level of care and concern, regardless of their appearance, behavior, level of education, and economic status. Not everyone will look, act, behave, or even smell as you would like. They will not all express appreciation for your efforts. People who feel sick may be irritable and cranky. The satisfaction you obtain from your work must be based on what you can give to others, not on what you receive from them.

Good health care practice is based on the principle that all human beings deserve to be treated with respect and dignity. The need to treat all patients equally and fairly has been recognized and endorsed by professional organizations such as the American Hospital Association (AHA). The AHA formalized this belief in "The Patient Care Partnership" mentioned in Chapter 1. Specifically, it states that patients have the right to "be treated with compassion and respect."

It is also important to demonstrate respect toward your supervisor and co-workers. The quality of work produced in any organization depends on the quality of the relationships among the people who work there, and good relationships are based on mutual respect.

Guidelines for Respectful Behavior

- Be courteous. Many observers today have noted that as a society we are moving away from the practice of common courtesy. Many people fail to use expressions like "please" and "thank you." These are powerful words that improve the quality of both personal and professional relationships.
- Maintain professionalism. As a student and on the job, it is important to display maturity and competence. Examples of inappropriate communication behaviors are chewing gum, arguing, swearing, and yelling.
- Acknowledge the other person. No one likes to be ignored. If you are busy working with someone else

or talking on the telephone when a patient arrives, use eye contact and a quick nod to let the person know you are aware of his or her presence.

- Don't interrupt. Avoid breaking in when another person is speaking. Some people need extra time to compose their thoughts or express themselves. Avoid the habit of finishing sentences for others. This frustrates the speaker, and your assumption about what they planned to say may be incorrect.
- Show interest. Look at the other person when you are talking and listening. Show you are listening by nodding or using confirming sounds or phrases such as "uh, huh," "I understand," "okay," and so on. Don't turn your body toward the door as if to say, "Hurry up. I need to move on to something else."
- Guard privacy. This is good practice in your personal life. In health care, patient privacy is protected by law. It is illegal to discuss patient information with anyone who is not working directly with the patient. Make a habit of never sharing anything told to you in confidence by family members, friends, or classmates. (Patients must even give written permission before information can be given to insurance companies, other health providers, and so on.)
- Avoid gossip. Gossip can be a very serious problem in the workplace. It serves no useful purpose and can lead to hurt feelings, broken trust, and strained relationships. If it involves confidential patient matters, it can lead to a lawsuit.
- Remain calm. It is important to behave and speak calmly when you are dealing with situations such as emergencies and angry patients. A calm demeanor both reassures others and enables you to focus on doing what can best help the situation.

APPRECIATING DIVERSITY

"Commandment Number One of any truly civilized society is this: Let people be different."

David Grayson

The population of the United States is made up of people from all over the world. Immigration has increased dramatically in recent years, and Americans now more than ever represent a wide variety of races, religions, lifestyles, languages, and educational and economic levels. These variations are known as diversity.

Diversity also refers to differences not related to cultural background or race. These include age, sexual orientation, disabilities, and appearance. People who are different are sometimes ignored or treated inappropriately, sometimes even cruelly. This may not be done intentionally, so you must think about what you are doing and how it might be interpreted. For example, it is not uncommon for health care professionals to speak to younger relatives who accompany elderly patients as if the patients were not present. Other examples are using "baby talk" with the elderly or shouting at them if they were hard of hearing.

Our society can benefit from the contributions of people with different customs and ideas. By drawing from a variety of viewpoints, we increase our chances of solving the complex problems encountered in modern society. Learning from our differences can be beneficial. Many Americans, for example, find pain relief from the ancient Chinese practice of acupuncture, the insertion of very small needles into specific points on the body. Unfortunately, differences in values and beliefs about life can cause misunderstandings and even lead to violence. Learning to take advantage of the differences and to peacefully work out misunderstandings is one of the major challenges the world faces today.

Work in health care will give you opportunities to interact with people from many different backgrounds. Your personal actions and efforts to understand and serve others can contribute to a more harmonious society. The students in your school probably come from diverse backgrounds. Initiate communication with them. And if your own background is different from that of your classmates, you can serve as a source of information about your culture.

Promoting Understanding

When we learn about others, we also learn about ourselves and what it means to be human. You can enrich your life by accepting diversity and seeking opportunities to learn about different ways to view the world. Here are some suggestions to help people of all backgrounds better understand each other:

- **Put fear aside.** Many people are frightened by what they don't understand. Some are afraid that acknowledging differences among people will result in negative changes in society. In fact, the contributions of people from different backgrounds have resulted in the economic success and political stability of the United States.
- **Listen to other points of view.** Seek opportunities to interact with people whose backgrounds are different from yours. Encourage them to express their ideas and opinions. Listen carefully to what they say.
- **Ask questions.** Use questions to learn more, but not to challenge the other person. For example, instead of asking, "Why do you believe that?" you could say, "That sounds interesting. Could you tell me more about that?" Your goal is to learn and understand, not to imply that the other person is wrong.
- **Avoid stereotypes.** Don't make assumptions about people because of their age, race, gender, or other categories. Consider each person as an individual with a unique set of characteristics.
- **Don't judge people by their appearance.** Outward appearances do not always represent who people are.

To truly know people, you must talk with them and observe their actions. If you immediately dismiss them based on how they look, you may lose the opportunity to form a friendship or a beneficial working relationship. Assuming that patients "are what they look like" may detract from the care you give them.

- **Explore different cultures.** Many schools and communities sponsor activities that highlight the cultures represented in the local population. Check your local library and the Internet for other sources of information about the backgrounds of your classmates and future patients.
- **Learn about other value systems.** People are defined by their values and beliefs about how they should live. Culture is much more than typical foods and daily customs. Develop a deeper level of knowledge and understanding through conversation and by learning about the religions and important beliefs of the people in your area. See Table 4-1 for examples of cultural and personal beliefs.
- **Look for commonalities.** As human beings, we share many of the same needs, concerns, and goals for our lives. Explore what you have in common with people who seem different.
- **Offer to help others.** Expand your attitude of caring by looking for ways to help others. For example, offer to help a classmate who has trouble speaking or writing English. Or if English is your second language, offer to teach your language and customs to others.
- **Learn another language.** You may not have time now to study another language formally, but you can learn a few key phrases of any major cultural groups in your area. This can increase your effectiveness as a health care professional and your worth to an employer.

PERSONAL REFLECTION

1. Which cultural groups are represented where you live?

____

____

2. How much do you know about their customs and beliefs?

____

____

3. How can you learn more?

____

____

DIVERSITY ON THE JOB

Everything we do is influenced by our cultural background. Being aware that differences exist can help you to better understand the people you will encounter on the job. Beliefs that many of us take for granted, such as, "It is important to always be on time," are not important to everyone. Making assumptions can result in misunderstandings. Let's look at an example. A patient has to wait 15 minutes before you can perform his lab test. In an effort to respect his time and not add to the delay, you keep conversation to a minimum and complete the procedure as quickly as possible. You believe you have been considerate. The patient, from a culture that does not consider time in the same way, is insulted. His interpretation of your behavior is that you obviously have more important things to do than work with him, so you are rushing along. The "right thing" in your eyes was the "wrong thing" in his. Of course, it is impossible to know and accommodate every cultural difference that you encounter. You can, however, be aware of what types of differences exist and strive to be sensitive to them. Ask questions if you are unsure about a person's feelings or understanding of a situation. Table 4-1 lists common areas of differences among cultures.

EXPERIENCING EMPATHY

"Don't judge a man until you've walked a mile in his shoes."

Empathy means attempting to see the world through the eyes of other people in order to understand their feelings and experiences. Prescription for Success 1-6 in Chapter 1 asked you to imagine yourself as a patient with a broken arm. Putting yourself in the place of someone else is an important part of experiencing empathy. This is not always easy to do because we are all influenced by our own beliefs, values, and previous experiences. Being empathetic requires listening carefully to others without judging what you hear. You then think about what you hear and, if necessary, ask for clarification or more information. What is the person trying to communicate or trying to hide? What clues are you getting from the person's body language? What is important to this person?

Health care professionals must have empathy with patients to understand their needs and learn how best to help them. Being empathetic sends the message, "You are important and worth my time and respect. I will make every effort to know who you are and what you need."

A key part of empathy is letting the other person know that you are trying to understand his or her experience. It is best, however, not to say that you know exactly how he or she feels. This sounds insincere because, in fact, it is impossible to know precisely how another person feels. In trying to be helpful, we may be tempted to share and compare our own stories—for example, saying, "Oh, I know just what you mean. The same thing happened to me..." and then launching into a detailed explanation about what happened to us. This shifts the focus to us and away from the person who needs the attention.

Learning to experience empathy improves all interpersonal relationships, including those with friends, family

TABLE 4-1	Examples of Cultural and Personal Beliefs
Time	It is important to always be on time for meetings and appointments. Appointment times are just estimations of when they might take place. Time is valuable and should not be wasted. Time is not a resource over which we have control. It just is. Planning and using time productively are important. If something is important, it will eventually get done; there is no reason to rush. The present is more important than the future. The present should be used for planning and preparing for the future.
Personal Space	The distance comfortably maintained when people are talking ranges from a few inches (when you can feel the breath of the other person on your face) to over a foot away.
Age	Youth is valued. People should try to maintain a young appearance and lifestyle as long as possible (exercise, wrinkle creams, and hair dyes). Older people are valued for their wisdom and are shown great respect. When elderly people are no longer able to care for themselves, it is appropriate to place them in nursing or retirement homes. Older people should live with and be cared for by family members until they die.
Touching	Shaking hands is okay for everyone. Only members of the same sex can shake hands with one another. Hugging is okay for everyone, even members of the same sex. Kissing is okay between women. When meeting a new person, only a slight bow is permitted, not touching.
Gender	A woman cannot be treated by a male physician. Women and men are equal. Men are dominant. Women act as the head of most families. Women have no economic or political power.
Eye Contact	Direct eye contact is a sign of sincerity, honesty, and interest in the other person. It is a sign of disrespect. Sustained eye contact communicates hostility and aggression or sexual interest.
Personal Control	Each person is in control of his or her own life. Luck, fate, or the will of God determines how things turn out.
Spiritual Practices	There is one God. God helps those who help themselves. God punishes those who sin. God answers all prayers. There is uncertainty about the existence of God. There is no God. Witchcraft and magic can both help and hurt us.
Definition of Success	Personal and professional achievement. Acquiring material possessions. Living a spiritual life. Achieving inner peace. Raising many children. Being a kind person and helping others.
Health Care Beliefs	Disease is caused by germs, environmental conditions, and personal habits such as smoking. Good health is a gift or reward from God. Illness is a punishment sent by God. Illness happens when the body's energy or humors get out of balance. Science has the best answers for preventing and curing disease. The body can heal itself naturally. Herbs are the best remedies. Only God can heal. Good health is a balance among the mind, body, and spirit. Individuals are responsible for their own health and healing.
Beliefs About Death and Dying	Death is a natural part of the life cycle. Death should be avoided at all costs. Dying is up to God. Death means the health care system has failed. Autopsies destroy the soul. Cremation frees the soul. Everything possible should be done to save life. People who are terminally ill or suffering should be assisted to die if this is their wish. Families should take care of the dying. Hospitals or other health care facilities should take care of the dying.

members, classmates, instructors, co-workers, and supervisors. Your relationships can be more harmonious when you make an effort to see the views of others. Here are some ways to increase your practice of empathy at home and in school:

- When you talk with your classmates, listen carefully. How are their views different from yours? What experiences have they had that explain these differences?
- Are there students who exhibit poor behavior? Why do you think they behave in this way? What are some clues that might explain their actions?
- Why do family members sometimes "act out"?
- What kinds of experiences have shaped the opinions of your friends?

ORAL COMMUNICATION: CREATING THE PEOPLE CONNECTION

Many people believe they are good communicators because they are friendly and like to talk. But the ability to speak is only one part of effective communication. There are four other essential parts of effective communication: listening, thinking, requesting feedback, and using and interpreting nonverbal communication (body language, expressions, and gestures). Successful oral communication takes place when the receiver (listener) receives and understands the intended message of the speaker. We all know this is not always the case! Let's look at how you can increase the effectiveness of your communication.

Speaking

Speaking consists of creating and sending messages. The first step in creating a clear message is to determine your purpose. In Chapter 7, we discussed the importance of determining your purpose when writing. It is the same with speaking: you need to know your communication goal.

Effective messages match the purpose of the speaker with the needs of the receiver. These needs are determined, in part, by the characteristics of the receiver.

Success Tips for Sending Effective Messages

- Speak from a base of sincerity, caring, and respect for others.
- Choose a level of language that is appropriate for the receiver. If a person is heavily medicated, for example, use simple words and short sentences.
- Choose appropriate vocabulary. Using medical terminology is an effective way to be precise when speaking with co-workers, but it can be confusing for patients. They may hesitate to tell you they don't understand because they don't want to seem dumb. However, ensuring that patients understand your questions and explanations is critical for their health outcomes. The inability to understand health care providers is a major patient complaint.
- Avoid slang and nonstandard speech. These are often characteristic of certain age and social groups and can cause misunderstandings with people outside those groups. Speech that is appropriate among friends and at social gatherings may not be correct for school and work. For example, the current use of the word "goes" to mean "says" is understood by many young people but may be confusing to others.
- Speak clearly and at a moderate speed—not so quickly that you are difficult to understand or so slowly that the receiver's mind wanders. (We hear and comprehend many times faster than we speak.)
- Avoid speaking in a monotone. Speak naturally, but with expression in your voice. Make sure it is appropriate for your message. For example, speak with respect when asking questions in class, friendliness when greeting a new student, reassurance when calming fears, and firmness when giving instructions that affect patient safety.

ACTIVE LISTENING

"To listen well is as powerful a means of communication as to talk well."

U.S. Supreme Court Chief Justice John Marshall

Active listening, as was discussed in Chapter 6, should not be confused with hearing. Listening requires effort, whereas hearing is more passive. To listen well, you must pay attention, focus on the speaker's words, and reflect on what you hear. Active listening demonstrates respect for the speaker. It is an essential skill for the health care professional because all patients want to work with someone who listens to them and makes every effort to understand their needs. In fact, patient satisfaction surveys show that patients highly value providers who are excellent listeners and take what they say seriously.[1]

Think for a moment about your own listening skills. Do you sometimes catch your mind wandering and thinking about other things? Do you think about what you are going to say next? Do you argue mentally when you disagree? These habits can interfere with your attention and prevent you from hearing the speaker's message. Look over the following checklist of techniques designed to improve listening skills. Are there any you'd like to try?

- Prepare yourself mentally to listen by clearing your mind of other thoughts.
- Control the noise level of your environment as much as possible. Turn off the radio or television, look for a quiet place to talk, or move out of the busiest part of the office.

- Focus on the other person and concentrate on following what he or she is saying. Sometimes when we think we are listening, looking at the speaker, and perhaps even nodding in agreement, we are actually thinking about something else. Practice being aware of where your attention is directed.
- If you disagree with what you are hearing, try not to engage in mental arguments. Internal self-talk interferes with your ability to listen. It is usually easy to understand people we agree with. It takes more effort to hear people we disagree with, but only by listening carefully can we begin to understand another's point of view.
- Practice making quick mental notes about points you need to clarify Work on being able to do this without losing track of what the person is saying.
- Focus on what is being said rather than how it is said. Move beyond the speaker's appearance, manners, language level, or even odor. Try not to let unpleasant factors about the person interfere with your ability to concentrate on what he or she has to say.
- Acknowledge the person even if you are taking notes or performing a test or procedure while he or she is talking. Look at the person from time to time and make eye contact.

Listening effectively is one of the most valuable skills you can develop for both personal and professional success. It can increase your learning, your effectiveness in helping others, and even your popularity. At the same time, it is a skill many people neglect because they assume they know how to listen. Working to improve your listening skills is one of the most important actions you can take to work well with others.

FEEDBACK

Feedback is a communication technique used to check your understanding of what a speaker says. Even when you listen carefully, there may be times when what you hear is not what the speaker intended. We have all experienced the misunderstandings that occur when we assume we understand the speaker's message—and then learn that the intended message was quite different!

There are several methods for giving and requesting feedback. Here are three of the most common kinds of feedback:

1. **Paraphrasing.** This means saying what you heard in your own words so that the speaker can confirm or correct your statement.
2. **Reflecting.** This is similar to paraphrasing, but you repeat what the other person says using words as close as possible to his or her own words. This gives the person the opportunity to confirm or add additional information.
3. **Clarifying.** This means asking the speaker to explain what he or she means.

ASKING QUESTIONS

"No man really becomes a fool until he stops asking questions." *Charles P. Steinmetz*

Scientific discoveries and technologic advances are the result of people asking questions. What causes...? What would happen if...? How can we...? Asking questions is a powerful tool for learning. You can increase your knowledge and understanding in school by asking questions. Yet many students sit through hours of classes and never ask a single question. Take advantage of your opportunities to learn and get ready to ask good questions in class. Here are some tips to get started:

- **Prepare ahead for class.** If you haven't read the assignment or completed the other homework, you won't have the background information on which to base a question.
- **Write questions down.** Suppose you did the reading and remember that there were several points you didn't understand, but you didn't write them down, and now you can't remember what they were! Don't let this happen to you. During lectures, write down questions as you think of them so you can ask them at the appropriate time.
- **Don't be embarrassed.** No one wants to ask what they think is a dumb question. But if you already knew everything, you wouldn't be in school, right? Instructors welcome questions in class and are usually pleased when students take an interest in the subject. (Exception: You don't pay attention in class and/or don't read the assigned material and then ask lots of questions that force the instructor to repeat what he or she just finished saying.)
- **Ask the questions later.** If all the class time is taken up with the lecture or the instructor never gets around to your lab group, arrange a time to ask your questions later. Be willing to make the extra effort to get the information you need.
- **Be brave.** Have you ever found yourself so confused in class you can't even phrase a question? This is exactly when you should ask a question. Try something like, "I'm lost here. Could we go back to...?" Avoid waiting until you're so far behind that you don't have a chance of catching up.

Types of Questions

There are four basic types of questions, as follows:

1. **Closed-ended.** Can be answered with a "yes" or "no" or in one or two words. They are used for getting specific facts.

2. **Open-ended.** Require a longer answer and request explanations, descriptions, examples, and other details.
3. **Probing.** Based on what the other person has already told you. The purpose is to acquire additional information.
4. **Leading.** Question is worded to provide a possible answer. These questions should be used with great care because they may encourage the other person to simply agree because he or she doesn't really understand the question or thinks you have provided the correct answer. Leading questions can be helpful with people who find it difficult to communicate because of injury, language barriers, shyness, or other problems that make communicating difficult.

Success Tips for Asking Effective Questions

- **Choose the right place.** Some important questions are personal, embarrassing, or potentially difficult to answer. A question for the instructor about a low grade you believe to be unfair is best asked in private, not during class. An interview with a patient with acquired immunodeficiency syndrome (AIDS) must be conducted out of the hearing of others.
- **Choose the right time.** Asking your supervisor a question about your performance when he or she is ready to leave the office isn't fair to either of you.
- **Avoid challenging or judgmental questions.** Your choice of words and tone of voice can communicate the negative message, "You are wrong, and I demand an explanation." For example, questions like, "Why did you do that?" or "What were you thinking?" may draw a defensive reaction or no response at all. A major goal of communication should be to encourage discussion so that issues can be resolved.
- **Know what not to ask.** There is a difference between showing interest in others and asking questions that are too personal and may offend. To show concern without prying, you can say something like, "You seem really upset. Is there some way I can help?" This allows the person to reveal as much information as is comfortable. If you must ask potentially embarrassing questions, explain why you are asking them and how the information will be used. Assure patients that anything they say will remain confidential, as required by law.
- **Know what's legal.** Some questions, especially when asked in hiring situations, are illegal. These include asking about age, marital status, number of children, and other matters that are not related to job performance. (See Chapter 12 for more information.)
- **Allow silence.** Some people need more time than others to think and prepare a response. Unless it is obvious they don't understand the question, don't feel that you must speak to fill the silence.

NONVERBAL COMMUNICATION

More than half of the content and meaning of our messages is communicated nonverbally through our movements, posture, gestures, and facial expressions. In fact, nonverbal communication is often more revealing than verbal communication because we are usually not aware we are doing it—it is not completely under our control. For example, telling a friend that you are "fine" when you have a worried expression on your face sends a mixed message. The friend is more likely to believe your face than your words. Nonverbal communication can either emphasize or distort the content of verbal messages.

Use the following questions as a starting point for becoming more aware of your own nonverbal language.

1. Do you have nervous habits, such as jiggling your leg or playing with your hair, that distract from or distort your messages? These habits can give the impression that you would rather be somewhere else.
2. Is your general posture upright or slouching? Do you face the person you're talking with or partially turn away, as if looking for escape? Leaning slightly toward the other person communicates interest.
3. Do you assume an accepting body position? Crossing the arms, for example, can be a sign of being closed to what the other person is saying.
4. Do you use gestures to emphasize or add meaning to your words? Or are they routine habits that add nothing to your message? Gestures are especially helpful when used for demonstrations and to communicate with people who have limited ability to understand spoken language. Examples include very young children, non-English speakers, and the hearing impaired.
5. Does your face express interest or boredom? In class, do you usually face the instructor or look out the window? When an activity is announced, do you roll your eyes and exchange pained looks with other students? Poor attitudes are easy to read and can negatively affect the quality of the class by annoying the instructor or putting him or her on the defensive. Learning to control facial expressions is important because as a health care professional you will need to maintain expressions that convey caring and reassurance even in difficult situations.
6. Do you smile when it is appropriate? Does your face send the message "I'm glad to be here talking with you"?
7. Do you maintain appropriate eye contact? Failing to look at the other person while you are speaking tends to communicate a lack of sincerity, interest, or respect. (Exceptions to this include cultures that interpret eye contact in different ways.)

In addition to monitoring your own nonverbal communication, practice observing it in others. This will be important when working with patients who may be unable or unwilling to fully communicate with you verbally. Learn to "listen between the lines." Do the speaker's words and actions match? Are there nonverbal signs of confusion, fear, or anger that you should take into account? Does your instructor give any of the nonverbal messages, discussed in Chapter 6, that communicate what is most important for you to learn?

Ask for clarification if verbal and nonverbal messages seem to conflict. Use the feedback and question techniques discussed previously. Be willing to take the time and make the effort to get the true message. You can improve the interpersonal relationships in all areas of your life by combining an understanding of nonverbal communication with active listening and feedback.

GIVING PRESENTATIONS WITH CONFIDENCE

Many students find speaking in front of a group to be a frightening experience. This is a fear worth conquering, because the ability to speak with confidence can increase your opportunities to grow professionally and advance in your career. Proper preparation and a lot of practice can take the terror out of public speaking.

Preparing an oral presentation requires some of the same skills you use when writing, such as conducting research and organizing your material. It is said that an excellent way to learn something is to explain it to someone else. Try making oral presentations positive experiences by focusing on how you can learn from them.

Preparation

The six steps for preparing a presentation listed here are similar to the suggestions given in Chapter 7 for writing a paper.

Step One: Choose your topic early. It should be something you want to know more about or something you have strong feelings about. (Note: If you must speak on a topic with which you disagree, as sometimes happens in a debate on a controversial subject, this is a chance to practice seeing other points of view and experiencing empathy.)

Step Two: Be clear about your purpose: inform, persuade, demonstrate, encourage people to take action, entertain.

Step Three: Find out about your audience. What is their background? How much do they know about the topic? What are their beliefs? What is their interest level?

Step Four: Identify what you need to find out, and then do your research. Make sure you have accurate, up-to-date facts. Health care is constantly advancing and changing. Start now to develop the habit of verifying all information you use or distribute to others. In this sense, preparing for a presentation is like preparing for a test: master your material so you'll "know that you know."

Step Five: Organize your information using one of the techniques suggested in Chapter 7 for use when writing. These include idea sheets, note cards, the brain dump, questions, and mind maps.

Step Six: Divide your presentation into the following three parts:

1. **Part One: Introduction:** "Tell the audience what you're going to tell them."
    - Engage your listeners with an interesting story or fact. Give them a reason to pay attention. Why is this topic important to them? What should they know about it? How does it relate to their lives? Approach your audience with the attitude that you have something to offer them. This helps put both you and them at ease.
2. **Part Two: Body:** "Tell them."
    - This part takes up the most time. In it you explain and develop your ideas; give supporting facts, details, and examples; narrate events; and tell stories. This is the "meat" of your presentation.
    - Put the body of your speech together so it flows smoothly. For example, you might number your major points. Tell your audience how many points there will be and then announce each one as you come to it, for example:
    - "The kidneys have five important functions. The first is the regulation of fluid and electrolytes." (You then explain how they do this.)
    - "The second function is regulation of blood pressure." (More explanation.)
    - "The third is..." (etc.)
3. **Part Three: Conclusion:** "Tell them what you've told them."
    - Briefly review your major points, show how they tie together, and summarize why they are important. Tell the audience what action you want them to take or how they can use what you have told them.

It is especially important that oral presentations be put together in a logical, organized way. With written material, readers can take their time and go back if they miss a point or don't understand something. Listeners don't have this advantage. You continue talking whether they are following what you're saying or not. You can lose them entirely if you jump from topic to topic, fail to support your ideas, or don't provide clear and complete explanations of the material.

Memory Joggers. It is usually a bad idea to read directly from your paper when giving an oral presentation. You may be tempted to look only at your paper instead of at the audience. Presentations that are read lack the warmth of human interaction and are less interesting for the audience. It is better to become familiar with your material and then use one of the following prompts to help you remember what you plan to say:

1. *Note cards* with key points.
   A. **Advantages:** Small and easy to handle. Prevent you from reading directly from your paper. Encourage you to practice beforehand and become familiar with the material.
   B. **Watch out for:** Having too many cards and getting them confused. Failing to number the cards and getting them out of order. Fiddling with them, which can distract the audience. Not including enough information on them and forgetting what you meant to say about each point.
2. *Outline* on full sheets of paper.
   A. **Advantages:** Includes more information than note cards and may increase your confidence in remembering what you plan to say.
   B. **Watch out for:** Rattling the paper while you speak. Looking at the paper instead of the audience. Holding the paper with both hands and failing to use natural gestures while you speak.
3. *Mind map* with major topics and supporting points in graphic form.
   A. **Advantages:** Easy to see major points at a glance. Especially helpful if you are a visual or global learner and don't need a lot of notes to remember what you plan to say.
   B. **Watch out for:** May be less room on the page to include detail, so be sure you know your material. Sometimes mind maps have words written at angles and are difficult to read quickly. Make sure you set it up in an easy-to-read format so that you don't get lost. Nonvisual learners are not likely to find mind maps helpful as memory prompts.
4. *Key points* written on PowerPoint slides, overhead transparencies, or charts or listed on the board.
   A. **Advantages:** You and the audience are working together and sharing the experience of looking at the same materials. Listeners may become more involved if they are both listening and seeing. This technique also helps visual learners (the majority) follow your presentation. Take care, however, to explain each point, rather than simply reading the list. The audience can do this for themselves!
   B. **Watch out for:** Poorly prepared visual aids that have too much information or lettering that is difficult for the audience to see. Equipment failures such as a balky computer, burned-out light bulbs, or no extension cord (or discovering at the last minute that the equipment you need is being used by another class!). Prior planning and consulting with the instructor are critical to prevent being tripped up during your presentation.

Practice

"The audience is not the enemy. Lack of preparation and practice is."

Give yourself the best chance possible to make a smooth presentation by practicing it a few times in advance. Run through your presentation in front of a mirror, and then try it on friends and family members. Use the materials that will serve as your prompts to make sure they are clear and easy to follow. Time yourself to find out if you need to lengthen or shorten your presentation. Rehearsing will give you the reassurance that comes from being familiar with your materials and knowing you have anticipated potential problems before you stand in front of an audience.

Should you memorize what you plan to say? Unless you are entering a formal speech contest or it is part of the assignment, this is usually not necessary or even a good idea. First, it is time consuming. Second, it can make you sound stiff and unnatural. Finally, and perhaps most important, if you forget a line or lose your place, it can be hard to get back on track. Rather than continuing to talk as you would with natural speech, you are in the uncomfortable position of trying to remember exactly where you are. The resulting long pause is very uncomfortable for both you and your audience.

Whenever possible, check the room where you'll be giving your presentation for details like the following:

- Is there a place to set down your cards or outline, or will you have to hold them as you speak? If you are short (like me), can you see over the podium?
- Do you know how to operate the computer or overhead projector? In which direction should the transparencies be placed? How do you adjust the image? Is the machine in working order? Are there extra bulbs available? Can the people in the back row read the material?
- Is there chalk or a pen available for the blackboard or white board? Will you have time to write out what you need? Is there an eraser?
- Is there a place to hang your charts, graphs, and other illustrations? Will you need tape, tacks, and so on?
- If you have models, samples, or other objects to show, is there a place to set them? Will the audience be able to see them? Will you pass them around?

Success Tips for Making an Oral Presentation

- Before you start to speak, take a breath, smile, and look at your audience. Even if you don't feel glad to be there, act as if you are. Try putting yourself and everyone else at ease.

- Look at the audience while you are speaking. Make eye contact with them. Look around the audience, not just in one direction. Catch the eyes of people who appear to be listening attentively and are "with you" to increase your feelings of support.
- Pause briefly if necessary. Some speakers even use pauses for dramatic effect. If you need a moment to gather your thoughts, stay calm. It is better to pause than to nervously ramble on or repeat filler words ("uh") that, if overused, are distracting. Pauses also give the audience time to reflect on what you have said.
- If you do lose your place or blank out a whole portion of your talk, stop and take a breath. Try not to panic. Acknowledge the audience with a smile or a nod (they may be as nervous as you are), and then concentrate on getting reorganized.
- Shift your focus from yourself to the audience. Remember that you have prepared well and have something of value to share. The audience needs this information, and you are being of service by sharing it with them.
- An old trick used by speakers is to imagine the audience in a funny situation: dressed in silly costumes, wearing big fake noses, standing on their heads—anything to change your perception of them as a threat.
- Consider organizing a buddy system. If you are already in a study group with classmates, that might do the trick. Practice your speeches with each other and offer constructive suggestions. Ask them to "cheer you on" by making eye contact when you are speaking, signaling when your time is almost up, and letting you know if you need to speak louder. Ask them to help you with handouts or visual aids. You will feel less alone.

DEVELOPING YOUR TEAMWORK SKILLS

If you are in a study group like the one suggested for giving speeches, you are already working on a team. Modern health care delivery relies on specialized professionals who work together. Look through the help wanted ads for health care jobs and you will see "team player" and "teamwork" mentioned in many of them. Teamwork refers to the efforts of individuals to coordinate their work to achieve common goals. High-quality patient care depends on how well people communicate and function as team members.

People do not always work together easily and naturally. Competition, rather than cooperation, is built into many aspects of our educational system. As a student, for example, you may be competing for grades, especially on tests that are scored on a curve. On the job, there can be competition for pay raises, bonuses, and recognition by the supervisor. But competition can get in the way of providing good care. The focus in the workplace must be on serving patients, not on competing with co-workers. Teamwork is so important in health care that National Healthcare Foundation Standards 8 is devoted entirely to teamwork criteria.[2]

President John F. Kennedy's famous statement is often quoted: "Ask not what your country can do for you, but what you can do for your country." Kennedy encouraged Americans to work together to reach goals that ranged from establishing the Peace Corps to putting a man on the moon. Americans achieved both, proving that when people work together, they can accomplish amazing things.

You can begin practicing teamwork in school. Group activities assigned by instructors and lab sessions provide excellent opportunities to prepare for real work situations. You can practice cooperating in study groups. Many students report disliking group activities, saying they much prefer being responsible for their own work. If you feel this way, be aware that learning to work together and knowing how to encourage group members who fail to do their part are essential job skills. Welcoming opportunities to work with others while you are still in school is a good strategy for future career success.

Differences among Team Members

When team members support one another, work becomes a pleasant experience. On the other hand, teams in which members don't get along can slow down the work process and make life difficult for everyone. People have differences that can interfere with communication, cause hurt feelings, and disrupt the workflow. Understanding and taking advantage of these differences can help teams flourish rather than fight.

Just as we all have different learning styles, we also have different work styles. Identifying and taking advantage of the styles of each team member can help prevent misunderstandings and allow each one to make useful contributions. There are no right or wrong work styles. Ignoring styles, however, can decrease the effectiveness of the team and reduce the satisfaction of the people on it.

Here are some common work preferences. As you read the list, check the ones that apply to you.

- Work methodically and complete one task or part of a task before moving on to the next.
- Work on several projects at the same time.
- Work alone and are responsible for your own work.
- Work with others in situations in which cooperation determines the success of the project.
- Work with details. Enjoy striving for accuracy and neatness.
- Think of ideas, but prefer to let someone else carry them out.
- Receive assignments with clear deadlines.
- Know exactly what is expected.
- Receive general instructions and a final due date. Figure out yourself how to get it done.

- Generate new ideas, products, and ways to work. Like to be creative.
- Receive a lot of guidance. Have someone check and approve your work as it progresses.
- Work with little supervision. Ask questions when you need help.
- Prefer quiet and order.
- Find noise and activity stimulating.

After reading this list, you can see how work styles are not only different, but even contradictory! It is not surprising that people sometimes find it difficult to work together. Attempting to understand the views and needs of your co-workers and supervisors is part of empathy, discussed earlier in this chapter. Applied in the workplace, empathy contributes to establishing good relations among staff members and creating a positive work environment.

Success Tips for Being an Effective Team Member

- **Understand the ground rules and agreements.** These may not be formally stated or written down, but they are important for keeping communication open and preventing misunderstandings.
- **Be clear about the purpose and goals of the group.** Everyone should know what is to be accomplished. Have you been assigned a specific project? Or is the goal an ongoing effort related to your role as a student or an employee?
- **Do your part—and then some.** Follow through and complete any work you have been assigned or have volunteered to do. Let the group know if you run into problems. Ask for help. Someone may be willing to pick up the slack. Letting things go can result in serious consequences, such as affecting the group's grade, endangering patient safety, or costing the facility money.
- **Listen to what others have to say.** What can you learn from them? What are their ideas about how to accomplish the work? What are their needs? What can they contribute?
- **Speak up.** Share your ideas and opinions.
- **Take advantage of differences.** Maximize group efficiency by assigning tasks that are appropriate for each member.

UNDERSTANDING ORGANIZATIONS

Organizations, such as schools and dental offices, have their own personalities, just as individual people do. These personalities are known as **organizational cultures,** and they include the goals, rules, expectations, and customs of the organization as a whole. Schools have cultures, too. For example, some are very formal and emphasize respect for authority. Students are required to address their instructors by title and last name. Uniforms must be worn, and rules are strictly enforced. At other schools, the atmosphere is more casual, with students and instructors on a first-name basis. At some health care facilities, people eat lunch together, celebrate birthdays and holidays, and meet after work. At others, there is a clear distinction between work and social life. Some organizations stress orderliness, engage in detailed planning, and have clear work assignments. Others move at a fast pace, with informal job descriptions and planning done "on the run."

It is important to be aware of the culture you are in—or plan to enter—to see if it matches your preferences or if you can at least adapt to it. Sometimes we can learn from a culture that has values we would like to develop in ourselves. For example, if you have poor study habits and find yourself in a strict school, this can be a great opportunity to get the encouragement you need to develop new habits.

UNDERSTANDING YOUR INSTRUCTORS

We have discussed how people have different learning and working styles. Another factor that can influence your academic success is teaching and classroom management styles. Instructors are individuals who have their own ideas about education, teaching methods, and the proper roles of teachers and students. Understanding what is important to your instructors will help you benefit fully from your classes. You will use these same skills to identify the characteristics of your future supervisors so you can work with them more effectively.

Following are some common characteristics of instructors, along with suggestions for what you can learn from each:

1. **Strict.** Rules are emphasized. They are clearly explained, and there are consequences if they are broken.

   You learn: Good habits for health care work situations in which rules must be followed to ensure patient and worker safety.
2. **Value appearance.** Students must be neat, with clean, pressed uniforms and polished shoes. Points may be deducted from grades for infractions. Students who arrive out of uniform are sent home to change. (In a work environment, improperly dressed employees may also be asked to leave.)

   You learn: To practice the habits of excellent hygiene and correct professional appearance that are critical in health care work. (Remember: Your professional career began when you started school.)
3. **Believe students should be responsible for their own learning.** Instructors with this philosophy may allow you to go all term without ever mentioning that you haven't handed in all your homework assignments. You interpret this as meaning that it's not important and are shocked to receive a final grade of D or F.

Never assume that no nagging means "not important." The same can happen at work. An employee may not be told about unsatisfactory work performance until the day of a formal evaluation or the initiation of a disciplinary process.

You learn: To take responsibility for yourself and what you must do. On the job, supervisors won't have time to remind you constantly about your tasks. It will be up to you to get them done.

4. **Believe they must monitor students closely.** Some instructors believe it is their responsibility to prompt students to complete their work. They give constant reminders, check their progress frequently, call students who are absent, and generally provide "super-support." They are like those supervisors who are very organized and nurturing and are willing to tell employees what's to be done. They provide a lot of feedback.

   You learn: To work with frequent deadlines and a hands-on manager and how to meet deadlines and avoid falling behind in your work. Be careful, however, that you don't become dependent on continual help, because you can't always count on it being there for you.
5. **Value order.** The classroom is neat and tidy, lectures follow a clear pattern, and class activities are well planned.

   You learn: To practice orderly habits when necessary. Although your home may be comfortably chaotic, order is necessary in the health care environment. Forms must be filled out in a very specific way, tests performed in a prescribed order of steps, and disinfecting procedures carried out precisely. Tidying up the classroom or lab before you leave is a good habit to develop, and your instructor will certainly notice and appreciate your efforts.
6. **Value creativity over order.** Classes may seem disorganized. Lectures are mixed with interesting stories and don't follow an orderly plan. Group activities and creativity are emphasized over doing things the instructor's way.

   You learn: To be creative and think for yourself, to work with classmates, and to practice the teamwork skills discussed in this chapter.

The teaching styles chosen by instructors are often reflections of their own learning styles or the way they remember being taught themselves. Instructors may rely on lectures to teach because they are auditory learners or because they believe that their role is to tell students what they know. You can take advantage of different teaching styles to help you improve your weak areas. For example, if an instructor uses a lot of group activities and you prefer to work alone, you now have an opportunity to increase your ability to work with others, something you might not choose to do if it weren't required.

If you have difficulty with an instructor, the first step in resolving the problem should be to speak privately with him or her. If you go straight to a school administrator, neither you nor the instructor has a chance to explore the problem and try to work out a solution. Furthermore, the administrator doesn't have personal knowledge of the situation. The problem has been moved away from its source. If speaking with the instructor fails to resolve the situation, inquire about the proper procedure to follow at your school. If you have problems with your supervisor at work, it is expected that you speak with that person first.

When meeting with an instructor or supervisor to discuss a problem, it works best if you are prepared in advance. Think about what you want to discuss. It might be a good idea to prepare some notes in advance of the major points you want address. At the meeting, let the other person know that your goal is not to complain, but to resolve the issue. Find out their views and listen carefully and nondefensively. Express your own view of the situation, and then discuss the problem in terms of possible solutions.

Most instructors decide to teach because they want to share what they have learned about their profession. They are motivated by concern for their students. This does not necessarily mean they strive to be liked by their students, because this is not the purpose of teaching. Their job is to train students to be excellent health care professionals. You may not like all your instructors, but given a chance, they all have something of value to share with you. And although you may not like all your supervisors, you can still find satisfaction in your work.

DEALING WITH DIFFICULT PEOPLE

"One of the best ways to persuade others is with your ears—by listening to them."

Dean Rusk

People problems cannot be avoided entirely. There will be classmates who annoy you, who don't do their share of the work on a group project, or who take up a lot of class time with questions because they never read the assignments. Family members may criticize you because they are upset about the amount of time you spend studying. Friends may be jealous of your future career possibilities. Some of your future patients, clients, co-workers, and supervisors will be challenging, too. Learning to get along with difficult people helps make life more pleasant and productive.

In difficult situations, do your best to separate your health care role from you as a person. It is often your position with which the other person has a problem. For example, your family may be annoyed with your role as a student because of the time it takes away from them. Or a patient may take his anger out on you as a representative of the clinic with which he has a problem.

Empathy, which we discussed earlier in this chapter, can help. Listen carefully to the other person. Try to see the world from his or her point of view. What might explain the behavior? Might there be personal problems you don't know about? Is there a chance you have unintentionally done something to hurt his or her feelings? It can be helpful to acknowledge the other person's feelings without agreeing to feel the same way. For example, you might begin your discussion like this: "I can see why you feel that way, but..." and then state your view. Recognizing the validity of the other person's feelings often decreases the negativity. Remain calm and courteous. Reacting negatively only makes the situation worse. (This does not mean you have to take verbal or physical abuse. If this occurs, seek the assistance of your instructor, other school personnel, or your supervisor.)

Seek solutions to interpersonal problems by being honest and "up front." Tell the other person what you see as the problem and explain how it affects you. For example, with a lab partner who is never prepared to practice the assigned procedures, you might say, "I feel really frustrated when you continually come unprepared. I'm worried that I'm losing the chance to learn, and I can't afford to do that." Simply venting or arguing won't solve the problem; it might even make it worse. Work for a mutually acceptable agreement. Using the lab partner example, you could ask, "Can you agree to come to class prepared?" When there are serious consequences at stake, such as your grades or work performance, let the other person know what you plan to do if the situation is not resolved. Tell your lab partner, "If I can't depend on you to come prepared to work with me, I'll have to ask the instructor to let me change lab partners." As you attempt to find a solution, try to keep a positive attitude. Recall from our discussion about attitude in Chapter 3 that it doesn't make sense to give an unpleasant person the right to ruin your day. Do what you can to seek a positive solution and then move on.

We learn and develop professionally when we engage in all types of relationships, both positive and negative. Expressing kindness toward a troublesome classmate or giving an instructor the benefit of the doubt are signs of maturity. It's easy to be professional when things are going well. True professionals can also deal effectively with challenging situations.

Dealing with Criticism

Criticism and constructive suggestions about your work present you with opportunities to learn. In school, you are paying for instruction that includes correction of your work. Your teachers would not be acting responsibly if they awarded inflated grades or withheld criticism to avoid hurting students' feelings. It would be unfair to allow students to perform work incorrectly, because this would only set them up for failure on the job, where the consequences are more serious.

You may receive criticism for behaviors or work results when you are on the job. This might come from your supervisor, a co-worker, or even a patient. No one likes to be criticized, and it is natural to react strongly. Dismissing the criticism as unfounded, becoming angry, or taking the criticism to heart and feeling worthless are common reactions. These feelings are natural but not very helpful. A more constructive response is to pay attention to the message, examine the criticism, and consider it carefully. Then decide if any or all of it actually applies to you. If it does, you can choose to benefit from it and engage in self-improvement. If it does not, consider talking over your feelings with the person who gave the criticism to see where the misunderstanding lies.

If you receive criticism that seems harsh, try to focus on the content and not on the way it is delivered. Not all instructors and supervisors are skilled at giving suggestions. If you don't understand what you did incorrectly, ask for clarification. It is your responsibility to learn as much as possible. Feelings must be put aside, if necessary, to ensure that you attain the skills necessary to be a competent health care professional.

Giving Constructive Criticism

The purpose of constructive criticism is to provide the person receiving the criticism with the means for improvement. It is based on the assumption that behavior can be changed for the better. It is important, when giving constructive criticism, to focus on the problem behavior rather than on the person. Suppose you have a co-worker who frequently fails to return equipment to its designated storage space, causing you to waste time looking for needed items to do your work. State the problem behavior clearly: equipment is not being returned and this is affecting your efficiency. Avoid negative statements about the other person such as that she is inconsiderate, a poor co-worker, disorganized, and so on. Judgmental statements about personal characteristics tend to put people on the defensive and make them less willing to examine their behavior and make positive changes.

Here are a few more suggestions for giving criticism that helps rather than hurts:

- Choose a private location to talk, and allow enough time for the other person to respond and ask questions.
- Use empathy and show respect for the other person's feelings.
- Include positive statements along with the criticism.
- Be clear when explaining the problem. Give specific examples that illustrate the problem.

Neither giving nor receiving criticism is easy, but done well and taken in the spirit in which it is intended, it contributes to our learning and growth.

To Learn More

Hildebrand V, Phenice LA, Gray MM, Hines RP: *Knowing and serving diverse families,* ed 2, Upper Saddle River, NJ, 2000, Merrill, Prentice-Hall.

This book offers a good introduction to diversity, then covers a different ethnic group in each chapter. In addition, a variety of family structures are discussed, including single teenage parent and step families. Recommendations are given for serving each group.

Luckmann J: *Transcultural communication in health care,* Clifton Park, NY, 2000, Thomson Delmar Learning.

From this book you can learn about the cultural values and beliefs of a wide variety of people, including Latinos, Muslims, Native Americans, and Hasidic Jews. The author's purpose is to help students increase their self-awareness and become more sensitive to cultural differences.

Mears P: *Healthcare teams: building continuous quality improvement,* Boca Raton, 1994, St Lucie Press.

Although written for group facilitators, this book can help you understand the importance of teamwork in health care settings.

Milliken ME: *Understanding human behavior: a guide for health care providers,* ed 6, Clifton Park, NY, 2004, Delmar Cengage.

This reader-friendly book gives practical information to assist health professionals understand and effectively work with their patients.

Purtilo R, Haddad A: *Health professional and patient interaction,* 7th ed., Philadelphia, 2007, Saunders.

Good discussions and examples of how to empathize and communicate with patients.

Tamparo CD, Lindh WQ: *Therapeutic communications for health care,* ed 3, Clifton Park, NY, 2008, Delmar Cengage.

Easy to read and full of specifics and examples.

REFERENCES

1. Anderson R, Barbara A, Feldman S: What patients want: a content analysis of key qualities that influence patient satisfaction. www.drscore.com/press/papers/whatpatientswant.pdf (Accessed 2/9/09)
2. National Consortium on Health Science and Technology Education: National Healthcare Foundation Standards and Accountability Criteria. www.nchste.org/cms/wp-content/uploads/2008/03/foundation_standards_ac_rev_01_08. (Accessed 2/13/09)

PRESCRIPTION FOR SUCCESS 4-1 | **SHOWING RESPECT**

1. List three ways, in addition to those listed in the text, you can show respect to others.

____

____

____

2. Describe a situation in which someone made you feel that you were respected. How was respect communicated to you?

____

____

____

3. Explain why showing respect to patients is an important part of providing good health care.

____

____

____

PRESCRIPTION FOR SUCCESS 4-2 | GETTING TO KNOW YOURSELF

The first step toward understanding others is knowing ourselves. Fill in the chart below with your own beliefs about each concept. You may use any of those listed in Table 4-1 or you can write your own.

Concept	My Beliefs
Time	______
Personal space	______
Age	______
Touching	______
Gender	______
Eye contact	______
Personal control	______
Spiritual practices	______
Definition of success	______
Health care beliefs	______

PRESCRIPTION FOR SUCCESS 4-3 | YOUR HEALTH CARE BELIEFS

1. What is your personal definition of "health"?

______

______

2. How much responsibility do you believe people should have for their own health?

______

______

3. What do you believe are the main causes of health problems?

______

______

4. What are the best ways to take care of health problems?

______

______

5. How do you think your own beliefs about health may influence your future work?

______

______

PRESCRIPTION FOR SUCCESS 4-4 **WHAT WOULD IT BE LIKE TO BE . . . ?**

Answer the questions that follow for patients in the following conditions:

- Paralyzed
- In pain
- Unable to work
- Blind
- Mentally ill
- Poor and without health insurance
- Elderly and living alone
- Unable to speak English
- Being terminally ill

1. What emotions might they be experiencing?

2. What might be their concerns and fears?

3. What are their major needs likely to be, both physical and emotional?

4. How are their conditions likely to affect their quality of life?

5. How could you learn more about each person?

PRESCRIPTION FOR SUCCESS 4-5 | RATE YOUR COMMUNICATION SKILLS

1. Do any areas need improvement?

   a. ____________________ Sending clear messages

   b. ____________________ Listening actively

   c. ____________________ Requesting feedback

   d. ____________________ Asking good questions

   e. ____________________ Understanding nonverbal communication

   f. ____________________ Demonstrating appropriate nonverbal communication

2. If so, what can you do to improve them?

   ____

   ____

   ____

3. What resources, including people, can help you improve your communication skills?

   ____

   ____

   ____

CHAPTER

5

Identifying the Three Levels of Understanding

READING WITH A PURPOSE

As students in the health care professions, you quickly discover the great amount of reading that you are required to complete. It is necessary that you accomplish these reading tasks as efficiently as possible. This means that you get as much understanding as you can during each of your study sessions. You cannot afford to waste time by performing at less than your best each time you sit at your desk and read. An excellent strategy that guarantees that each reading session will be successful is to read with a purpose. When you read with a purpose, you create a goal that you wish to accomplish each time you read. Having a goal to reach will keep you focused and involved in your reading. Your comprehension will be improved by reading with a purpose.

INTRODUCING THE THREE LEVELS OF UNDERSTANDING

There is more than one way to understand what you are reading in your textbook. The goal or purpose you set for yourself as you read will determine the level of understanding required for comprehension of the reading material.

- The first level of understanding is called **literal understanding**. This level of understanding requires that you know what the subject of your reading is and the most important points being made about the subject. For example, when you need to learn important terms, names and functions of different parts of the body, or steps in a procedure from your textbook, you use literal understanding.
- The second level of understanding is called **interpretive understanding**. This level of understanding requires that you draw conclusions about what you are reading by examining the facts that are presented. For example, when you are reading to learn how to schedule patients according to the seriousness of their complaints, reading to learn how to decide on the proper medical insurance forms to fill out for a patient, or reading to learn how to examine stained smears for the presence of certain microorganisms, you use interpretive understanding.
- The third level of understanding is called **applied understanding**. This level of understanding requires that you see how ideas are similar so that you can use ideas from one situation in another related situation. For example, when you are asked to read a chapter about focusing the microscope and then you use one correctly in the laboratory or when you memorize from your text the proper hand-washing technique and then use it when you handle patients, you use applied understanding. Again, your goal or purpose for reading will determine which level of understanding you need to use when reading your textbook.

Literal Understanding

When you read for literal understanding, you are reading for facts and information. You are trying to determine what the passage is saying in a basic, straightforward way. The strategy to use for literal understanding is to identify the topic and main idea of the selection you are reading. Finding the topic and main idea of a passage will give you a purpose for reading and will help you to concentrate on the essential points in the selection that you need to learn.

Identifying the Topic of a Passage. The topic is the key subject of the passage. To find the topic, you ask:

- What is this passage mostly about?

The answer will be the topic or subject of the passage and should be stated as briefly as possible.

Identifying the Main Idea. The main idea of a passage is what the passage is all about. The strategy to use to identify the main idea is to ask,

- What is the most important point being made about the topic?

The answer will be the main idea and should be stated in sentence form.

Interpretive Understanding

When you read for interpretive understanding, you are reading to figure out something unstated in the passage. The strategy you use for interpretive understanding is to examine the facts or details in the passage and to use your own experience and background knowledge to draw a conclusion about the meaning of the passage. Drawing the correct conclusions about what you are reading will allow you to understand better what the writer really means and will allow you to function better in your workplace.

Details as Clues. When you use interpretive understanding, you need to go beyond the literal meaning of the passage and reason out in what direction the facts or details are leading. This requires that you infer or make a judgment about the meaning of the details. In other words, your responsibility when using interpretive understanding is to examine the details and use them as clues to help you form your own logical conclusions. In addition, you need to rely on information you have learned from your other classes and from your own life in order to come to the right explanation of the passage.

Applied Understanding

When you read for applied understanding, you are reading to learn ideas from your textbook so you can use these ideas in school or in the workplace. The strategies you will use for applied understanding include the strategies you use for literal and interpretive understanding.

- In order to apply information, you must first learn the facts. This will require that you learn and remember ideas literally. Finding the topic and the main idea will help you focus on what is important.
- In order to apply information, you must be able to interpret what you are reading. This will require that you have some background knowledge of the subject and of the situation to which you will be applying the information.
- Finally, in order to apply information, you must use good judgment. You must be able to recognize the similarities and differences between the facts you read and the situations in which you will be applying these facts. You must be able to judge when and where it is appropriate and correct to apply these facts. This judgment requires that you know your facts and have experience. Following is an example adapted from Bird and Robinson (p. 478) of how one dental assistant student thought through an emergency situation and successfully used applied understanding in the workplace.

REVIEWING THE LEARNING STRATEGIES

To Learn	Use this Strategy
Literal understanding	Identify the topic of the passage by asking What is this passage mostly about? Identify the main idea of the passage by asking, What is the most important point being made about the topic?
Interpretive understanding	Examine the facts and details. Use your own experiences and background knowledge to draw conclusions.
Applied understanding	Learn the facts for literal understanding. Use experience and background knowledge to interpret situations. Use your best judgment to determine when it is appropriate to apply facts to a new situation.

Exercise 5–1

Directions: Your instructor gives you assignments to learn different types of information.

These assignments are listed below. If the assignment requires literal understanding, write "L" in the blank next to the assignment. If the assignment requires interpretive understanding, write "I" in the blank next to the assignment. If the assignment requires applied understanding, write "A" in the blank next to the assignment.

Assignment 1: You are asked to memorize the names of the important parts of the human brain. _____

Assignment 2: You are asked to make up a patient chart following a model chart that the instructor has created. _____

Assignment 3: The instructor asks you to retype a document that has been corrected and marked with proofreading symbols. _____

Assignment 4: You are asked to figure out what the different tail positions of a cat mean. _____

Assignment 5: You are given a chart of the components of blood and are asked to label the different parts. _____

Assignment 6: The instructor hands you a study sheet describing the different plural endings of medical terms. You are asked to use the plural endings for every medical term in a report you are writing. _____

Assignment 7: After successfully completing Chapter 9 in your textbook, you are expected to be able to fill a syringe. _____

Assignment 8: You are expected to spell all the important words in the first chapter of your health care textbook. _____

Assignment 9: You are asked to list the six sections of the Food Guide Pyramid. _____

Assignment 10: You need to determine whether a patient's diet includes all sections of the Food Guide Pyramid. _____

Let us now take a closer look at each of the different levels of understanding and see how each level suggests a strategy for improving reading comprehension.

CHAPTER 6

Taking Notes

NOTE-TAKING FOR SCHOOL SUCCESS

Taking good notes combines the art of listening and the act of selective writing. Many students report having trouble taking good notes, but it is a skill that can be mastered. Be optimistic about developing your ability to learn to take good notes. You actually have a big advantage because you can take in words much faster than your instructors can speak!

The most common teaching methods for health care courses are lectures, instructor demonstrations, and hands-on activities in the lab or at the clinical site. The first two require students to take notes they can use as study aids. You will have many opportunities to practice this important skill, and note-taking will serve you now and later on the job.

Some students wonder why they should even bother taking notes. Why not just look in the textbook later and find the information? There are a number of important reasons for taking notes in class in addition to learning to take good notes because it is an important health care skill:

1. Taking notes forces you to attend class, pay attention, process the material mentally, and selectively write down what you hear. It converts you from a passive to an active listener. Increasing the number of ways you interact with new material greatly increases your chances of understanding and remembering it, so hearing and writing it down in class give you a head start in learning.
2. Your instructors are likely to present more information than what appears in your textbook. They may have examples and additional techniques from their work experiences or new information from a seminar they just attended.
3. Some of the information in your textbook may be outdated. Although publishers do their best to ensure that textbooks contain the very latest information, it usually takes over a year from the time a book is written to get it ready for distribution to students. In a fast-changing field like health care, there is a continuous flow of new developments, and your instructors can provide you with the latest updates.
4. There may be information in your textbooks that does not apply to your geographic area. The scope of practice of professionals varies across the country. For example, some states allow medical assistants to take an active role in taking x-ray films. Therefore many medical assisting textbooks include information about positioning patients when taking x-rays. In some states, however, only graduates of approved x-ray programs who have also passed a state exam are allowed to perform these procedures. Classroom instructors give you the rules and regulations of the area in which your school is located.
5. Your instructors can help you understand difficult sections of the textbook, presenting the material in a way you better understand. They may break it down into manageable chunks, provide examples, or explain it in different words. You can ask instructors questions, a definite advantage over textbooks.
6. Health care programs cover vast amounts of information. Your instructors' lectures can help you identify the most important points and give you clues about what will be included on tests.
7. You boost your personal efficiency. Taking notes saves you the time of looking up the information discussed in class that does not appear in your regular textbook and would require you to go to other sources.
8. Notes serve as powerful tools for studying and mastering important information needed for school and job success. In this chapter you will learn techniques for converting your notes into study aids.

Active Listening: Prerequisite for Good Note-Taking

Good note-taking requires good listening habits. You can't record what you don't hear. It is sometimes difficult to pay attention in class when you're tired, there are distractions, the instructor speaks too quickly or not clearly, or you don't find the subject matter interesting. However, listening is one of the most essential skills for the successful health care professional. In fact, poor listening skills can doom your professional life to failure. Patient surveys report that the failure of the health care professional to listen is a major cause of dissatisfaction.[1] The classroom provides the perfect opportunity to learn information and an essential life skill at the same time.

Success Tips to Develop Good Listening Skills

- Develop a positive attitude toward listening. Listening well increases your chances for success in life. Review your goals and think about how being a good listener will help you achieve them.
- Leave your mental baggage at the classroom or health care facility door. Try to go in with a clean slate for listening and learning. If you are having a bad day or your mind is distracted, look at class as an opportunity to focus, learn, and have a productive experience.
- Sit where you can both see and hear the instructor. Avoid sitting near people who talk or continually ask you questions during class. The distraction will disrupt your attention and can make you tense. (And don't you be the talker!)
- Concentrate on the content of the lecture, not the way it is delivered. It's easy to let the appearance, mannerisms, and voice of the instructor distract you from what is being said. Learning to focus on content is an important health care skill because patients will come to you with all kinds of physical and emotional conditions, and each merits your full attention.
- Reel in your wandering mind. Do your best to stay with the instructor mentally. If you think of something important, jot a quick note to yourself so you can take care of it later. This frees your mind to be in the moment and focus on the class.
- Keep your mind open and suspend judgment. It is common to stop listening when we disagree with something we hear. A better strategy is to write down the point of disagreement. After listening to the remainder of the presentation, ask the instructor to clarify the point. There may be several "right answers" or ways to perform a technique. Perhaps you heard or interpreted the information incorrectly. If the instructor did make a mistake, show respect. Enjoying "being right" in front of the class is unacceptable classroom conduct. On the job, it could be perceived as insubordination with a supervisor, and this behavior is generally not tolerated.

Learning Styles and Listening. Obviously, auditory learners have the edge when it comes to lectures. They can, however, get caught up in the listening and find it difficult to take adequate notes. This can be a problem because even good listeners won't remember every important point presented.

Visual learners may have more difficulty paying sustained attention and comprehending long lectures. If you are a visual learner, here are some techniques to help you get the most from lectures:

- Complete any reading and assignments related to the lecture before going to class. Knowing something about the topic, rather than starting out cold, provides a framework to guide your listening.
- Avoid sitting near visual distractions, such as a window with an interesting view or pictures and displays not related to the topic being discussed.
- Watch the instructor. Note movements, gestures, and facial expressions and see how they reinforce the material being presented.
- Pay attention to anything shown on the board or through other visual aids to help you better visualize and understand the material.
- Ask the instructor to write down any words or phrases you cannot understand orally.
- During lectures, refer to the sections of your textbook or handouts that relate to the material.

If you are a kinesthetic (hands-on) learner, you can benefit from the physical activity of writing when you take notes. Additional suggestions to improve your listening include the following:

- Think of applications for ideas you hear during lectures. (But be careful not to get too carried away and miss the next thing the instructor says!)
- Imagine yourself interacting physically with the topic: performing procedures, touching things, or operating a machine.
- Make slight movements that do not disrupt others: count off steps on your fingers, stretch your legs slightly, take occasional deep breaths, or move your hand down the page of your text or handout as the material is being explained.
- Take enough notes to keep busy, but not so many that you miss the important points as the instructor moves on.

Advance Preparation for Taking Good Notes

Preparing for classes is an important part of listening and taking good notes. Advance preparation, according to many instructors, is the key to benefiting from class sessions. If you forget about class between meetings and just show up each time as the instructor begins to speak, you will lose out on a good part of your educational investment. To obtain maximum benefit from your in-class experiences, try the following suggestions:

- Complete any assigned reading and other homework. There is nothing more frustrating than trying to follow a lecture in which the instructor assumes you know something about the subject—and you know nothing! Give yourself every advantage by anticipating what the lecture might cover.
- Review your notes from the previous lecture. This gives you an opportunity to set the stage for a con-

tinuation of the subject and to recall questions or points you want to have clarified.

- Arrive at class a few minutes early. This gives you a chance to choose an appropriate seat, quickly look over your notes from the last class, and prepare yourself to take notes.
- Set your attitude for learning. Make the decision to get as much benefit as possible from every class. Be positive and expect to acquire useful information.
- Take all necessary supplies to class: a binder with extra paper, pencil or pen, textbook, and handouts. (Make sure they're in the "big bag" discussed in Chapter 3. If books and binders get heavy, consider using a flight bag on wheels to prevent stress on your shoulders.)

PERSONAL REFLECTION

1. Are you satisfied with your note-taking skills?

____

____

2. Does your note-taking system need improvement?

____

____

Note-Taking Materials

There are a variety of ways to take and organize notes, and these will be discussed in the following sections. When choosing the best one for you, consider your learning styles and personal preferences, your instructors' lecture styles, and the number and type of handouts distributed in your classes.

Taking notes in class is the first step in creating a personalized learning tool. Your notes are not completed when the instructor finishes the lecture. You still need to edit them to increase their value as a learning tool and then review them regularly.

Notes are useless, however, if you cannot find or identify them, so good organization is essential. Loose-leaf binders receive the highest marks from instructors for keeping notes together because they are the most flexible and easiest to organize and keep in order. You can add new information in any order you wish, something you can't do with spiral notebooks. Binders allow you to insert class notes, revisions of your notes, handouts, assignments, reference sheets, and skill check-off sheets. Binders also offer the best protection against weather and keep papers flat and neat. Portfolios and other types of folders with pockets tend to tear and get messy.

You can purchase several binders with thin vinyl covers and use one for each class. Or you can divide a large binder with indexed dividers. Each class can also be subdivided for class notes, handouts, reading notes, and assignments. Periodically review and tidy up your binder as needed.

Regardless of how you organize your binder, the important thing is to keep your notes for each class together and in order. Label the outside cover with the name of the class or classes. If you are using more than one binder, color-code or mark them in such a way that you never arrive at anatomy class only to discover you have your pharmacology notes! Label the individual pages with the name of the class and the date.

The Cornell System

The Cornell system is a method for laying out, editing, and studying from your notes to get the most benefit from them. It was devised by Professor Walter Pauk, who wanted to help his students improve their study habits. A key feature of the system is leaving enough blank space on the page to add specific kinds of information when you review and edit your notes. To do this, set up each page on which you will take notes by drawing a line about 2½ inches in from the left side. Then draw a line about 2 inches from the bottom. Figure 6-1 shows this page layout.

The large space in the center is for recording notes during class. The left side is used after class to write key words, headings, questions, and other notes. The bottom space is reserved for writing short summaries of the contents of the page. We will discuss how to use these spaces later in this chapter.

Deciding What to Record

Instructors can say a lot during a lecture, and sometimes it's difficult to decide what to write down. If this happens to you, you're not alone. Students report this to be the hardest part of note-taking. This is especially true when a subject is new and you don't have the background to help sift the must-know from the interesting-to-know. You need to write down enough to understand your notes later. But if you try to record every word, you're likely to miss half of what the instructor says. There are a number of things you can do to get the most important content from class lectures.

As mentioned before, and it is worth repeating, do the reading and assignments before going to class—even if it is not required. This will give you an overview of the topic. Your textbook has headings and other ways of emphasizing the major points of a subject. Use these to develop a mental outline. If you find the subject especially difficult and have the time, prepare a written outline of the chapters before the lecture.

In class, listen for the main ideas. Your prereading is an excellent way to help you identify what these might be. Listen carefully to your instructors. They may list

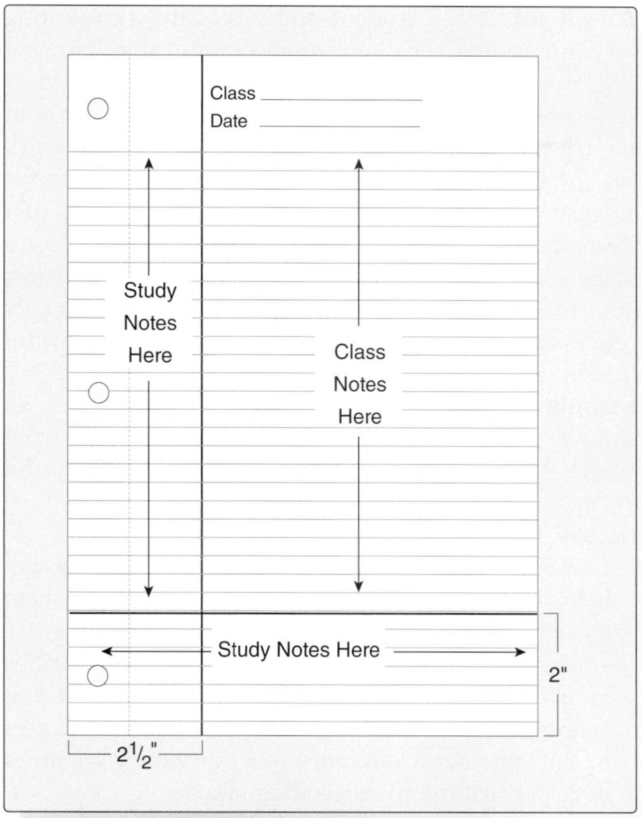

FIGURE 6-1 Example of setting up a page when using the Cornell note-taking system. After class, write additions and revisions on the reverse sides of the pages.

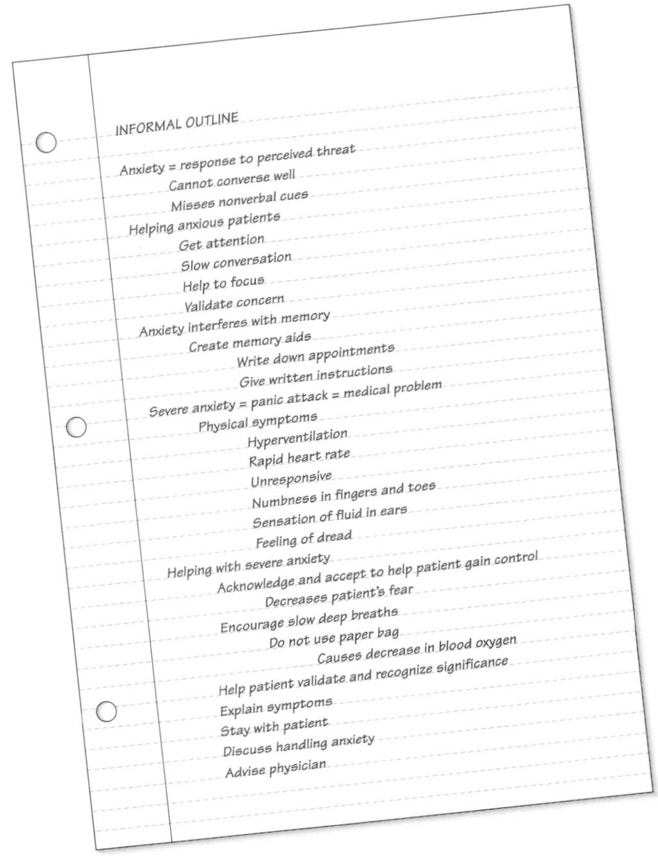

FIGURE 6-2 Example of notes using an informal outline. This is probably the most commonly used method. (*Data from Bonewit-West K, Hunt S, Applegate E:* Today's medical assistant: clinical and administrative procedures, *St. Louis, 2009, Elsevier.*)

important points, introduce them and provide details and examples, and/or tell you what is most important. As you become familiar with the material and health care topics in general and take quizzes and tests, you will find it easier to identify the major points.

Clues from Instructors. Listen and watch for clues from the instructor. Instructors plan their lectures to help students learn the subjects they are teaching. They want you to succeed, so many of them provide clues, both consciously and unconsciously, about what is important in their classes. Here are some common instructor behaviors that say, "Write this down!"

- Saying, "This is important" or "You must know or be able to do this when you are working in the field" or "Write this down" or "This will be on the test." (They really do say these things. This is what you might miss if you are absent from class or daydreaming when you *are* there.)
- Emphasizing certain words or concepts by saying them loudly, writing them on the board or overhead, or repeating them. (It is a good idea to copy everything the instructor writes down.)
- Expressing extra interest or enthusiasm. This may indicate an area the instructor believes to be especially important.
- Illustrating points with stories and anecdotes.
- Asking questions of students during the lecture. These are usually points the instructor considers to be important.

A technique to keep yourself on track is to mentally ask yourself questions, based on the topic, and then listen for the answers during the lectures. Here are some sample questions:

- Why is this important?
- How does it work?
- What are the main parts?
- Why is it done this way?
- How is it done? How will I do this? When will I do this?
- How will I apply this in my work?
- How will this knowledge help me be a better health care professional? How will it help me to help patients?

If you continually miss the major points of lectures, see your instructor outside of class. Ask for suggestions to improve your listening, follow the style of lecturing, and take better notes. Ask if the instructor has lecture outlines you might have, so you can follow along in class. If English is your second language and you have difficulty understanding spoken and/or written English, seek help from your instructor or school advisor.

Deciding How to Record Your Notes

There are several ways you can organize lecture content as you record it. When choosing formats to try, consider your learning style, the instructor's style of lecturing, and the subject matter. You may like one method and decide to use it in all of your classes. The important thing is to become proficient so that when you are in class, you can focus more on content than on how you are recording it. Four of the most common methods for taking notes, described in the following sections, are:

1. Informal outline
2. Paragraphs
3. Key words
4. Write it all

The description for each method is written in the format being presented to show what the methods look like.

Informal Outlines

How to use
    Create indentations to organize ideas
    Write phrases
    Don't use numbers or letters
When to use
    Student is linear thinker
    Lecture is easy to follow
Advantages
    Helps you organize thoughts
    Keeps materials in logical order
Disadvantages
    Difficult if lecture is disorganized, rambling
    May distract from lecture content
        Trying to make neat outline
    Holistic thinkers need time to formulate outline

Paragraphs. Writing in paragraphs helps when lecture hard to follow. Use phrases. Create paragraph for each main idea. Mark important points during lecture. Organize later by creating outline.

Difficult for some. Must write quickly and neatly. Must decide what to write. Advantage for kinesthetic learners—involves activity. Lots of writing.

Key Words

Main ideas only
Relationships
Supporting facts
Auditory learners
Reminders
Fill in later
Difficult material—may miss facts
Easy to forget!

Write it All. A few students are successful with writing everything down. They are more comfortable knowing they haven't missed anything the instructor says. Must use shortened sentences, phrases, and abbreviations, but they try to record all that instructor says. Might work well for kinesthetic learner, who needs activity, or for students who have trouble concentrating and find that this method helps them concentrate. Method not recommended for most students because if you don't write fast you can get behind and get very frustrated. Usually unnecessary to write everything down. Lose important ideas in details.

Examples of Note-Taking. Figure 6-2 contains an example of notes based on the lecture segment from *Today's Medical Assistant* by Bonewit-West, Hunt, and Applegate[2].

Success Tips for Taking Great Notes

- Creating your own symbols and abbreviations can help you take notes more quickly and can make them more useful. Creating abbreviations can help increase your note-taking speed. Try standard abbreviations or invent your own—or use a combination. If you create your own set of abbreviations, it's a good idea to put together a directory to keep with your notes in case you forget your coding system.
- Be there! Do your best to be present for both the beginning and end of class. Introductions and conclusions often contain valuable information about what the instructor considers to be most important. Conclusions may clarify points that seemed fuzzy or unrelated earlier in the lecture.
- Leave some blank space on your pages between the major ideas or clusters of related information so you can make additions when you edit and review. If you get lost and have gaps in your notes, leave extra space to fill in later.
- Write out examples, definitions, formulas, and calculations.
- Write on only one side of the paper so you can lay the pages out and see all your notes at once. Some students use the blank facing pages to create additional study notes.
- Do your best to write down words you don't know. Guess at the spelling and circle the words so you can look up their meanings or ask the instructor.
- Write as neatly as possible. If necessary, practice improving your handwriting or try printing if it doesn't slow you down too much. Aim for a balance between speed and legibility. Recopying notes to make them neater takes time you could use more productively. There are, however, a few circumstances in which rewriting, typing, or word processing notes is recommended. If you have strong keyboarding skills, you may find that this process serves as a good review of the lecture. If you are a kinesthetic learner, you may benefit from the activity of keyboarding or rewriting. Finally, on those occa-

sions when your notes are a total disaster, it may be worth your time to clean them up.
- Erasable pens are good for taking notes, although regular pens can be used if you make corrections neatly. Pencils can break or need sharpening, and the writing tends to fade and smudge over time.

Make Your Notes Work for You

It takes work to take good notes in class. Now let them work for you. Start by reviewing them as soon as possible after class. Try not to wait more than 24 hours because the average person forgets more than half of what was said during a typical class lecture within that time. Even a quick review will help create memory pathways for the new information.

Begin your review by reading over your notes and filling in any missing words or abbreviations with meanings you might forget. Next, fill in ideas or reorganize your notes, as needed. If there are gaps where your mind wandered or you did not understand well enough to take clear notes, look in your textbook, ask a classmate, or make a note to ask the instructor for help.

Consider rewriting your notes if they are extremely disorganized or if you think a different format might help you better learn from them. For example, if the topic emphasizes relationships and you wrote paragraphs, create a mind map. If the lecture was organized by classifications, put together a chart that lays out the various categories.

Use a highlighter or colored pen to mark key words and phrases. You can also personalize your notes with drawings, arrows to show relationships, pictures from magazines, or anything else that helps you focus on and better understand the material. Auditory learners might record their edited notes for reviewing.

Reviewing Productively. The most important thing you can do with your notes is to review them often, at least twice a week. If your classes last for less than 1 month, review your notes even more often. As we discussed in Chapter 3, the key to long-term memory is repetition over time. Your review sessions don't have to be long, but make them a regular part of your study schedule. Keep in mind you are not simply learning to pass a test but are accumulating knowledge to apply when you are working as a health care professional.

Engage your mind actively when you review. Passively reading and rereading your notes will not store them in your mind. Use the review column to the left of your notes to prompt recall of the information. Cover the notes you took in class, and explain the key words or answer the questions you wrote. This is the most effective part of the review because it forces you to think and helps transfer the content of your notes into your long-term memory.

Think about your own past experiences and how what you are learning relates to them and to what you already know about the topic. This gives you reference points and makes new information more meaningful.

Use what you know about your learning styles when studying from your notes. Here are a few ways to do this:

- Visual: Picture the words and concepts in your mind as you review; label drawings from memory; draw sketches. Rough ones are fine—no one is grading the art!
- Auditory: Review out loud, even if you must speak in a soft voice. Have someone read your key words and questions and check your answers as you give them out loud. Listen to recordings of your notes.
- Kinesthetic: Stand up, move around, re-create the lecture. Or teach someone else by explaining one on one. Use movement and gestures to emphasize important points. If the content concerns a procedure or something that involves movement, act it out or actually perform it as much as possible.
- Interactive: Exchange notes with a study partner or group. Discuss and quiz.
- Global: Write out concepts, then create a list of supporting related details.
- Linear: Look for logical patterns in the material.

Finally, create practice tests based on your notes. You can write your questions to the left of your notes or on a separate page. You can also record them. Don't take your "test" for at least 3 days. Here are some suggestions for questions:

1. What is the definition of ______________________?
2. What is the meaning of ______________________?
3. What are the steps in performing a ______________?
4. What is important to remember about ___________?
5. Why must you ______________________________?
6. What are the principal parts of _________________?
7. How does ________________________ function?
8. What is the purpose of ______________________?

READING TO LEARN

"To read without reflecting is like eating without digesting."

—Edmund Burke

Reading, along with listening and taking notes, is one of the most important ways you will acquire information as a student. Like effective listening, reading to learn requires you to pay attention and participate actively. It should be approached purposefully because you must work at understanding, remembering, and applying new material. If you were reading instructions about how to perform a medical procedure, you would ask yourself, "Do I understand this? What, exactly, am I supposed to do?" and then you would read carefully to make sure you got it right. The goal when reading your textbooks is also to comprehend and think about what to do with your new knowledge. You will spend a great deal of time reading textbooks, so it makes sense to learn how to gain the most benefit from your efforts.

Earlier in this chapter, we discussed why you should take notes. You might wonder why you have to read and take notes. There are several reasons, as follows:

1. The more ways you take in information, the more likely you are to remember it. Paths are worn over time by many walkers. If no one uses them, they disappear. Your memory paths are also created and maintained by repeated use. Even if a subject is discussed in class, reading gives you one more encounter with it.
2. As we suggested in the section on taking notes, reading will give you background information for class lectures. It also reinforces what you hear in class.
3. Textbooks provide a permanent means of saving information. You can refer back to them over and over as needed.
4. Books usually contain more supporting details, examples, graphics, and organizational aids than lectures.

Getting Ready to Read

There are several prereading activities you can do to make your reading easier and more beneficial. The first is to clear your mind of clutter. Reading requires concentration, and this is difficult when you have unfinished business on your mind. If something is bothering you that can be handled quickly, take care of it before you start studying. (But try not to let "urgencies" be an excuse to put off getting together with your books indefinitely.) If it will take more than a few minutes of your attention, write it down (your planner would be a good place) so you can deal with it later.

Next is to find a place that encourages reading rather than sleeping or daydreaming. Many people find that a straight-backed chair at a desk works best (you will be doing some writing as you read). Give your back good support, and make sure the lighting is adequate. An uncomfortable environment can tire you and cut your reading time short.

You need more than just your textbook to read actively, so gather your tools: notebook, pen or pencil, highlighter or colored pen, and dictionary. Develop the habit of gathering needed supplies before you start studying. This is an important health care practice, too. You would not want to interrupt a patient procedure because you forgot to bring something from the supply room. Your study time is valuable, too, and should not be interrupted while you look for the dictionary.

Previewing

"Advice worth repeating: Work smarter, not harder."

Many methods have been developed to help students gain maximum benefit from their reading assignments. Some methods have many steps and others just a few, but they all recommend that you preview before you start reading. Using our medical procedure example, you would never perform a treatment on a patient without taking a few preliminary steps: (1) identify the patient, (2) introduce yourself, (3) verify the procedure, (4) gather the necessary supplies, and (5) put on gloves. Previewing in reading means that you look over the entire selection, learn any new vocabulary, pay attention to the headings, and use clues in the text to anticipate and think about the content. Fortunately, most textbooks are set up to help you and contain many features to guide your previewing and reading.

Anatomy of a Textbook. When you get a new textbook, take a few minutes to look it over carefully. Don't wait until the end of the course to discover something that could have made your life easier. Every textbook contains at least a few of the following useful features:

1. **Preface:** An introductory section at the beginning of the book. It typically contains a statement of the author's purpose and an overview of the book's content and structure. Some prefaces include information of special value to students, such as how to use the different features, study tips, and career ideas.
2. **Table of contents:** Some books supplement the usual list of chapter titles with a complete listing of chapter sections. This detailed format gives you a good overall view of the topics covered.
3. **Appendices:** Extra materials placed at the back of the book. Their contents are based on the book's subject and vary widely. Look these over when you first begin using the book, because you may discover valuable resources to help you understand both the textbook and the subject. There may also be sources of career information and reference guides. Examples from recent editions of health care textbooks include guidelines for infection control, important abbreviations, a metric conversion chart, Spanish translations of common health care phrases, laboratory test values, and a Celsius-Fahrenheit conversion scale.
4. **Index:** An alphabetical listing of all the topics in the book and the page numbers on which they appear. The items included are much more specific than those listed in the table of contents. The index is located at the back of a book and is very useful when you need specific information or are reviewing.
5. **Bibliography and/or references:** A list of source materials used by the author and/or recommended

readings for students who want to learn more about the subject. Each chapter may have its own bibliography, or there may be one list at the end of the book. Bibliographies can be excellent resources for expanding your knowledge of specific areas in which you are interested.

6. **Glossary:** An alphabetical list of words with their definitions, usually located at the back of the book.
7. **Vocabulary or key terms:** Lists of new words, often placed at the beginning of each chapter. Because reading is based on understanding words, learning new vocabulary before you begin to read is essential for comprehension. Take a few minutes to study the terms listed before you read the chapter, marking any words you find difficult. Word lists may also contain clues about what the author considers to be most important.
8. **Objectives:** These are statements telling you what you should learn or be able to do as a result of studying and applying the information in the chapter. Knowing the chapter objectives gives structure and purpose to your reading. Objectives are also useful to check your understanding after reading the material. Here are some examples of objectives:
   - Describe the steps in the communication process.[2]
   - Identify key differences between law and ethics.[2]
   - List and describe the three stages of a fever.[2]
   - Explain the advantages of outpatient intravenous (IV) therapy.[2]
9. **Chapter introductions:** In addition to giving an overview of chapter content, these often contain explanations of why the material is important and how it relates to your career.
10. **Section headings:** Words or phrases that divide and identify sections of text. Headings give you an idea of the content that follows. An important part of previewing is going through the assigned reading page by page and reading the headings. You will see they are organized like an outline, often with several levels of subheadings. Some books distinguish the levels with different colors and lettering styles. The following example of headings comes from a chapter entitled "Interacting with Patients" in *Today's Medical Assistant*[2]:

Communicating with Patients
Verbal and Nonverbal Communication
Interference with Communication
Listening Skills
Nonverbal Measures to Facilitate Communication
Interviewing Techniques
  Closed Questions
  Open Questions
  Keeping the Conversation Going
  Drawing Out Patients
  Avoiding Responses That Inhibit Communication

Headings provide a logical structure to guide your reading. In the example, you learn three things before even reading the chapter: (1) interviewing techniques are used when communicating with patients; (2) there are at least two kinds of questions; and (3) some types of responses interfere with good communication.

One effective way to increase learning is to relate new information to what you already know. After reading the headings, but before reading the material, take a few moments to think about what you know about the topics.

You may be thinking that previewing is a waste of time and that it would be better to just jump into the reading and get it done. Not true! You are not "just reading." You are engaging in a learning activity, and previewing increases your ability to comprehend and remember the information presented in your textbooks. Previewing is actually an excellent investment of your time.

Success Tips for Reading

- Look up unfamiliar words as you come to them by using the book's glossary, a general dictionary, or a medical dictionary. You can write the definition in your book, in your own glossary you keep in your notebook, and/or on flash cards. (An exception to this for English-as-a-Second-Language [ESL] students is explained in Chapter 2.)
- Take advantage of illustrations, charts, lists, and boxed text. These are designed to give you examples and additional opportunities to master the material. Boxes often provide summaries of text content and serve as handy review aids.
- Read through procedures carefully, paying special attention to the rationales. It is important for health care professionals to understand the reasons behind their actions because nothing in health care is routine. You must think through every action and know why you are performing it.
- Read in short sessions. Depending on the difficulty of the material, you may find you are able to read and absorb for only 20 to 30 minutes without a short break. Experiment to see what works best for you. Just don't wander off too far or get involved with a 2-hour movie on TV!
- Don't worry about your reading speed. Health care textbooks contain lots of technical and detailed information. Your goal is not speed; it is comprehension. Read at a rate that keeps your attention and also allows you to understand the material. One way to prevent getting bogged down is to avoid saying each word, even if you are only doing this mentally. Try to read in phrases. When you drive a car, you see and act on many things at once. The same is true for reading, and with practice, you can see and process several words at a time.

DOING RESEARCH TO LEARN

Research is not limited to finding information for a paper you have to write. We do research all the time, such as when we investigate which car to buy, how to find the best auto insurance, and how to change a tire. Research simply means finding sources of reliable information and obtaining what you need from those sources.

Library

Your school's library may be large and contain thousands of books and loads of other material, or it may be small and focused on the specialized materials needed to support the programs offered at the school. You should get to know both your school library and your local public library. If there are other schools of higher education nearby, inquire whether they allow the public to use their libraries. Some give checkout privileges for a yearly fee. Hospitals and clinics often have libraries for employees. It is possible you will have access to these during your clinical experience.

Today's libraries have many resources in addition to books and journals. Most offer Internet services, videos, DVDs, and other multimedia materials. Every library is different. Walk around and explore. Look for informational brochures and how-to guides, and ask the librarian for help.

Internet

The Internet, a connection of many millions of computers throughout the world, is a valuable source for all kinds of information. Literally anyone or any organization can create a website on the Internet for everyone to access. Following are a few examples of what is available:

- Articles from newspapers and magazines
- Informative articles by researchers
- Directories
- Dictionaries
- Opportunities to communicate with experts
- Job postings and applications
- Information about diseases and injuries for both patients and health care professionals
- Career advice from professional organizations
- Photographs
- Video presentations
- "Stores" from which you can order almost any product or service imaginable

If you don't own or have access to a computer, check with your school to find out what is available. A complete discussion on how to search the Internet is outside the scope of this book. However, it is easy to use and doesn't require a significant amount of computer experience. If you don't have much experience searching the Internet, online tutorials are available and can be accessed by entering the key words "Internet tutorials" or "online search tutorials."

You can find information on the Internet in several ways. The first is by using a website address. All sites have one, just like houses. If you know the address, you simply type it in. If you do not know which sites have the information you are looking for, you can use a program called a *search engine*. You simply enter key words and the search is on! Here are the three general search engines recommended by the University of California (UC), Berkeley[4]:

- Google: www.google.com
- Yahoo!Search: www.search.yahoo.com
- Exalead: www.exalead.com/search

Some search engines are limited by subject area, such as the following:

- fealth! is limited to health: www.fealth.com
- Scirus is limited to science: www.scirus.com

General subject directories contain information categorized by topic, including health. The following two examples are recommended by UC Berkeley[4]:

- Infomine: www.infomine.ucr.edu
- About.com: www.about.com (for resources limited to health: www.about.com/health)

Evaluating Websites. A word of caution—the Internet is not controlled by any organization or agency that checks on content or keeps the connections up-to-date. For serious research, be sure to check the credibility of the information supplier. Here are some questions you should ask about a website:

1. Who is the sponsor? Universities, government agencies, professional organizations, research institutes, and established publishers are usually good sources. (This is not to say that commercial sites do not contain excellent information. Just note whether their purpose is to inform or advertise a product.) The endings of the web address indicate sponsorship:
   university: .edu
   government: .gov
   professional organization: .org
   commercial enterprise: .com
2. Who is the author? He or she should have education and/or experience in the subject matter. Can you contact the author?
3. What is the purpose of the website? Many sites are designed to sell products or persuade viewers to believe in a cause. The material provided may be biased and/or not well researched.

4. How are claims supported? Check for statistics and references to original sources of information.
5. How current is the information? Are dates given? Advances and changes in health care and its delivery occur continually.
6. What is the purpose of the document? To present facts? To give an opinion? To sell a product or service?

Examples of Health Care Sites. The Internet is a relatively new technology. Websites close down, merge with others, or change their addresses, and this can be a source of frustration. The following are examples of reliable sites that have a wealth of information about health topics:

- Agency for Healthcare Research and Quality
  www.ahrq.gov
- Centers for Disease Control and Prevention
  http://cdc.gov
- Family Doctor
  http://familydoctor.org/
- Healthy People
  http://healthypeople.gov
- MedlinePlus, sponsored by the National Library of Medicine and the National Institutes of Health
  http://medlineplus.gov
- National Institutes of Health
  http://health.nih.gov
- University of Iowa Hospitals and Clinics
  www.uihealthcare.com/topics/catindex.html
- Web MD
  www.webmd.com

Health care professional organizations have websites. Appendix A contains a list of many organizations with their contact information.

To Learn More

Dartmouth College Academic Skills Centers
www.dartmouth.edu/~acskills/videos/index.html
Although created for college students who live on campus, the videos on note-taking and reading contain useful information for all post-secondary students.

Pauk W, Owens R: *How to study in college*, ed 9, Clifton Park, NY, Cengage.
Professor Pauk developed some of the most successful study techniques, which are still being used by students today.

Study Guides and Strategies
www.studygs.net
This website has been a public service since 1996 and contains hundreds of helpful strategies categorized by topic.

Study Skills Help Page: Learning Strategies for Success
Middle Tennessee State University (MTSU)
http://frank.mtsu.edu/~studskl
Created for students at MTSU, this site contains dozens of helpful study tips.

REFERENCES

1. Anderson R, Barbara A, Feldman S: *What patients want: a content analysis of key qualities that influence patient satisfaction*. www.drscore.com/press/papers/whatpatientswant.pdf (Accessed 2/9/09)
2. Bonewit-West K, Hunt S, Applegate E: *Today's medical assistant: clinical and administrative procedures*, St Louis, 2009, Elsevier.
3. Wahlstrom C, Williams BK: *The commuter student: being your best at college and life*, Belmont, Calif, 1997, Wadsworth Publishing.
4. University of California, Berkeley: Teaching Library Internet Workshops. Available at: www.lib.berkeley.edu/TeachingLib/Guides/Internet/SearchEngines.html. (Accessed 2/14/09).

PRESCRIPTION FOR SUCCESS 6-1 | MY LISTENING HABITS

You can start improving your listening skills by practicing awareness. One way is to listen to the news or other programming on the radio for several minutes at a time. Pay attention to when your mind wanders or you lose track of what is being said. (You can try the same technique in your classes if you don't have time to listen to the radio and only if it does not distract your attention further from the lecture.)

1. Think about your listening. Is there a pattern to the breaks in your concentration? (For example, you are distracted by something visual or your private thoughts, you don't understand everything being said, it is difficult to follow long periods of speech.)

2. How might you improve your listening habits?

PRESCRIPTION FOR SUCCESS 6-2 | WHAT WORKS FOR YOU?

1. Choose or create a note-taking method you believe might work well for you.

____

2. Try it during the next few class lectures you attend, and report on how it works. For example, did it make it easier or harder for you to take notes?

____

____

____

____

3. If this method didn't work well for you, choose or create another one to try.

____

____

____

____

____

PRESCRIPTION FOR SUCCESS 6-3 | BOOK REPORT

Look over your current textbooks. Which of the following features do they contain?

__________ Preface

__________ Detailed table of contents

__________ Appendices

__________ Index

__________ Bibliography

__________ Glossary

__________ Vocabulary or key terms

__________ Objectives

__________ Chapter introductions

__________ Headings

__________ Other

PRESCRIPTION FOR SUCCESS 6-4 | CHECK OUT THE LIBRARY

Visit your school and/or local public library to learn about and create a list of the services offered.

____

____

____

____

____

Go to the Source

Choose a topic in which you have an interest, and locate five different sources of reliable information. Briefly describe each source and state why you believe it to be reliable.

Topic:

	Name of Source	Description of Source	Why Source Is Reliable
1.			
2.			
3.			
4.			
5.			

CHAPTER

7

Writing Strategies

YOUR WRITING ABILITY: A KEY TO PROFESSIONAL SUCCESS

Good written communication is critical for the delivery of high-quality health care. Notes on patient charts and entered onto computers, letters to insurance companies, and printed instructions for patients must be written clearly and accurately. Consistency of care, reimbursement for services, and good relations between health facilities and the public they serve depend on the quality of written documents. You may think you won't do much writing in your future work. Not true! Almost every job in health care today involves paperwork and some writing tasks.

Your writing is like a personal advertisement, representing who you are. It influences the opinions of other people about you and your work. Writing is a form of permanent communication. Unlike speaking, which can be revised and corrected so your listener understands what you are saying, you have only one opportunity to express yourself in writing. Readers must rely on what they see on the page and may question your competence if you make grammatical and spelling errors or organize information poorly. How well you write makes an impression on potential employers when you are applying for jobs. Once you are hired, it reflects on your employer and the health care facility where you work. In short, writing is an important skill to master. Written communications skills are included in the National Health Care Standards and Accountability Criteria:

- 2.31 Recognize elements of written and electronic communication (spelling, grammar, formatting, and confidentiality).
- 2.32 Describe techniques for planning and organizing written documents.[1]

Contrary to what you might think, the computer age has actually increased the importance of good writing skills. E-mail, in which you correspond electronically over the computer, is replacing a lot of the communication that until recently was conducted over the telephone. Although e-mail messages tend to be informal and often use phrases instead of complete sentences, they must be expressed clearly and in an organized fashion to be useful to the receiver. The growing use of electronic health records also requires the ability to record information clearly and accurately. Technology is actually increasing, rather than decreasing, the need for you to develop your writing skills.

Many students find writing difficult and dread assignments in which they have to write more than a few words. Maybe this applies to you. Perhaps you thought your previous English classes were boring or you were never required to do much writing. Or maybe English is not your first language. Whatever the reason, it is not too late to upgrade your skills. Although a complete writing course is beyond the scope of this book, this chapter contains information about the basics of good writing and includes suggestions to help you write more effectively. The main goal is to encourage you to care about your writing skills and motivate you to improve them, if necessary.

WRITE ON! DEVELOPING GOOD WRITING SKILLS

There are two components to good writing: content and form. Content refers to *what* you write: the information and ideas. Form is *how* you present it: grammar, spelling, and formatting. You must pay attention to both content and form in order for your reader to receive your intended message. Employers today rank this as an important job skill.

Content: Determine Your Purpose

The first step when starting to write is to think about what you want to accomplish. Your purpose determines what you say and how you say it, so it needs to be clear in your own mind. It will be based in part on who your audience is. (Identifying and addressing the needs of readers will be discussed later in this chapter.)

The following examples illustrate common writing goals of students and health care professionals.

1. **Demonstrate your knowledge and/or inform your readers.** This is one of the reasons why instructors ask you to write research papers (also called "term papers" or "reports") and answer essay test questions. They use these assignments to assess what you have learned about a subject. To do well on papers and tests, you must know about your subject, state information clearly, and provide accurate facts to support what you write. When your purpose is to show what you know, it is important not to pad your writing with repetition or statements that add nothing meaningful to the content. Although instructors often assign papers by numbers of words or pages, a common mistake of students is to use many words to make it look as if they've said a lot when they really have said very little.
2. **Persuade your readers.** A common class assignment is to write a paper about a controversial topic in which you must convince the reader to accept your point of view. Outside of class, you may have opportunities to write with the goal of influencing the reader to take certain actions. For example, you may write application letters to include with your resume when you are looking for employment. The purpose of these letters is to convince prospective employers to interview you. Persuasive writing can be used on the job to present your ideas about how the facility might run more smoothly or to request a promotion or a pay raise. Supervisors often ask that you submit these ideas and requests in writing, so it is important to know how to write convincingly.

   There are various ways to persuade readers. One is to present facts that support your arguments. In the case of the letter to a prospective employer, you could list the ways you can be of benefit and can help provide great service to patients. Another method is to appeal to readers' emotions. For example, if you want to convince them to take action against cigarette advertising aimed at children, you could point out the need for adults to express their love for vulnerable children by protecting them from potential health hazards. It is generally most effective to use both facts and emotions so they support each other and strengthen your case. In the argument against cigarette advertising, you could cite the number and ages of children who start smoking each year, along with statistics about diseases and deaths caused by smoking.
3. **Make a request.** This is related to persuasive writing, but it is usually more direct and has the goal of initiating a definite response. Although writing a request is not a common school assignment, you might use this form for tasks at school outside of class. For example, some schools require you to submit a written request if you need a leave of absence. Or you may fill out an application for a scholarship or write a request for information about your student loan. During your job search, you may submit requests to health care facilities for information about their application procedures. Once on the job, you may submit requests to vendors for information about their products, compose letters to physicians asking them to send you patient records, or write to insurance companies requesting action on unpaid claims.
4. **Provide an explanation.** Some school assignments, such as exercises in workbooks, ask you to explain the steps in a procedure or explain why something is done a certain way. Test questions that require short answers are often requests for explanations. On the job, you may write instructions for patients or directions for co-workers. It is important that this type of writing be very clear and organized in a logical order. Including information about why something should be done or why it should be done in a specific way strengthens your writing because people tend to be more willing and able to follow instructions when they understand the reasons behind them.
5. **Narrate a story or event.** If you take an English or a writing class, writing an original story may be one of your assignments. Although stories are not commonly used in workplace writing, they can add interest and provide examples in persuasive or explanatory works. The main considerations in story writing are to use your imagination and to write good descriptions. An example of the use of creative writing in the workplace would be writing a story to help children overcome their fear of the dentist. A word of caution: stories used in the workplace should be directly related to the situation. And it is inappropriate, even dangerous, to share work stories based on real people and events outside the facility.

Many pieces of writing have more than one purpose, and these can be combined so they reinforce each other. For example, when preparing instruction sheets for patients, they can be more effective if you include persuasive language that encourages the patients to follow their special diet or perform their exercises every day.

Content: Gather Information

Writing sometimes requires research and always requires thought. This may sound obvious, but many people simply start writing without any preparation or in-depth thinking. The result is a collection of words and sentences that don't say much. There are many sources of information, and the first one may surprise you—your own knowledge and experience. Start by writing down what you already know in whatever format you find most useful, such as lists of key ideas and facts, a mind map, or an outline.

After assessing what you know, identify what you need to find out. If the instructor has assigned a topic about which you know very little, consider developing a list of questions to help guide your research. For example, if you are to write about infectious diseases in the world today, your questions might include the following:

- What are the major infectious diseases?
- What are the symptoms?
- What causes these diseases?
- How are they spread?
- How are they treated?
- How widespread are these diseases? How many people are affected each year?
- What is the annual mortality rate?

If you know very little about the topic, start your research with resources that provide definitions and general information. Examples of these resources include encyclopedia and journal articles, textbooks, nontechnical books for the general reader, and websites for the general public. Once you have an overall view of the topic, you can narrow your research to specific areas of interest. Your instructors may require you to consult certain types and numbers of resources beyond your textbook. They may also have good suggestions for additional sources of information.

As you consult each resource, record the important facts and ideas. Some people like to use note cards. Try using a separate card for each topic or subtopic. If you need more than one card for each topic, number or mark them in some way to keep them organized. Another method is to take notes on sheets of paper (one side only), organizing by resource rather than topic. You may have several pages for each source. When it's time to organize, you can cut up the papers and sort the pieces by related information. Other methods are to leave the sheets whole and color-code the different topics or write key words in the margins to identify the various topics. You can then quickly scan the pages for needed information as you write. You can also take and organize your notes using the computer.

Whichever way you take your notes, you also need a system to keep track of your resources so you can create your bibliography or reference list. This includes all the books, journal and magazine articles, brochures, websites, and any other resources you have used. See Table 7-1 for examples of what information to record about each kind of source. There are several standard styles you can use for organizing your bibliography, so check with your instructor to find out which one you are to use. Even if your project does not require a bibliography, it is a good idea to write down your sources so you can find them later if you need them. One way to keep track of your sources is to create a numbered list and then write the corresponding number on each card or page of notes.

TABLE 7-1 Information Needed for Various Sources

Source	Facts You Need
Book	Author(s) or editor Title of the book Publisher Location of publisher (city) Year published Edition
Journal or magazine article	Author(s) Name of the journal or magazine Title of the article Volume number of journal Issue number Page numbers of the article
Newspaper article	Author(s) Name of the newspaper Title of the article Date of the newspaper Page numbers of the article
Website	Author(s) or creator(s) of site, if available Title of the site or "home page" if no title Name of any organization associated with the site Date site was created or latest update Date you accessed the site Complete site address

Content: Organize Your Information

"Since it is not possible to think about everything all at once, most experienced writers handle a piece of writing in stages."

—Diana Hacker

When you are assigned a research paper or have a report to prepare for work, it can be difficult to decide how to get started and then how to organize what you want to say. Some instructors require students to prepare an outline as the first step in writing. If you find it difficult to think in outline form (you're just not linear) or you just don't know where to start, outlining can be as intimidating as writing the paper itself. Don't despair. There are some other ways to tackle the problem of getting things in order and getting started. Suppose you are assigned to write a paper about electronic health records. Here are some ways you can gather and organize your information:

1. **Questions.** List questions you would like answered. Your information falls into place as you research and find the answer to each question.
2. **Idea sheets.** As you think of major ideas, write each one at the top of a separate sheet of paper. Then list all related and supporting ideas on the pages. To organize, lay the sheets out and move them around until you find the best way to order them.
3. **Note cards.** Dave Ellis, writer of popular student success books, recommends the use of note cards for

generating creativity and promoting organization.[2] List all your ideas, both major and supporting, on 3 × 5 cards, one idea per card. Sort the cards by topics or categories, and then arrange them in logical order. You can lay them out on a flat surface or pin them to a wall or large bulletin board.

4. **Mind maps.** Mind maps are diagrams drawn freehand that link and arrange words and ideas around a central key word or idea. Mind maps can be helpful if you don't have a clear idea of the order you want for your material. Some people find mind maps useful when brainstorming because they don't require ideas to be organized in a linear way. The result is a "map" illustrating how ideas relate to and support one another. If you have several major ideas, you can make a series of maps.

Who Are My Readers?

Effective writers consider the needs of their readers. This is especially important in health care, where safe and consistent care depends on how well health care professionals communicate with patients and with one another. Whenever you write, take into account the readers' ages, cultural backgrounds, knowledge of health issues, and purpose for reading the material. Remember that you will not usually be present to clarify information, answer questions, or see from their facial expressions that they do not understand or agree with what you have written. This is why it is so important to write clearly and organize your text so readers can follow it easily. If you are addressing a mixed audience, plan your writing for the readers who are most likely to have difficulty understanding. When writing class assignments and tests, your instructor is the audience. He or she wants you to demonstrate what you know about a subject and how well you express yourself. There may also be specific requirements about the form of writing you are to use.

Organize Content for Your Readers. Everyone prefers to read material that is easy to follow. Good writers achieve this by organizing material logically, and you can do this too. How you organize your content is based on the type of document you are writing. Letters, research papers, and long essay answers are easier for the reader to follow if they are divided into sections:

1. **Introduction.** Present your major points. Tell what you are writing about. State your purpose.
2. **Middle or body.** Develop, support, and explain your ideas. You may have several sections, one for each topic or idea.
3. **Conclusion.** Show how everything you have written pulls together. Give your "final word" on the subject. Summarize your points. State what you have attempted to prove with your information. Tell the readers what action you hope they will take as a result of your writing.

Short answers to test questions and brief letters and notes require tight organization to cover all necessary material in a small space:

1. Give your answer or state your purpose or main point in the first sentence.
2. Give supporting details in one or two paragraphs.
3. Limit your conclusion to one or two sentences.

Instructions and directions can be organized into lists of steps or activities in the order in which they should be performed or in order from most to least important. Rationale or purpose (reasons why something should be done) can be included just before or after the step or action to which it relates.

Starting to Write

Don't aim for perfection on your first draft. Many people find a piece of blank paper very intimidating, even professional writers. A good way to beat the blank-paper monster is to just start writing. Begin with a rough draft, and don't worry about how rough it is. Writing creatively and writing perfectly and correctly require different intellectual skills that can actually cancel each other out. Peter Elbow, a professor who wrote a very helpful book about how to write, says that trying to write perfectly the first time is "dangerous writing" because you can't generate good ideas and be critical of your work at the same time.[3] He recommends that you spend half of the time on a project **freewriting** the rough draft and the other half revising. (This is a good argument for starting your writing assignments well in advance of the due date!)

When freewriting, don't worry about starting with the introduction because this can put unnecessary pressure on you to start out "just right" with good opening sentences. You may not even know at this point how your piece is going to turn out because writers develop and come up with new ideas throughout the writing process and you may add or delete topics. Go ahead and start with the middle section if that works for you. (An exception is when you are writing answers to essay questions on timed tests. State your answer at the beginning and spend the rest of the time supporting it.)

A technique called "brain dump" can work when you're really stuck getting started. It works like this: Get out some paper and just start writing, using the information you have gathered. This will be easier if you have used one of the techniques described earlier: outline, idea sheets, questions, and so on. Write quickly, and get as much down on paper as possible. Then go back and look for ideas and themes you can put in logical order. Although this is not always the fastest method for completing a paper or report, it can get you started when you find yourself with a bad case of writer's block. You may end up with a jumble of ideas that has to be unsnarled, but at least you have something on paper, and the chances are good you'll have something you can use. Many writers use brain dump to promote creativity and get ideas flowing.

Once you have completed your first draft, let it rest for a couple of days (or hours, if the due date is directly ahead). Then assume the role of your readers and try to imagine you are reading the piece for the first time. Read it aloud to hear how it sounds. Better yet, have someone else read it so you can listen for the following points[4]:

- Do you have an introduction?
- Is your purpose clear?
- Do your ideas flow smoothly, one to another?
- Have you supported your ideas?
- Is there enough information about each topic or idea?
- Have you included unnecessary details that should be left out?
- Do you repeat yourself unnecessarily?
- Does the conclusion summarize your information?
- Do you achieve your stated purpose?

Form: Attending to the Details of Writing

Your content may be important, interesting, and well organized, but poor **grammar** and spelling can cause your readers to misunderstand what you have written and even to question your competence. You may believe that worrying about grammatical details is unimportant. However, work in health care demands that you attend to details every day. Performing accurately and following exact procedures are valuable health care skills. In many types of written and electronic health care **documentation,** the contents are strictly controlled by federal and state laws as well as by nongovernmental regulatory agencies. For example, California law requires that reports prepared to document patient home care visits be written on the day of the visit, contain specific information, use certain abbreviations, show any corrections made in a specific way, and record the time of the visit using the 24-hour system.

Written documentation is often the only proof to show that patients have received appropriate care. It is recognized in court and by **auditors** who perform compliance reviews of medical institutions. A standard rule in health care is "If it was not documented, it was not done." We might add "If it's written poorly, it's not documented properly and may not have been done properly!" Most patients are covered by some type of insurance, and payment to the health care provider depends on clear and accurate claims submitted by health care facilities. Even if your job does not include preparing insurance claims, your notes may provide the information on which the claim is based. Writing correctly and paying attention to details are skills that today's employers require.

First Aid for Grammar. All languages are organized into systems with rules that determine how words are organized. These systems and rules help listeners and readers make sense of what they are hearing or reading because they know what to expect. Comparing the structure of different languages is one way to illustrate the role grammar plays. Let's look at word order. In English, we usually place describing words (adjectives) in front of the words they describe (nouns). If a friend said to you, "I live in the house blue with the trim white," it might take you a few moments to figure out what she was talking about. You are not accustomed to this word order. But in Spanish, this would be correct. Spanish speakers expect to first hear the noun before the adjective.

Another example is the methods used in language to let you know who the subject is; that is, who is doing the action. In English, we use pronouns such as "I," "we," and "they" to tell who this is: I swim, we studied, they will graduate. Again, using Spanish for our comparison, these words are not always necessary because the last letters of verbs change to indicate the subject: estudi*o* = I study; estudi*amos* = we study; estudi*an* = they study.

There are many differences among the thousands of languages spoken the world over. The point is that each has its own grammar, the purpose of which is to help people communicate effectively. Mastering the grammar of the language(s) you use improves your ability to communicate. Correct grammar is especially important in writing. Listeners may not notice the mistakes we make when we are speaking. If something is unclear, listeners can ask us to repeat or explain what we mean. Written material, however, must stand on its own. If it is unclear, the reader is not likely to have an opportunity to ask for clarification. Worse yet, readers may follow directions incorrectly, and this can result in costly mistakes when dealing with matters of health. In addition to helping ensure safety, proper grammar results in writing that reflects competence and professionalism.

If you need to improve your writing skills, ask your instructors about other resources and find out whether your school offers English classes and/or has tutors. Many good books and websites with information about grammar and writing exist. (A few examples are listed at the end of this chapter.) The extra time you spend now will help you in valuable ways on the job.

A couple of notes about grammar references: First, many professional organizations have preferred styles for writing. For example, the American Association of Medical Assistants' book of style states that abbreviations for time should be written in lower case using periods: "a.m." for morning, "p.m." for afternoon and evening). Other references suggest using uppercase to show time: A.M., P.M. Find out if there are style books or references for your profession.

Second, a word about grammar checkers on word-processing software. I am writing this book using a popular computer program. To my surprise, most of the suggested changes have been incorrect. In many cases, making the "corrections" would result in sentences that don't make sense. At the same time, many obvious errors are not caught. Although word-processing software has made writing and making corrections easier, the final judge is still the human writer.

First Aid for Spelling. Many people, even good writers, have difficulty with spelling. English is a combination of many languages and contains silent letters, different ways of pronouncing the same letter, different ways of spelling the same sound, and other irregularities. There are a few rules, but the spelling of many words simply must be memorized. Developing a good learning system for spelling will be helpful when you are learning medical terminology. Spelling medical terms correctly is critical because errors can negatively affect patient care. Some medical words look alike and can be confused. Here are a few common examples:

- ilium—part of the hipbone
- ileum—part of the intestine
- alveoli—tiny air sacs in the lungs
- areola—brown pigmented area around the nipples

Begin now to practice good spelling habits by learning everyday English words.

Success Tips for Spelling

- Try the memory techniques suggested in Chapter 3.
- If you have children in school, make spelling a family activity.
- Work on spelling in a study group: quiz one another, have contests, give small prizes, and make learning fun.
- Start your own dictionary and spelling list to keep in your notebook or on your computer.
- Make flash cards to quiz yourself.
- Put cards on the bathroom mirror and other places where you'll see them every day.
- Spell aloud.
- Create a "mental movie screen" on which you visualize the words spelled out in large colored letters.
- Create hints and ass ociations.
- Write the words over and over. Try using colored pens and/or writing larger than you usually do.
- Record practice words to listen to at home or in the car.

Q&A With a Health Care Professional: Dolores Michaels

Dolores, a nurse in a large California medical clinic discusses the importance of good writing skills in the medical field.

Q Is being able to write well really that important for a health care professional?

A Absolutely! In fact, in our clinic written communication is central to everything. We have individuals who take phone messages from patients. These messages get passed on to doctors or to nurses like me who are responsible for reviewing them and getting back to patients. If we can't read or don't understand the message, we waste time checking back with whoever wrote it. In a fast-paced clinic, this can really create problems.

Q Do you have any examples of problems that resulted from unclear writing?

A Well, the other day I got a written message that said, "Patient has planteritis." This was a mystery because there's no such thing as "planteritis." I didn't want to call the patient without having some idea of the problem, so I had to take time to find the person who wrote this. Turns out the patient had "plantar fasciitis," which is inflammation of the tissue in the bottom of the foot. I have to say that good spelling is really critical. Another problem is with abbreviations. When we're in a hurry we tend to use them, but they can cause problems. The other day a nurse wrote on a chart, "Will call tom for a dressing change." The other staff then wasted time looking for someone named Tom who the patient was supposed to call. It turned out that "tom" was an abbreviation for "tomorrow." Totally different thing.

Q So abbreviations can really be a problem?

A Yes. You have to be really careful when using them. An interesting example is the shortcut for "shortness of breath." This is a common condition, but if someone simply writes "patient is sob," the meaning is open to interpretation. If this were the only sentence on a chart with no context, it could be really inappropriate! So you really have to be careful.

The idea is to save time, but if abbreviations aren't clear, they can waste time. One day a doctor wrote "brbpr." I had no idea what this was and had to take time to find the doctor. It turns out it meant "bright red blood per rectum," but there was no way I was going to figure this out.

Even when everyone agrees on a facility abbreviation, it can be confusing to personnel who move from department or facility to another as fill-ins. Something like "mltcb" means "message left to call back." But lots of medical personnel work in various departments and facilities, and this can be confusing.

Q It sounds like we're not talking about the kinds of writing that students think of as assignments, like papers and reports.

A No, I'm referring to things like memos and electronic notes. These aren't long, but they're extremely important. They must be clear and accurate because we need the right information to give appropriate patient care. It's important to be precise and include all necessary details. If you're describing a wound, for example, you need to note the location, size, condition—all the things that the next person who sees the patient can use to see if the wound is healing or getting worse.

What students also need to understand is that these are legal records. If there's a malpractice suit, for example, they can be used in court as evidence.

PERSONAL REFLECTION

What are some possible future effects on the job for students who passed their classes by cheating instead of studying?

____

____

____

____

____

To Learn More

Elbow P: *Writing with power: techniques for mastering the writing process*, New York, 1998, Oxford University Press.

This is one of the best books on writing I have found. It has many techniques to help you effectively put what you want to say on paper.

Hacker D: *A writer's reference*, ed 6, Boston, 2007, Bedford/St. Martin's.

This is an excellent, easy-to-use book that includes explanations and examples of grammar, sentence structure, punctuation, and organization of content.

Pauk W: *How to study in college*, ed 7, New York, 2005, Houghton Mifflin.

Professor Pauk developed many original and practical ideas to help students study more effectively.

Purdue University's Online Writing Lab.

http://owl.english.purdue.edu

Purdue offers information on dozens of topics related to writing of all types in its award-winning writing lab.

REFERENCES

1. National Consortium on Health Science and Technology Education: *National Healthcare Foundation Standards and Accountability Criteria*. Available at: www.nchste.org/cms/wp-content/uploads/2008/03/foundation_standards_ac_rev_01_08. (Accessed 2/13/09)
2. Ellis D, Toft D, Mancina D, McMurray E: *Becoming a master student*, ed 12, Boston, 2009, Houghton Mifflin.
3. Elbow P: *Writing with power: techniques for mastering the writing process*, New York, 1998, Oxford University Press.
4. Palau SM, Meltzer M: *Learning strategies for allied health students*, St Louis, 2007, Elsevier.
5. Fry R: *How to study*, ed 6, Franklin Lakes, Clifton Park, NY, 2004, Delmar Cengage.
6. Pauk W: *How to study in college*, ed 7, New York, 2005, Houghton Mifflin.

PRESCRIPTION FOR SUCCESS 7-1 WHAT'S THE PURPOSE?

List What do you think would be the major purpose of each of the following writing projects?

1. A three-page report about a skin disease that includes the causes, methods of diagnosis, and treatment.

____

2. An instruction sheet explaining how patients with leg casts can take a shower without getting the cast wet.

____

3. An essay in which you explain why quitting smoking can improve the quality of and increase the length of a person's life.

____

4. A letter asking for a transfer to a job at your facility that requires more experience than you currently have but for which you feel you are qualified.

____

5. A letter of recommendation for a co-worker who is moving to another state.

____

6. A letter to your local newspaper in which you express your ideas about the lack of affordable medical care for the poor.

____

7. Directions for using the office copy and facsimile (fax) machines.

____

PRESCRIPTION FOR SUCCESS 7-2 WHAT WORKS FOR YOU?

1. Which of the organizational techniques presented do you think best fits your learning style?

____

2. Explain why.

____

____

3. Describe any other organizational or writing techniques that have worked for you.

____

____

____

CHAPTER

8

Improving Test Scores

TESTS: PART OF SCHOOL, PART OF LIFE

Taking tests is not limited to your life as a student. Much of what the health care professional does every day is a kind of test. Let's compare some typical classroom test questions with the performance of a procedure on a patient.

Test for A Class	Performance of A Procedure
Supply definitions	Know when to use the procedure
List items needed to perform the procedure	Gather equipment and supplies for the procedure
Recall information	Create mental checklist of steps
Write explanations	Provide patient with clear explanation and instructions Perform procedure correctly
Write short answers to questions	Record results accurately on patient chart

Using Tests to Your Advantage

Classroom tests and work on the job both involve interpreting sets of instructions (questions and job tasks), performing within time limits (class session and appointment schedules), following given standards (instructor criteria and facility protocols), and being measured by indicators of the level of performance (grades, patient satisfaction, evaluations, and raises). In reality, performing on the job is more serious in terms of requirements and consequences than any classroom quiz or final exam. Students can repeat a test—or a class, if necessary—but correcting a medical error, winning back an unhappy patient, or reversing the poor opinion of your supervisor is more difficult. At the extreme is the possible damage done by an incorrect procedure or inaccurate medication dosage.

The intention here is not to terrorize the future health care professional, but to put the subject of tests in the classroom in perspective. Tests are a fact of life, and if approached with the right attitude, classroom tests can provide you with opportunities to increase your learning. For example, tests encourage students to study. Most of us perform best when there is a consequence for our actions. In Chapter 3 we discussed how "good stress" can stimulate us physically and mentally to be alert and take appropriate actions. In the same way, you can harness the anxiety experienced when thinking about future tests to energize yourself and focus your efforts on learning. You can use tests to mark your progress toward achieving your long-term goal of becoming a competent health care professional—which is, after all, the real reason for learning.

Tests also teach you to work under pressure, which is a daily reality for health care professionals. You can never take your tasks for granted, and classroom tests provide practice for working calmly and efficiently when it counts. Planning and preparing ahead, thinking about what you are doing, and performing to the best of your ability are habits that apply to both test taking and work.

Finally, test results give you opportunities to improve and advance your learning. Answer sheets and scores are not for the exclusive use of your instructors. And contrary to what you might believe, assigning you a grade is not the only purpose of tests. Take advantage of them to help you as a student. They identify what you know and don't know. Review your answers to discover which material you haven't mastered. What did you not understand? What do you need to ask the instructor? What should you review again? Fill the gaps in your knowledge now, while you are still in school. Don't brush off wrong answers and hope the knowledge all comes together on the job. Remember why you are in school: to learn the basics of your profession. Sometimes you will make mistakes, a fundamental student right. Learning from your mistakes is a fundamental student responsibility.

What Tests Are—and Are Not

"Think of a test as a challenge instead of a threat."
—Walter Pauk

Tests can turn otherwise sensible individuals into quivering masses of anxiety. For many students, the grades earned on tests influence their feeling of self-worth. You may be worried about appearing stupid and wonder if you have the ability to learn. Or you may feel insecure about your test-taking skills. In reality, your own personal experiences may be helpful in dealing with tests and other stressful situations. Although there is no denying that tests are used as indicators of progress by both instructors and students, understanding more about tests and their purpose can help you control them rather than letting them control you.

Good tests measure your knowledge and ability in specific areas. They can also measure how much you have packed into temporary memory as a result of last night's cram session, so they may or may not indicate the extent of true learning or your ability to perform effectively on the job. Tests, however, are never a measure of your value as a person. You can be an "A" in life even if you do not receive straight As in the classroom.

Preparing Effectively for Tests

The best way to prepare for tests is the same way you prepare yourself for career success: Start preparing early and study to learn because being prepared for tests means mastering the content of your courses. Let's review a few study techniques that lead to successful test taking:

- Manage your time so that studying is a priority.
- Identify and use study techniques that correspond with your preferred learning styles.
- Use learning techniques that help move information into your long-term memory.
- Take good notes in class and review them often.
- Read textbooks actively and review them regularly.
- Seek help early if you are having trouble.

In addition to practicing good study habits, there are specific steps you can take to prepare for important tests.

1. Find out as much as possible about the test. Gather your notes and handouts and ask the instructor for suggestions on how to best prepare. Suggested questions to ask your instructor: "What type of questions will be asked (such as multiple choice and true-false)?" "Will there be a time limit?" "Will it be given at the beginning or end of class?" "Will you review first?"
2. Quickly review your notes, textbook, handouts, and any other class materials to check your comprehension. Is there anything you don't understand or can't remember, even after reviewing? Write a list of questions about the subject to ask in class. (This is why you start your review early, not the night before the exam!)
3. Make a schedule, and divide what you have to review over the time you have available so you won't run out of time before you have a chance to review everything (another good reason to start reviewing a few days before the test).
4. Review your textbook and use any supporting materials that came with it such as a companion website or CD.
5. Use the study tools you developed when you reviewed throughout the class—or create some now! Here are a few ideas:
   - Keywords or questions to prompt recall of notes and text.
   - Outlines, charts, or mind maps to help you organize the material and make it meaningful for you.
   - Flash cards to practice recall. Put aside the ones that you know well and concentrate on the ones you have the most difficulty remembering. Your goal is to move all cards into the "know-these" pile.
   - Saying aloud or writing answers to your prompts and practice questions.
6. Identify and concentrate on the material you find most difficult and have the most trouble remembering. Don't keep restudying material that you know. (Except when you are deliberately overlearning, as discussed in Chapter 3.)
7. Use the practice questions and quizzes you created from your class notes and from your reading. This may be the single best way to ensure you are prepared for classroom tests.

The Anxiety Monster

You have studied throughout the class, you have reviewed for the test, and you feel pretty secure about your knowledge of the material, but you are panic-stricken by the idea of your final exam. You just know you'll freeze up and won't be able to remember a thing. You may even feel physically ill when you enter the classroom on test days. There just doesn't seem to be any way around it—you just "can't take tests." This is a real problem for many students, and solving it is an important step toward achieving your professional goals. Following is a list of actions to help you manage test anxiety:

- Evaluate your study habits and test-review methods. Can you improve them? Are you really using your study time efficiently? For example, some students spend a lot of time reading notes over and over but never actually quizzing themselves without looking at the written information. They think they know it, but without their book or notes, they can't remember very much.
- Think about your actual test preparation. It may seem like you are spending a lot of time reviewing because you feel worn out by it. In reality, if you engage in a marathon review session the last 2 days before the test, you may feel as if you studied a lot but are too tired to remember much of the material.
- Be honest with yourself. Do you have trouble understanding in your classes but don't ask for help because you are embarrassed? Remember that instructors are there to help you, and asking for help is not nearly

as embarrassing as failing a test or finding that you lack information needed to perform your job. Have you been an active participant in class? Do you lack the time after class to stay for extra help? Is there another reason? If you are serious about achieving your career goals, you must decide to make school a priority and organize your life so that you can study when and as much as needed.

- Don't let your classmates freak you out. If you worry about competing with them, such as finishing the test first or earning a higher grade, you can get distracted from focusing on your own performance. Your education is not a race with winners and losers; the goal of a health care program is for everyone to win by graduating as a competent professional. Although the awarding of grades tends to set up a competitive environment, modern health care is delivered by teams of individuals who must work cooperatively, not competitively. Some classmates are even more anxious about tests than you. These people often express their nervousness by talking a lot and predicting total gloom and doom. Be upbeat with them rather than letting their negative talk increase your own anxiety. Avoid participating in "ain't it awful" conversations around test time.
- Join forces with positive students. Organize a small group to review, share ideas, quiz one another, and cheer one another on. Have each person make up a few test questions and quiz the others. Seek out classmates who are dependable and will contribute to the group. Keep the number small (three to five) so that everyone can make a contribution. If the group is too large, it can be very difficult to plan meetings that accommodate everyone's schedule.
- Use visualizations and positive self-talk to promote learning and good test performance.
- Practice good health habits and the stress management techniques described in Chapter 3. Remember that physical exercise releases endorphins, the body's natural tranquilizers. Do your best to get enough sleep before major tests so that you're not exhausted and more subject to anxiety. Finally, the relaxation exercise described in Chapter 3 is effective just before taking a test. Take deep breaths to help quiet the mind. Help your body work for instead of against you.

If you review thoroughly and try the suggestions for relieving anxiety, but still find yourself freezing up during exams and feeling as if even dynamite couldn't blast facts out of your brain, you can try a technique called "desensitization." This is a treatment developed for people who have anxieties that interfere with their daily lives. It works by providing exposure to small doses of the source of the fear and then gradually increasing the size and number of exposures.[5] Develop a plan to increase your exposure to tests. Have a friend or family member make up and give you tests, starting with short quizzes. Make them as realistic as possible. For example, set and stay within a time limit. Ask your instructor to give you practice tests. Find out if you can take these in a classroom under conditions as close to those of a real test as possible. Many sponsors of professional exams have sample tests you can take. These techniques may seem like a lot of work and even a little embarrassing, but if test anxiety is running your future career off track, desensitization is worth trying.

Tripping Yourself Up

Some students procrastinate in preparing for tests (and starting other projects, such as term papers) because they are afraid of failing. Their fear causes a kind of paralysis that prevents them from taking positive steps to prepare. For other students, not studying creates an excuse for failure. After all, if they try their best and still fail an exam, this might mean they lack ability. Another problem is feeling overwhelmed. Students who feel there is just too much to learn may decide to give up without really trying. If any of these behaviors sound familiar, make a deal with yourself to try something new. Study throughout the course, use the suggestions in this chapter on preparing for tests, ask for help, and work with a study group. The chances are very good you will experience success, and that can be habit-forming!

The Day of the Test

Okay, it's the day of the test and you feel reasonably prepared. You certainly don't want to perform poorly because you fail to follow some common sense test-taking guidelines. Here are some helpful hints you can apply to any test situation:

- You deserve a good start, so plan to arrive early. Don't stress yourself out by rushing in late, scrambling to find a seat, and missing the introductory instructions.
- Bring your supplies, including books, notes, and a calculator (if these are allowed). An erasable pen (blue or black ink) works well because you can make corrections neatly and your instructor will be able to read your answers.
- Read and/or listen to all instructions. Ask the instructor to explain anything you don't understand. This is not the time to be shy. You have a right to know exactly what is expected.
- Quickly review the *entire* test before starting. Read *all* directions on every page. If you have questions and the test has begun, go to the instructor and ask them quietly.
- If there are different types of questions, note which ones will take the most time to answer and/or are worth the most points. Then quickly plan how to divide your time among the different parts of the test.

- If the test is longer and/or more difficult than you expected, do *not* panic. Take a deep breath, follow the guidelines, answer the easiest questions first, and focus on doing your best.
- Give yourself a boost by answering the easiest questions first. When there are different types of questions, it is usually best to move from the shortest to the longest answers: true-false, multiple-choice, matching, fill-in, short essay, long essay. This is like giving yourself a warm-up. Also, the questions that have the answers provided for you to choose from may give you ideas for questions in which you must supply the answers from recall.
- Limit the time you spend on questions you find very difficult or don't know. Mark them and return later after you complete the rest.
- Proofread your answers before you turn in your test. Did you answer all the questions? Mark the correct boxes on the answer sheet? Follow all directions correctly? Check for spelling errors, words left out, and other careless errors.
- Use all the time allowed if you need it. You don't earn extra points by finishing early, and hurrying may cost you a few correct answers.

Specific Test-Taking Techniques

A message repeated throughout this book is the importance of mastering the knowledge and skills presented in your classes. The well-being of patients depends on what and how well health care professionals learn. The purpose of studying is to learn for the future, not just to pass tests. And the *best* way to prepare for tests is to know your material well.[6] That said, it is also true that learning about commonly used test formats can help you be more effective in showing what you know. Students who are unfamiliar with question formats can waste time and energy figuring them out.

It is important to keep in mind that some of the techniques suggested for answering test questions would be downright dangerous if applied to work in health care. For example, most study skills books recommend that if there is no penalty for incorrect answers, go ahead and guess. With true-false questions, you have a 50-50 chance; with most multiple-choice questions, the chance is 25%. But there is no room in health care for a 50-50 chance of correct performance. Some tasks, such as administering medications, must be 100% correct. There is no guesswork allowed here!

The suggestions given in the following sections are based on the experience of many students. However, they are only guidelines and do not substitute for knowledge.

True-False Questions

Purpose. Test your recognition of correct facts, statements, and cause-and-effect relationships, as well as your ability to distinguish fact from opinion.

Examples. *Read each of the following statements. If the statement is true, circle the T. If it is false, circle the F.*

T F 1. Classroom tests are always good indicators of how well students understand a subject.

T F 2. Test performance can be improved by cramming as much as possible the day before the test is given.

T F 3. Reviewing material regularly throughout the course is the best way to do well on tests.

Suggested Techniques for Answering

- Be sure that every part of the answer is correct. If any part of it is false, the entire answer is false.
- Watch out for words like "always" and "never." Few things in life are that final, and statements with these words are often false. (There are exceptions, however. For example, there are safety rules in health care that must always be followed and legal rules, such as those concerning the release of patient records, that can never be violated.)
- Answers with middle-of-the-road words like "usually," "sometimes," and "often" tend to be true (except as previously noted).
- Do not spend a lot of time on true-false questions you really don't know, especially if they are at the beginning of a test that also contains more time-consuming questions
- Guess only as a last resort (and only if there is no penalty).

Multiple Choice Questions

Purpose. Test your knowledge of terminology, specific facts, principles, methods, and procedures.

Examples. *Circle the letter to the left of the response that best answers each question.*

1. Which is the best reason for learning to spell correctly?
   A. Patients are impressed by correct spelling.
   B. Patient care can be negatively affected if words are misspelled on medical documentation.
   C. Students who spell correctly get better grades in school.
   D. It increases the chances of receiving a promotion at work.
2. The Cornell note-taking system has proven helpful to students because it:
   A. prevents them from having to review notes after class.
   B. helps them record everything the instructor says.
   C. provides a format that encourages review.
   D. teaches specific active listening techniques.

Suggested Techniques for Answering

- Read the instructions and questions carefully. If the question asks you to identify the "best" answer, it is possible that more than one is correct. In the first sample question, all answers are good reasons for spelling correctly. So you need to think about which is the most important reason, and that is patient safety. Therefore B is the correct answer.

- If the direction states to select the correct answer (as opposed to the "best," "most complete," etc.), consider each statement separately and ask yourself if it is true or false. (Many professional exams, such as the Certified Medical Assistant exam, are multiple choice.)
- Read through all the answers before selecting one.
- Immediately eliminate answers that are obviously incorrect.
- If the answer requires a math calculation, do the problem yourself before you look at the answers.
- Match each answer to the question rather than comparing the answers to each other.
- If you are guessing, choose an answer that has information you recognize.
- You can sometimes eliminate choices by using logic. For example, if two answers say basically the same thing, they must both be incorrect. As with true-false answers, if any part of a statement is wrong, the entire answer must be wrong. If the answer is silly or farfetched (instructors sometimes like to have a little fun), eliminate it immediately.
- If you are allowed to write on the test, circle or underline key words in the question to focus your attention when you read the answers.

Matching Questions

Purpose. Recognize definitions of terms and identify correct facts based on simple associations.

Examples. *On the line to the left of each number in Column A, write the letter from Column B that explains one of its uses.*

	Column A	Column B
_____	1. Comma	A. Substitutes for letters that are dropped when contractions are formed
_____	2. Semicolon	B. Indicates a change of thought within a sentence
_____	3. Colon	C. Connects two sentences into one long sentence when a connective word is used
_____	4. Apostrophe	D. Follows the greeting in a formal business letter
_____	5. Dash	E. Connects two sentences into one long sentence without the use of a connective word
		F. Is placed at the end of a sentence

Suggested Techniques for Answering

- Read the instructions carefully. Note whether any item can be used more than once.
- Quickly count each column to see if both columns have the same number of items. Sometimes they do not. It is possible that an item may be used more than once.
- Read through both columns before you write in any answers.
- Do the ones you know first.
- Some students find it easier to read the longer answers first (usually placed in the right-hand column) and then look for the shorter match. See which method works best for you.
- Mark or cross out each item as you use it, if you are allowed to write on the test paper.

Fill-in-the-Blank Questions

Purpose. Test your ability to recall terminology, facts, and procedures and to interpret information.

Examples. *Fill in each blank with a word or phrase that correctly completes the sentence.*

1. The huge group of interconnecting computers located around the world is called the ___________________.
2. Learners who are both visual and global sometimes find that ___________________ is a useful note-taking technique to record information in a way that clearly shows relationships.
3. An explanation of why a procedure is performed in a certain way is called the ___________________.

Suggested Techniques for Answering

- Read the entire statement before attempting to fill in the blank(s).
- Write answers that fit the form and content of the words around them. For example, if the last word before the blank is "the," you know the answer is a noun.
- It sometimes helps to convert the phrase into a question in which the answer is the correct fill-in.
- The length of the space may be a clue to the answer, but there is a chance the person who typed the test didn't even know the answers and randomly chose the lengths. This is not a reliable way to select an answer.

Short-Answer Questions

Purpose. Recall facts and definitions or write explanations that demonstrate your understanding.

Examples. *Write a short answer to each of the following questions using the spaces provided. Some questions have several parts. Your answers do not need to be complete sentences.*

1. List three reasons why many educators recommend using a three-ring binder to keep your notes and class materials in order.
2. Explain why previewing is a critical part of the reading process.
3. Describe four ways of starting to write a paper when you are having trouble determining exactly what to write and/or how to organize it.

Suggested Techniques for Answering

- Read the instructions to find key words that tell you exactly what is expected in the answer. Are you asked to explain? Give two examples? List five reasons? Define? Give the steps?
- If you are asked to write several sentences, answer the question as directly and completely as possible without padding with unnecessary information.
- If you don't know the entire answer, write down as much as you do know. You may receive partial credit.

Essay Questions

Purpose. Demonstrate ability to select, organize, relate, evaluate, and present ideas. These questions provide an opportunity to show what you know about the topic.

Example. *Write a well-organized essay at least one-page long explaining the meaning of this statement: "Study skills are career skills." Support your answer with examples and references to SCANS and the National Health Care Skill Standards. You will be graded on how well you demonstrate understanding of the concept, as well as on spelling and grammar.*

Suggested Techniques for Answering

- As with the short-answer questions, read the instructions to find out what you are supposed to include in your answer. Provide evidence for your response? Give examples to illustrate? Give the sequence? Explain reasons and purposes? Defend your answer? Compare and contrast?
- Don't write answers that are too short. Even if the question does not specifically ask for examples or evidence, you should fully explain or defend your answer.
- Don't spend time with a lot of words that don't really mean anything, such as repeating the question or writing a long introduction. Answer questions directly.
- If you have trouble organizing an answer in your head, quickly jot down a few key ideas, an outline, or a mind map.
- Use the rule journalists use when they write a newspaper article: state the most important information first by answering the question as quickly as possible. Use the rest of the time to develop your answer, write examples, provide evidence, and so on. This way, if you run out of time, you know you have included the most important information.
- Include the principal ideas of the course, as appropriate, especially ones the instructor emphasized.
- Use the principles of good writing discussed in this chapter.

After the Test

Much as you'd like to forget about the test you just took, don't. Just like athletes who analyze each game to learn which plays worked and which didn't, you can use debriefing to your advantage. As soon as possible after finishing the test, review your notes and books to find the answers to the questions you were unsure about or just didn't know.

When the test is returned in class, try not to react emotionally. If you earned a top score, give yourself credit. Continue to review the material from time to time to reinforce and retain important facts and information. If you did poorly, don't lose heart. Instead, try the following:

- Listen to any review the instructor gives of the test.
- If you have to return it to the instructor, take notes on a separate sheet of paper.
- Pay special attention to the questions you missed and write down the correct answers.
- If the instructor explains information, be sure to take notes.
- Ask questions about anything you don't understand.
- If your instructor does not discuss the test with the class and you did poorly, make an appointment to discuss it privately.

At your earliest opportunity, review your notes and the marks you made in your books. Did you miss some of the major points? Study the wrong material? Not really understand it? What can you do to improve your performance next time?

A WORD ABOUT PROFESSIONAL EXAMS

Many health care professions have exams you must pass to work in the field. The purpose of professional exams is to ensure high standards for practitioners by testing for knowledge and competence. These exams may be administered by a governmental agency or a professional organization. Passing them allows the professional to use one of several special designations such as "licensed," "certified," or "registered." Most exams require a fee. Your school may have included this cost in your tuition or fees. The school may also assist you in applying to take the exam. Some exams are given year round, others only on certain dates. Find out whether professional exams are required for your occupation. Learn as much as possible about the exam(s) while you are still in school.

Some professions do not require formal approval (certification, licensing, etc.) for graduates to work. At the same time, voluntary testing is available and recommended for many careers. For example, most states do not have licensing requirements for medical assistants. (States do regulate what procedures medical assistants can and cannot perform.) Many physicians, however, prefer to hire only certified or registered medical assistants, designations earned by passing professional exams administered by the American Association of Medical Assistants and the American Medical Technologists, respectively. Some medical insurance companies require physicians to hire only credentialed professionals.

Success Tips for Passing Professional Exams

- Start preparing early (note the word is "prepare," not "worry"). This suggestion is not intended to add further stress to your already busy class and study schedule. It is a reminder that if you prepare over a period of time, you will learn more and experience less stress when the time comes to actually take the test.
- Keep your notes, handouts, and textbooks organized so you can find and use them for review before the exam.
- Pay attention to any information and advice your instructor gives you about the content of professional exams.
- Some textbooks refer to specific exams and requirements of professional organizations, and the authors of the textbooks design their content and review questions to help students prepare throughout their courses. Take advantage of these features!
- Find out if there are any review books available in your school library or for purchase or online materials to help you focus your studies on mastering the material likely to appear on the exam.
- Practice tests are available for many exams. Check with your professional organization.
- Find out whether review workshops are available in your area.
- Plan to take the exam as soon as possible after you become eligible. This is usually on graduation from your program, although some occupations also require work experience. You are less likely to forget information and lose your confidence if you do not wait too long.
- Think of the timed tests you take in school as opportunities to practice taking an important exam under pressure.

SOME HONEST TALK ABOUT CHEATING

Health care professionals must follow high ethical standards. High-quality patient care and safety depend on their actions, and there is no room for cheating in any form. Furthermore, governmental regulations have increased, and audits of health care facilities are common. The consequences for fraud, taking shortcuts, and even trying to just "get by" are severe, including costly fines and closures of health care facilities.

You may believe cheating on tests in school isn't as serious as cheating on the job, but this is not true. Health care graduates who cheat to pass their classes, instead of learning what they need to know on the job, may become dangerous practitioners. You are in the process of becoming a professional, and what you do now is setting the groundwork for your future actions. Integrity (honesty, sincerity) is an essential characteristic of the health care professional, and cheating undermines that integrity. Cheating is an unsatisfactory and potentially destructive way of approaching your education. It converts the opportunities offered by tests to develop effective study habits and to learn what you need to know into unacceptable behaviors.

Even if you do not cheat yourself, helping others to do so promotes incompetence in the health care system. Would you or one of your family members want to be treated by "professionals" who cheated to pass their classes? Do you want to carry the load at work for a co-worker who is used to taking the easy way out? Helping friends cheat allows them to avoid taking responsibility for themselves. This can lead to the habit of dependence and unsatisfactory performance on the job, resulting in negative consequences for everyone.

PERSONAL REFLECTION

What are some possible future effects on the job for students who passed their classes by cheating instead of studying?

____

____

____

____

____

To Learn More

Elbow P: *Writing with power: techniques for mastering the writing process*, New York, 1998, Oxford University Press.
This is one of the best books on writing I have found. It has many techniques to help you effectively put what you want to say on paper.

Hacker D: *A writer's reference*, ed 6, Boston, 2007, Bedford/St. Martin's.
This is an excellent, easy-to-use book that includes explanations and examples of grammar, sentence structure, punctuation, and organization of content.

Pauk W: *How to study in college*, ed 7, New York, 2005, Houghton Mifflin.
Professor Pauk developed many original and practical ideas to help students study more effectively.

Purdue University's Online Writing Lab.
http://owl.english.purdue.edu
Purdue offers information on dozens of topics related to writing of all types in its award-winning writing lab.

REFERENCES

1. National Consortium on Health Science and Technology Education: *National Healthcare Foundation Standards and Accountability Criteria*. Available at: www.nchste.org/cms/wp-content/uploads/2008/03/foundation_standards_ac_rev_01_08. (Accessed 2/13/09)
2. Ellis D, Toft D, Mancina D, McMurray E: *Becoming a master student*, ed 12, Boston, 2009, Houghton Mifflin.
3. Elbow P: *Writing with power: techniques for mastering the writing process*, New York, 1998, Oxford University Press.
4. Palau SM, Meltzer M: *Learning strategies for allied health students*, St Louis, 2007, Elsevier.
5. Fry R: *How to study*, ed 6, Franklin Lakes, Clifton Park, NY, 2004, Delmar Cengage.
6. Pauk W: *How to study in college*, ed 7, New York, 2005, Houghton Mifflin.

PRESCRIPTION FOR SUCCESS 8-1 MAKE TESTS WORK FOR YOU

Describe five ways you can use tests to your advantage as you prepare for a career in health care.

1. ______________________________

____

2 ______________________________

____

3. ______________________________

____

4. ______________________________

____

5. ______________________________

____

PRESCRIPTION FOR SUCCESS 8-2 STUDYING FOR A TEST

1. Choose at least three study techniques to use when you prepare for your next test. List the ideas here.

   Technique 1: ______________________________

   Technique 2: ______________________________

   Technique 3: ______________________________

2. Create a plan for using these ideas, including the actions you will take and a study schedule.

   ____

   ____

   ____

   ____

3. After you have taken the test, write a paragraph describing how the techniques worked for you.

   ____

   ____

   ____

   ____

CHAPTER

9

Math Strategies

MULTIPLICATION

Multiplication is the fast way of adding similar numbers over and over again. You can recognize a multiplication problem when you see the ·sign. To do multiplication problems well, you must memorize the multiplication tables. As an example, the multiplication table for 3 looks like the following:

$$0 \times 3 = 0$$
$$1 \times 3 = 3$$
$$2 \times 3 = 6$$
$$3 \times 3 = 9$$
$$4 \times 3 = 12$$
$$5 \times 3 = 15$$
$$6 \times 3 = 18$$
$$7 \times 3 = 21$$
$$8 \times 3 = 24$$
$$9 \times 3 = 27$$
$$10 \times 3 = 30$$
$$11 \times 3 = 33$$
$$12 \times 3 = 36$$

You can create similar multiplication tables for any number. However, there is a better strategy for learning the multiplication tables—making and learning the multiplication chart (see Table 9-1).

The method for using this chart is as follows:

- You are asked to figure out how many ounces of medicine Ms. Grande takes per week. You know that she takes 3 ounces a day.
- In your mind you see the problem as $7 \cdot 3 = ?$, where 7 stands for the number of days in a week and 3 stands for the number of ounces of medicine Ms. Grande takes per day.
- In the top shaded row, put your right finger on the number 7.
- In the shaded column to the left, put your left finger on the number 3.
- Slowly move your right finger down and your left finger to the right until they meet. The number at which both fingers meet is the correct answer.
- "21 oz." is the answer to this problem.

Although a multiplication chart is very handy, it does not substitute for learning the tables by heart. Memorizing the multiplication tables until you know them as well as your name will make your personal and student life easier. To help you learn the tables, try making flash cards or find a computer program that will make the learning task enjoyable.

DIVISION

Like multiplication, you use division to solve many common, daily arithmetic problems. You can write division problems two ways:

$$10 \div 2 = 5$$

In this example the number 10 is divided by 2. In other words, you always divide the number after the sign into the number that goes before the sign. The second way to write division problems looks like this:

$$2\overline{)10}\text{ with quotient }5$$

In this example, you divide the number that is inside the box by the number that is outside the box. If you have learned your multiplication tables well, you will have an easier time with division. You may have noticed in the first example that if you read the problem from right to left, it reads like a multiplication problem. Consider the following:

- Mr. Sheldon, a medical secretary, was asked to split a $3000 bonus among the three employees working in Dr. Joseph's office.
- Mr. Sheldon knows that $1000 \times 3 = 3000$.
- He reverses the procedure and divided 3000 by 3.
- Each employee will get $1000.

If you learn the multiplication tables thoroughly, you will be able to do more complicated multiplication and division problems.

TABLE 9-1 Multiplication Chart

x	1	2	3	4	5	6	7	8	9	10	11	12
1	1	2	3	4	5	6	7	8	9	10	11	12
2	2	4	6	8	10	12	14	16	18	20	22	24
3	3	6	9	12	15	18	21	24	27	30	33	36
4	4	8	12	16	20	24	28	32	36	40	44	48
5	5	10	15	20	25	30	35	40	45	50	55	60
6	6	12	18	24	30	36	42	48	54	60	66	72
7	7	14	21	28	35	42	49	56	63	70	77	84
8	8	16	24	32	40	48	56	64	72	80	88	96
9	9	18	27	36	45	54	63	72	81	90	99	108
10	10	20	30	40	50	60	70	80	90	100	110	120
11	11	22	33	44	55	66	77	88	99	110	121	132
12	12	24	36	48	60	72	84	96	108	120	132	144

Exercise 9–1

Directions: Spend some time learning the multiplication chart (Table 9-1). Then fill in the chart below. You may want to memorize one table at a time and then fill in the chart as you learn that table. Remember that learning the multiplication tables by heart will help you with both multiplication and division problems.

x	1	2	3	4	5	6	7	8	9	10	11	12
1												
2												
3												
4												
5												
6												
7												
8												
9												
10												
11												
12												

FRACTIONS

Fractions represent parts of a whole. You go to school 5 days out of 7 days. When this is written as a fraction, it looks like this:

$$\frac{5}{7}$$

In this example the number 5 on top is called the numerator. The numerator tells you how many parts of the whole. The number 7 on the bottom is called the denominator. The denominator tells you how many parts make up a whole.

This example of a fraction is called a **proper fraction.** A proper fraction is when the numerator is smaller than the denominator and has a value less than 1.

Consider this next fraction:

$$\frac{4}{2}$$

This is an example of an **improper fraction.** When the numerator is larger than the denominator, you have an improper fraction.

Sometimes you may see a whole number written with a fraction next to it. It will look like this:

$$13\frac{6}{12}$$

This is called a **mixed number.**

Reducing to the Lowest Term

Sometimes when working with fractions it is necessary to reduce them to their lowest terms. This means dividing the numerator and the denominator by the same number until you cannot go any further. Study the following problem:

$$\frac{50}{100}$$

What number is needed to divide both the 50 and 100 so that the answer comes out evenly?

Try 25. 50 divided by 25 is 2. 100 divided by 25 is 4. The answer so far looks like this:

$$\frac{2}{4}$$

Is it still possible to reduce this fraction? Is there still another number that can be divided equally into both the 2 and the 4?

Try 2: 2 goes into 2 once; 2 goes into 4 twice. The answer now is:

$$\frac{1}{2}$$

The lowest term for

$$\frac{50}{100}$$

is

$$\frac{1}{2}$$

Raising to a Higher Term

Similarly, any fraction can be changed to a higher term by multiplying both the numerator and the denominator by the same number.

$$\frac{9}{18} = \frac{27}{54}$$

$9 \times 3 = 27$ and $18 \times 3 = 54$

Adding and Subtracting Fractions

To add and subtract with fractions that have the same denominator, you add or subtract only the numerator and copy the common denominator to finish the problem.

$$\frac{5}{11}+\frac{3}{11}=\frac{8}{11}$$

$$\frac{9}{64}-\frac{1}{64}=\frac{8}{64}$$

However, if the denominators are different, you need to find the lowest common denominator. The lowest common denominator is the smallest number that can be divided evenly by the denominators of all the fractions in the problem. For example:

$$\frac{2}{3} \quad \frac{5}{6} \quad \frac{3}{9}$$

Think of the smallest number that can be divided evenly by 3, 6, 9.

$$3 \times 6 = 18 \quad 6 \times 3 = 18 \quad 9 \times 2 = 18$$

Or

$$18 \div 3 = 6 \quad 18 \div 6 = 3 \quad 18 \div 9 = 2$$

18 is the lowest common denominator. The problem now looks like this:

$$\frac{(2)}{18} \quad \frac{(5)}{18} \quad \frac{(3)}{18}$$

To finish the problem you must take one more important step. **Whatever you do to the denominator you must do to the numerator.**

In the first fraction, you multiplied 3 by 6 to get the lowest common denominator of 18. Now you must do the same to the numerator 2. $2 \times 6 = 12$. The fraction is now

$$\frac{12}{18}$$

In the second fraction you multiplied the denominator 6 by 3 to get the lowest common denominator of 18. Now you must do the same to the numerator 5. $5 \times 3 = 15$. The fraction is now

$$\frac{15}{18}$$

In the third fraction you multiplied the denominator 9 by 2 to get the lowest common denominator of 18. Now you must do the same to the numerator 3. $3 \times 2 = 6$. The fraction is now

$$\frac{6}{18}$$

The fractions now look like this:

$$\frac{12}{18} \quad \frac{15}{18} \quad \frac{6}{18}$$

These fractions are now ready to be added or subtracted.

Multiplying Fractions

To multiply fractions you simply multiply the numerators and then the denominators. For example:

$$\frac{4}{7}\times\frac{10}{10}=\frac{40}{10}$$

If you are working with mixed numbers, it is important to change them into improper fractions before multiplying or dividing. Look at the following:

$$2\frac{4}{8}$$

To change this mixed number into an improper fraction, first multiply the denominator by the whole number.

$$8 \times 2 = 16$$

Next add the numerator of 4 to the 16.

$$16 + 4 = 20$$

Finally copy the original denominator so the fraction now looks like this:

$$\frac{20}{8}$$

The mixed number has now been changed to an improper fraction.

Dividing Fractions

To divide fractions, you do the following two steps:

$$\frac{4}{16}\div\frac{5}{15}$$

First you reverse the second fraction. In other words, the 15 becomes the numerator and the 5 becomes the denominator.

$$\frac{15}{5}$$

Then you change the division sign to a multiplication sign and multiply the numerators and then the denominators to get the answer.

$$\frac{4}{16}\times\frac{15}{5}=\frac{60}{80}=\frac{3}{4}$$

Sometimes, if the numbers are large, you may want to reduce them in a multiplication or division problem. Remember to work on a diagonal across the signs.

$$\frac{10}{20}\times\frac{5}{40}\times\frac{1}{10}$$

$$\frac{\overset{1}{\cancel{10}}}{\underset{4}{\cancel{20}}} \times \frac{\overset{1}{\cancel{5}}}{40} \times \frac{1}{\underset{1}{\cancel{10}}} =$$

$$\frac{1}{4} \times \frac{1}{40} \times \frac{1}{1} = \frac{1}{160}$$

Exercise 9–2

Directions: Do the following fraction problems. Pay careful attention to the signs so that you perform the correct function. Remember to find the lowest common denominators if necessary and change any mixed numbers to improper fractions.

1. Reduce $\frac{12}{48}$
2. Determine the missing numerator: $\frac{2}{3} = \frac{?}{36}$
3. Change to an improper fraction: $9\frac{2}{14} =$
4. $\frac{9}{11} - \frac{7}{11} =$
5. $\frac{4}{28} + \frac{9}{28} + \frac{14}{28} =$
6. $\frac{1}{3} \times \frac{1}{2} =$
7. $\frac{1}{3} \div \frac{1}{2} =$
8. $\frac{5}{14} \times \frac{7}{25} =$
9. $4\frac{8}{10} \div \frac{4}{5} =$
10. $2\frac{2}{4} \times 1\frac{5}{20}$

DECIMALS

Decimal numbers are similar to fractions. They both describe parts of a whole number. However, there are two differences between decimals and fractions. The first difference is that denominators of decimals can be only 10, 100, 1000, etc. The second difference is that a decimal point or period is used to separate the whole number from the fraction. In the following example, note the difference between decimals and fractions of the same number.

$$\frac{2}{10} = 0.2$$

$$\frac{80}{100} = 0.80$$

$$\frac{425}{1000} = 0.425$$

$$\frac{734}{10000} = 7.0034$$

The way you read a decimal is determined by how many numbers are to the right of the decimal point. The first example, 0.2, is read "two tenths." The second example, 0.80, is read "eighty hundredths." The third example, 0.425, is read "four hundred twenty-five thousandths," And the last example, 7.0034 is read "seven **and** thirty-four ten thousandths."

Adding and Subtracting Decimals

When you add or subtract decimals, it is necessary to write the problem so that all the decimal points are lined up in a straight row. Then add or subtract decimal numbers the same way you would add or subtract whole numbers.

$$\begin{array}{r} 4.258 \\ 9.636 \\ \hline 13.894 \end{array} \qquad \begin{array}{r} 90.58 \\ 82.21 \\ \hline 8.37 \end{array}$$

If you are adding or subtracting decimals, use zeros to fill in the places without a number after you align the decimal points.

$$\begin{array}{r} 21.55 \\ +62.2\mathbf{0} \\ \hline \end{array} \qquad \begin{array}{r} 21.55 \\ 62.2\mathbf{0} \\ \hline 83.75 \end{array} \qquad \begin{array}{r} 9.4707 \\ -4.26\mathbf{00} \\ \hline \end{array} \qquad \begin{array}{r} 9.4707 \\ 4.26\mathbf{00} \\ \hline 5.2107 \end{array}$$

Multiplying Decimals

When you multiply decimal numbers, multiply the same way you would with whole numbers. Then count all the numbers to the right of the decimal point in both rows of numbers in the problem. Put the decimal point that number of places in the answer.

0.798	(3 numbers to right of decimal point)
×6.4	(1 number to right of decimal point)
5.1072	(4 numbers to right of decimal point)

Dividing Decimals

Dividing decimal numbers is similar to dividing whole numbers. If the number outside the box is a whole number, place the decimal point in the answer in the same decimal place as the number inside the box.

$$4\overline{)0.8} = 0.2$$

If the number outside the box is a decimal, change this decimal number to a whole number by moving the decimal point to the right of the last number. Use a **caret** (^) to show the new place of the decimal. If the number inside the box is also a decimal number, move the decimal point the same amount of numbers as you did the outside number. Also use a caret to show you have moved the decimal point. If necessary add zeros to get the same number of decimal places.

$$\begin{array}{r} 200. \\ .400\overline{)80.000} \end{array}$$

Notice that the decimal point in the answer is placed exactly over the new position of the decimal point of the number inside the box.

Changing Decimals to Fractions

To change a decimal to a fraction, write the numbers in the decimal as the numerator and write the name of the decimal (tenths, hundredths, thousandths, etc.) as the denominator. Reduce the fraction if necessary.

$$0.50 = \frac{50}{100} = \frac{1}{2}$$

Changing Fractions to Decimals

To change a fraction to a decimal, divide the numerator by the denominator. The dividing line of a fraction means "divided by." To divide the numerator by the denominator, it will be necessary to add a decimal point and one or more zeros to the numerator.

Carry the decimal point up to the answer.

$$\frac{1}{2} \qquad \begin{array}{r} 0.5 \\ 2\overline{)1.0} \end{array}$$

Exercise 9–3

Directions: Solve the following decimal problems.

Add the following decimals:

a. 5.439 + 7.63 + 1.257 =

b. 0.428 + 0.029 + 8.35 =

Subtract the following decimals:

c. 21.719 − 5.83 =

d. 103.8 − 62.45 =

Multiply the following decimals:

e. 943.27 × 0.5 =

f. 1.3294 × 0.566 =

Divide the following decimals:

g. 70 ÷ 0.25 =

h. 160 ÷ 0.40 =

Change the following decimals to fractions. Reduce the fractions if necessary.

i. 0.020 0.8 0.45

Change the following fractions to decimals:

j. $\frac{4}{5}$ $\frac{6}{80}$ $\frac{50}{250}$

PERCENTAGES

Percentage numbers, like fractions and decimals, represent a part of the whole. The percentage represents hundredths and is indicated by the percent sign (%). Thus 47 hundredths can be written as

$$\frac{47}{100},\ 0.47,\text{ or } 47\%$$

When doing percentage problems, you should change the percentage number to either a fraction or a decimal number and then solve the problem. Table 9-2 is a **conversion** chart of some of the more common percentages.

TABLE 9-2 Converting Percentages to Fractions and Decimals

Percent		Fraction		Decimal
25%	=	$\frac{1}{4}$	=	0.25
50%	=	$\frac{1}{2}$	=	0.5
75%	=	$\frac{3}{4}$	=	0.75
12.5%	=	$\frac{1}{8}$	=	0.125
37.5%	=	$\frac{3}{8}$	=	0.375
62.5%	=	$\frac{5}{8}$	=	0.625
87.5%	=	$\frac{7}{8}$	=	0.875
$33\frac{1}{3}\%$	=	$\frac{1}{3}$	=	$0.33\frac{1}{3}$
$66\frac{2}{3}\%$	=	$\frac{2}{3}$	=	$0.66\frac{2}{3}$
20%	=	$\frac{1}{5}$	=	0.2
40%	=	$\frac{2}{5}$	=	0.4
60%	=	$\frac{3}{5}$	=	0.6
80%	=	$\frac{4}{5}$	=	0.8
10%	=	$\frac{1}{10}$	=	0.1
30%	=	$\frac{3}{10}$	=	0.3
70%	=	$\frac{7}{10}$	=	0.7
90%	=	$\frac{9}{10}$	=	0.9
$16\frac{2}{3}\%$	=	$\frac{1}{6}$	=	$0.16\frac{2}{3}$
$83\frac{1}{3}\%$	=	$\frac{5}{6}$	=	$0.83\frac{1}{3}$

Changing Percentages to Fractions

To change a percentage to a fraction, use the number in the percentage as the numerator and put 100 as the denominator. Reduce the fraction if necessary.

$$35\% = \frac{35}{100} = \frac{7}{20}$$

Changing Fractions to Percentages

The easiest way to change a fraction to a percentage is to change the fraction to a decimal number first.

$$75\overline{)3.00}^{\,0.04} \qquad 0.04 = \frac{4}{100} = 40\%$$

Changing Percentages to Decimals

To change a percentage number to a decimal number, erase the percent sign and move the decimal point two places to the left.

$$51\% = 0.51$$

Changing Decimals to Percentages

To change the decimals numbers to percentage numbers, move the decimal point two places to the right and write in the percent sign.

$$0.76 = 76\%$$

Doing Problem With Percentages

To find a percentage of a whole number, change the percentage to a fraction or a decimal and then multiply by the whole number.

What is 25% of 500?

$$25\% = \frac{25}{100}$$

$$\frac{25}{100} \times 500 = 125$$

or

What is 8.5% of 250?

$$8.5\% = 0.085$$

$$0.085 \times 250 = 21.25$$

To find what percentage one number is of another number, turn the numbers in the problem into a fraction and change the fraction to a percentage.

5 is what percentage of 50?

$$\frac{5}{50} = \frac{1}{10}$$

$$\frac{1}{10} = 0.1 = 10\%$$

To find the whole number when a percentage is given, divide the whole number by the percentage. Change the percentage to a fraction.

10% of what number is 100?

$$10\% = \frac{1}{10}$$

$$100 \div \frac{1}{100} = \frac{100}{1} \times \frac{10}{1} = 1000$$

Exercise 9–4

Directions: Fill in the following chart. Check your work with the conversion chart in Table 9-2. Then solve problems 11 through 15.

Percent	Fraction	Decimal
1. 50%		
2.		0.125
3.	$\frac{1}{6}$	
4.		0.7
5. 60%		
6.	$\frac{2}{5}$	
7.		$0.66\frac{2}{3}$
8.	$\frac{3}{8}$	
9. 80%		
10.	$\frac{1}{4}$	

11. What is 8% of 75?
12. 18 is what percent of 16?
13. 40% of what number is 48?
14. 27 is what percent of 72?
15. 6.25% of 300 =

RATIOS

A ratio is a comparison of two numbers using division. A ratio can be written in three ways:

1. 16 to 32
2. $\frac{16}{32} = \frac{1}{2}$
3. 16 : 32

Regardless of how you write the ratio, you would read it as "16 to 32." Read the following and find out how you would solve a ratio problem.

Of Chloe's 28 teeth, 4 have crowns on them. Determine the ratio of crowned teeth to uncrowned teeth.

Use the 4 crowned teeth as the numerator and the total number of teeth as the denominator and reduce the fraction. $\frac{4}{28} = \frac{1}{7}$

$\frac{1}{7}$ of Chloe's teeth are crowned.

Exercise 9–5

Directions: Solve the following ratio problems. Choose any of the ways to express your answer. If necessary, reduce fractions to their lowest terms.

1. At the veterinary school there are 10 instructors for 400 students. What is the ratio of instructors to students?
2. Out of 25 typed pages, the medical typist had to redo 5 of them because of errors. What is the ratio of redone pages to correct pages?
3. The laboratory assistant discovered that 6 of the 54 microscopes needed repairs. What is the ratio of working microscopes to broken ones?
4. Of the 228 graduates of the medical assistant program, 19 found jobs immediately after graduation. What is the ratio of working graduates to nonworking graduates?
5. Prudence cleaned 15 of the rat cages out of a total of 50. What is the ratio of clean cages to dirty ones?

PROPORTIONS

A proportion is a statement that two ratios are equal. A proportion can be written in three ways:

1. 1 to 2 = 5 to 10
2. $\frac{1}{2} = \frac{5}{10}$
3. 1 : 2 = 5 : 10

All three of these proportions are read as "1 is to 2 as 5 is to 10." Below is what a **typical** proportion problem would look like. Determine the missing number in the following proportion:

$$\frac{?}{10} = \frac{3}{30}$$

To find the missing number, figure out what number you would multiply 10 by to get 30. The answer is 3. Earlier in this chapter you were told that whatever number you use to multiply in the denominator you must use for that numerator. So what number multiplied by 3 would equal 3? The answer is 1. The proportion equation now looks like this:

$$\frac{?}{10} = \frac{3}{30} \qquad \frac{1}{10} = \frac{3}{30}$$

Exercise 9–6

Directions: Write each of the following statements as a proportion.

1. 4 is to 12 as 1 is to 3.
2. 16 is to 40 as 2 is to 5.
3. 35 is to 30 as 7 is to 6.
4. 108 is to 24 as 9 is to 2.
5. 77 is to 99 as 7 is to 9.

Exercise 9–7

Directions: Solve the following problems by finding the value of the unknown number (?). Remember that the number that was used to determine the denominator should also be used to determine the numerator.

1. $\frac{4}{8} = \frac{?}{16}$
2. $\frac{5}{1} = \frac{35}{?}$
3. $\frac{45}{?} = \frac{5}{9}$
4. $\frac{?}{7} = \frac{18}{42}$
5. $\frac{7}{12} = \frac{?}{108}$
6. $\frac{40}{?} = \frac{4}{12}$
7. $\frac{18}{35} = \frac{108}{?}$
8. $\frac{51}{25} = \frac{?}{1000}$
9. $\frac{?}{76} = \frac{66}{228}$
10. $\frac{62}{909} = \frac{?}{1818}$

REVIEWING THE LEARNING STRATEGIES

To Learn	Use This Strategy
Multiplication and division	Memorize the multiplication chart
Fractions	Learn to recognize the numerator, denominator, proper and improper fractions, mixed numbers, lowest terms, and the common denominator
Decimals	Learn about place holding, reading decimal numbers, changing fractions to decimal numbers, and changing decimal numbers to fractions
Percentages	Learn about reading percentages and changing percentages to decimals or fractions

To Learn	Use This Strategy
Ratios	Learn the definition of *ratio* and to read and write ratios
Proportions	Learn the definition of *proportion* and how to read and write proportions

THE METRIC SYSTEM

The metric system is a system of measurements. Another system of measurements is called the English system. The United States is one of the very few countries that uses the English system of measuring. Most of the world, including the health fields, use the metric system of measuring. Therefore, it is very important to be familiar with the metric system. Table 9-3 shows how measurements in the English system and the metric system are equivalent. Since some of the equivalent numbers can be long and complicated decimal numbers, they have been rounded off.

To change from the metric system to the English system, multiply the amount of the metric measure by its equivalent in the English system. For example, to change 5 kilometers to miles, multiply 5 kilometers by 0.62 miles.

$$5 \times 0.62 = 3.1 \text{ miles}$$

To change from the English system to the metric system, multiply the amount of the English measure by its equivalent in the metric system. For example, to change 2 inches to centimeters, multiply 2 inches by 2.54 centimeters.

$$2 \times 2.54 = 5.08 \text{ centimeters}$$

Exercise 9–8

Directions: Study Table 9-3. Then answer the following questions.

Change the following liters to quarts:

1. 3 liters
2. 18 liters

Change the following square centimeters to square inches:

3. 9 square centimeters
4. 10 square centimeters

Change the following kilometers to miles:

5. 4 kilometers
6. 30 kilometers

Change the following yards to meters:

7. 7 yards
8. 45 yards

Change the following pounds to kilograms:

9. 18 pounds
10. 50 pounds

TABLE 9-3 Metric System and English System Conversion Chart

Metric Lengths	English Length
1 meter =	39.37 inches
1 meter =	3.28 feet
1 meter =	1.09 yards
1 centimeter =	0.4 inch
1 millimeter =	0.04 inch
1 kilometer =	0.62 mile
English Lengths	**Metric Lengths**
1 inch =	25.4 millimeters
1 inch =	2.54 centimeters
1 inch =	0.0254 meter
1 foot =	0.3 meter
1 yard =	0.91 meter
1 mile =	1.61 kilometers
Metric Liquid Measures	**English Liquid Measures**
1 liter =	1.06 quarts
English Liquid Measures	**Metric Liquid Measures**
1 quart =	0.95 liter
Metric Measure of Weight	**English Measure of Weight**
1 gram =	0.04 ounce
1 kilogram =	2.2 pounds
1 metric ton =	2204.62 pounds
English Measure of Weight	**Metric Measure of Weight**
1 ounce =	28.35 grams
1 pound =	0.45 kilogram
1 short ton (2000 pounds) =	0.91 metric ton
Metric Measure of Area	**English Measure of Area**
1 square centimeter =	0.155 square inch
1 square meter =	10.76 square feet
1 square meter=	1.2 square yards
1 square kilometer =	0.39 square mile
English Measure of Area	**Metric Measure of Area**
1 square inch =	6.45 square centimeters
1 square foot =	0.09 square meter
1 square yard =	0.84 square meter
1 square mile =	2.59 square kilometers

CHAPTER

10

Beginning the Job Search

THE SEARCH IS ON

"Employment is nature's physician, and is essential to human happiness."

—Galen

Congratulations! All the studying, assignments, labs, and clinical experience are about to pay off. You are now ready to focus on the job search and reaching your goal of working in the health care field. Completing your education and graduating represent important personal achievements. Your attitude played a large part in your success. In the same way, attitude will play an important role in helping you get the right job.

The Big A: Attitude

"Remember that your own resolution to succeed is more important than any one thing."

—Abraham Lincoln

Attitude is the single most important factor in determining whether a student finds a job. In Chapter 3, we discussed how we have control over our attitudes and noted that any situation can be approached either positively or negatively. For example, some people are nervous and fearful about looking for a job. They worry about lacking the qualifications needed by employers and see each interview as a chance to be rejected. A more positive approach is to look at the process from the employers' point of view. Think about it: health care facilities cannot function without good employees. Employers must fill positions with well-trained individuals who can help them serve their patients. *You* are a recently trained person ready to fill one of these positions.

You are now ready to begin marketing yourself to prospective employers. Knowing what skills and competencies you have is the first step in presenting yourself successfully as the person who fits an employer's needs. Students sometimes don't realize just how much they have learned. They tend to underestimate their abilities and the amount of practice they have had in applying their skills. Being aware of your accomplishments will build your self-confidence and help you present yourself positively at interviews. Take some time now to review what you have learned, your self-ratings in Prescription for Success 1-4, and to give yourself credit for what you have to offer.

Focus Your Search

"To find out what one is fitted to do, and to secure an opportunity to do it, is the key to happiness."
more important than any one thing."

—John Dewey

Knowing where to market yourself is the next step in carrying out a successful job search. This means identifying the type of job and facility in which you would prefer to work. In Prescription for Success 1-4 you began to identify your job preferences. As you worked through your educational program, you may have changed your work preferences.

As we discussed in Chapter 1, it is sometimes necessary to set short-term goals to achieve long-term career success. When seeking an entry-level position, you'll do better if you are open to a variety of possibilities. School career services personnel report seeing students lose good opportunities by setting limits that are too restrictive. For example, some students don't want to have long commutes. But passing up a good position at an excellent facility by refusing to consider jobs just outside your immediate area may not be a good career move. Driving an extra 10 minutes may, in the long run, be worth the inconvenience.

MAKING A COMMITMENT TO THE JOB SEARCH

"You can't try to do things; you simply must do them."

—Ray Bradbury

Obtaining a job has been compared to actually working at a job. It can take a lot of time and effort. You'll be most successful if you dedicate a portion of each day to your search and be on call to follow up quickly on leads.

Employment professionals recommend that job seekers spend between 20 and 40 hours per week on job-search efforts. In this and the following chapters, you will learn about the many activities necessary to conduct a successful search, such as the following:

- Preparing skill inventories and examples
- Networking
- Finding leads
- Conducting searches on the Internet
- Writing and revising your resume
- Assembling your portfolio
- Writing letters
- Contacting references
- Creating a reference sheet
- Preparing for and attending interviews
- Writing thank-you notes

Failure to spend adequate time on these activities is one of the major reasons why people fail to get hired. You can apply many of the time-management tools and techniques suggested in Chapter 3 to your job search.

Time Management Tips for Your Job Search

- **Prioritize.** The job search should be your main focus, apart from your family. Dedicate sufficient time and attention to achieving this goal. Looking for a job *is* your job. Determine which search activities are most productive, and spend the majority of your time on them.
- **Keep a calendar.** Missing—or even being late for—an interview is a sure way to lose a job even before you are hired. Take care to note all appointments and follow-up activities accurately, and check your calendar daily. If you haven't developed a calendar system yet, now is the time to start.
- **Plan a weekly schedule.** Decide what needs to be done each week, and create a to-do list to serve as a guide to keep you on track. It's easy to reach the end of the week and discover you've accomplished only half of what needed to be done.
- **Plan ahead.** This is very important. Suppose that one morning you are notified that a hospital where you want to work is scheduling interviews for later the same day. You don't want to miss out because you haven't completed your resume or don't have a clean shirt to wear. Being prepared leads to being hired. Make sure your car is in good running order or that you have other reliable transportation.
- **Plan for the unplanned.** The unexpected tends to strike at the worst possible moment. Keep an extra printer cartridge on hand. Have extra copies of your resume printed. Leave early for interviews in case you get lost. (Better yet, take a dry run a day or two in advance to learn the route. Check out alternate routes in case of traffic.)

BOX 10-1 Job Central Checklist

- Telephone
- Telephone directories, including Yellow Pages
- Computer, printer, and supplies
- Dictionary
- Good-quality paper for resume and cover letters
- Matching envelopes
- Extra copies of resume
- Note paper or thank-you cards
- Calendar, planner, or electronic planner
- Job-search notebook

SETTING UP JOB SEARCH CENTRAL

Create a personalized employment headquarters by designating a space for job-search activities. Save time and prevent the loss of important information by gathering your resources and supplies in one location. Check the list in Box 10-1 to see if you have what you need.

Your Job-Search Records

Each person's job search is unique. Creating personalized job-search records will help you focus your efforts and keep track of phone numbers, website addresses, and the name of the office manager at the clinic where you last interviewed. A three-ring binder gives you the flexibility to add pages and keep everything organized. If you prefer, create computerized folders and files. Choose content that will best support your efforts. The purpose of this resource is to save you time and effort. Here are suggestions for information you might find useful to include:

- List of professional contacts
- List of professional organizations (also from your Personal Reference Guide; see Appendix A for a list of health care organizations)
- Copies of Prescription for Success 10-1 and 10-2
- Resume Building Block forms from Chapter 11

Job Lead Log. A job lead log consists of pages, either paper or computerized, on which you record all job leads and contacts.

If you have more than one version of your resume (for example, different objectives to match specific jobs), indicate on your lead log which version you sent, place a copy of the resume on the next page in your binder, or refer to the computer file name. This way you'll know how to respond if you get a call for an interview. It will also ensure that you take the correct resume to the interview. (Chapter 12 contains more information about interviews and what to take with you.)

Students who prefer to use a computer for tracking can set up an Excel spreadsheet or other form, such as a table in Word, to record their job-search activities. Regardless of the method you choose, design something that is easy for you to use and be sure to keep it up-to-date.

Dialing for Jobs

The telephone provides a vital link with potential employers and job lead sources. The telephone can be one of the job seeker's best friends. It can also be a barrier if not used properly. Employers form an impression of you based on your telephone manners, so be sure they hear you at your best. The following suggestions for making calls will apply to your telephone habits on the job as well as during the search to get a job:

1. Be prepared with pen and paper for taking notes.
2. Prepare what you plan to say ahead of time, and be as brief as possible without rushing and speaking too quickly.
3. Be courteous, never pushy. If the receptionist cannot connect you to the person you wish to speak with, leave a clear message and ask for a good time to call back.
4. Speak clearly and distinctly. Don't mumble or use slang or nonstandard speech that the listener may not understand.
5. When making appointments or gathering important information, listen carefully and repeat (use feedback) to make sure that you have the correct date and time, address, suite or office number, and so on.
6. Always thank the other party and end the call graciously.

It is *critical* that your school, potential employers, and other contacts be able to reach you in a timely way. Be sure the telephone number you distribute is accurate and includes your area code. If you have an answering machine, call your number to make sure it is working properly. The outgoing message should be simple and professional. Avoid the use of music, jokes, and clever remarks, such as "You know what this is and you know what to do." (This also applies to your e-mail address. If it's too cute or strange, it may send the wrong message to any potential employer who sees it.) Instruct everyone who might answer the telephone about proper telephone manners and how to write down a message. Every contact represents you, and employers don't have time to deal with rude adults or untrained children. If you are away from the telephone during office hours and don't have a cell phone or an answering machine, give out an alternate number where someone reliable can take messages for you. You might consider getting an inexpensive cell phone with prepaid minutes. Don't lose out on jobs because you can't be contacted.

Communicating by Fax

Some employers want you to fax your resume. If you don't own a fax machine or a computer that has fax capability, find a print, postal, or business supply store that provides this service. Some schools will fax student resumes to potential employers. When sending documents by fax, the print on the original should be clear and dark for maximum-quality transmission. Be sure there is at least a 1-inch margin on all sides so nothing gets cut off.

When faxed resumes are requested, it is best to follow the employer's instructions. Mailed resumes may arrive too late to be considered. Demonstrate that you are resourceful and can follow instructions. If you don't hear from the employer in a couple of days, call to make sure your resume was received.

SETTING UP A SUPPORT SYSTEM

Your job search will be easier and more pleasant if you have people available who care about your success and are willing to help you. They can provide technical support or offer friendly encouragement. Could you use some help with any of the following tasks?

- Proofreading your resume and other written materials (more than one person should proofread).
- Role-playing with you to practice interviewing.
- Discussing postinterview evaluations. (Postinterview evaluations are covered in Chapter 12.)
- Acting as a cheerleader.
- Helping you to keep things in perspective and not get discouraged.

You may want to work with just one other person who is qualified to help you in many areas. Or you might enlist the help of several "specialists." Be sure the people you choose are qualified to spot spelling and grammatical errors and are comfortable giving you constructive feedback. They should know when you need a push and when you need a hug. Consider drawing from friends, family members, classmates, school personnel, and health care professionals. If you have a mentor, this person might be an excellent choice.

Most people will be happy to support your efforts to secure employment. Take care to keep your support system intact. Be considerate of everyone's time, be prepared when you have meetings with them, and show appreciation for their help.

The career services department at your school provides specific help and support to students as they conduct their job search. Find out what services are provided. In addition, some schools and communities have job clubs or support groups for people seeking employment. Consider using these resources to supplement your support system. They can offer additional viewpoints, encouragement, and helpful suggestions.

UNDERSTANDING THE JOB MARKET

Employment conditions vary from one geographic location to the next. And economic conditions change over time. Think about the following factors when planning your job-search strategies:

- Local employment customs
- Current economic conditions
- Current employment rate
- Trends in health care delivery
- Medical advances
- Changing government regulations

Local customs vary regarding what is considered acceptable dress for the workplace. In some parts of the country, health care providers dress casually, with men sporting long hair and even wearing an earring. In other areas, anyone who showed up for work looking like this would be sent home to change—or worse, sent home for good!

Local and national economic conditions affect the job seeker. When the economy is strong and unemployment is low, job seekers have the advantage. When the economy slows down, competition heats up and it becomes more difficult to find a position. At the same time, some health care occupations are experiencing of shortages of applicants, and this will make finding a job easier for qualified candidates.

Health care occupations are also affected by state and federal laws. The demand for certain occupations is influenced by the reimbursement (payment for services) policies of both government and private insurance carriers. Knowing what's happening in your local area as well as being aware of national trends is important when planning both your initial job search and your long-term career strategy. Your local newspaper is a good source of information. Look in the business section for articles about the economy and local employment trends. Health care trends and major facilities are often featured. For example, a state law that increased the required nurse-to-patient ratios in California hospitals was reported in the newspaper. The predicted result was (and will be for the next few years, at least) a shortage of registered nurses to meet employer needs. This information is valuable for the recent nurse graduate or a student who is considering nursing as a career. Articles about major health care employers can give you an edge when choosing where you want to work. Knowing about the facility to which you are applying enables you to present yourself at interviews as a candidate who has taken the time to learn about the employer.

Many newspapers publish a special weekly or monthly section dedicated to employment. These are good sources of information. They contain articles about resume writing, lists of local agencies that assist job seekers, and announcements of job fairs. News magazines such as *Newsweek, Time, U.S. News and World Report*, and *Business Week* contain many articles about health care topics. The Internet provides access to a wide variety of topics from literally millions of sources. For example, the Bureau of Labor Statistics maintains a website with reports on employment trends and the national labor market. Apply the research techniques discussed in Chapter 6 in conducting your job search.

LOCATING JOB LEADS

There are many ways to find job leads, ranging from talking with people you know to searching the Internet. You can increase your chances of finding the job you really want by using a variety of lead sources. Don't limit yourself to the one or two methods you find easiest or most comfortable to use. People who work in sales know that it usually takes many calls to make a sale. In the same way, the more sources you use in your job search, the greater your chances of finding the right job for you. Employment experts recommend that no more than 25% of your time be spent on any one job-search method.

When the economy is slow and there are few job openings, networking and developing personal contacts can be the most effective methods for finding a job. It's possible you won't find the "perfect job" under these economic conditions. Looking for an opportunity to gain experience may be the best strategy. When the economy is booming or there is a shortage of qualified workers in your field, you are likely to have a larger selection of opportunities. Under these conditions, you may find that responding to job postings and directly contacting potential employers are very effective methods. It is a sure thing that you will experience all types of job markets during your career. The economy and employment levels run in cycles, and you must be prepared to deal with changing conditions.

Career Services at Your School

The staff at your school wants you to succeed. The goal of health care educators is to train future workers, and a sign of *their* professional success is when a graduate becomes satisfactorily employed. Schools have special personnel who are trained to help students find jobs. These people work to develop relationships with local employers. Your school may be contacted about job openings before they are even advertised. It is time-consuming for employers to review resumes, set up appointments, and interview large numbers of applicants. The success of a health care facility depends on the quality of its employees, so it is important that they find and hire the right people. Considerable time, expense, and doubt can be avoided if employers know they can count on local schools to provide qualified candidates. So how can you be among those who are recommended by your school?

- Get to know the career services staff. Introduce yourself early in your program. Don't wait until you are beginning the job search. Seek their advice about how you can best prepare ahead for successful employment.
- Treat school staff with the same courtesy and respect you would an employer. They cannot risk the school's reputation with employers by recommending students who are rude or uncooperative.
- Maintain an excellent attendance record. Schools report that this is the question asked by nearly every employer about students. It ranks far above inquiries about grades. (Even great skills are no help to anyone if you aren't there to use them!)
- Participate fully in any career development classes or workshops that are offered. Attend every session and complete all assignments. Conduct yourself in practice interviews as if they were the real thing.
- Follow up on any leads you are given, even if you don't think the job is for you. Attend all interviews scheduled for you. Failure to show up embarrasses the school and may result in the employer refusing to consider candidates from your school in the future. Take advantage of all opportunities to meet potential employers. You will get valuable confidence-building interview practice. Even if the job isn't the one for you, the employer may know about one that is.
- Keep the school informed about how to contact you. If you move and career services can't find you, they can't help you.
- Let the school know when you are hired. Many agencies that regulate and accredit schools require annual reports to monitor graduation and job placement rates. These act as school report cards and are important for schools to stay in good standing. If the staff has taken the time to help you, return the favor by giving them the information they need to complete their reports.

Government-Sponsored Resource Centers

The government has established a program of "one-stop" resources for job seekers. These may be called One-Stop Resource Centers, County Career Centers, or possibly another name in your area. The U.S. Department of Labor sponsors them, and their purpose is to provide a wide variety of information and services for the public. Staff members are well informed about employment conditions, as well as specific employers, in their local areas. Ask your school about these resources or go to www.careeronestop.org for the location of your nearest center.

Direct Employer Contacts

Calling or visiting employers to inquire about job openings can be a successful strategy. These actions demonstrate motivation and self-confidence, the very qualities that can help win you a job. They are also a way to discover the estimated four fifths of jobs that are never advertised—the "hidden job market." There are two ways to make contact: in writing and by telephone. If you are sending a cover letter and resume, it is necessary to find the name of the person who makes the hiring decisions for his or her department. If you are calling a small medical office, this may simply mean getting the name—with correct spelling!—of the physician. In the case of a large facility, you may have to do more inquiring by phone to find the right person. When calling, use your best telephone manners.

Craft a letter that explains why you would be a good employee for this particular employer. The letter should demonstrate enthusiasm, interest, and a desire to help the employer. Of course, this means that you know something about the employer: specialty or services offered, typical patients, etc. Include your resume with the letter, which is directed to a specific person. Follow up in a few days with a phone call.

Calling employers by phone to inquire about job openings can be helpful if you are relocating. Phone calls provide an efficient way to contact a large number of employers. Explain that you will be moving and are unfamiliar with the area. If the facility contacted has no openings, ask whether they can refer you to anyone else in the area.

Dropping in on employers gets the word out that you are looking for a job. Visiting all the offices in a large medical facility can be a productive way to spend a day. It gives you a chance to introduce yourself to at least one staff member and personally distribute your resume. If the person who greets you has time, ask for information about the facility. If this is not possible, ask who does the hiring, leave your resume, and express your appreciation. Although you should be dressed as if you were attending an interview, *do not ask* for one at this time if you don't have an appointment.

Large medical facilities, such as hospitals, often coordinate hiring through their human resources office. All resumes and applications must be submitted to this office. It can be worthwhile to also contact or visit the department where you wish to work. Ask for the supervisor and, if he or she is available, let him or her know that you have applied for work through human resources and are very interested in working in that department. Explain why you want to work there and ask that your application be given consideration. If the supervisor is not available, ask to make an appointment. Don't be discouraged, however, if you are unable to make direct contact. Health care professionals today are extremely busy and simply may not have the time. If they don't, send a letter or e-mail that expresses your interest.

Networking

Many people learn about job openings and become employed through personal contacts. It is recommended that you start early to meet people in the health care field. Professional organizations were suggested as an excellent source of contacts. In addition to providing you with useful information about your occupational area, they can be a source of job leads and referrals. If you have already met people through professional networking, let them know that you are launching your job search. Don't be shy about asking for their advice about where you might apply, as well as about the job search in general. People who are successful in their careers are generally happy to help newcomers. Do show consideration for their time, and send a thank-you note when they put forth effort on your behalf. It is critical that you follow up on any leads given to you by professional contacts. Failure to do so is not only rude, it may result in the withdrawal of their support.

In addition to professional contacts, general networking can be an effective way to get the word out about your search efforts. I once learned about a job opening for a school director—a position I got and enjoyed for a number of years—from a friend who had seen the ad in the newspaper. Let the people in your life know you are seeking employment. By telling 10 people who each know 10 other people, you create a network of 110 people who know you are looking for a job. Of these 110, it is likely that a few work in health care. And most people use health care services. There is a chance that someone will know someone or something that can help you. Keep in touch with your classmates. Once they have jobs, they may be willing to pass on your name to their employers. When speaking with others about your career goals, present yourself positively and express enthusiasm about your field. People want to feel confident about passing your name along.

Your Clinical Site

Students who perform well during their clinical experience are sometimes offered jobs at the site. Some employers even create new positions for graduates who impress them with their attitude and skills. Although it is *not* appropriate to ask your clinical site for employment before completing your training there, you should work as if this were your goal. Even if the site is unable to offer you a position, your clinical supervisor can serve as a valuable reference and may recommend you to another employer.

Career and Job Fairs

Some schools, community agencies, and large health care facilities organize activities to connect job recruiters and job seekers. In a single day, you can meet dozens of potential employers. You can gather information, ask questions, and submit your resume. Check your local newspaper for events in your area. Inquire if large health care organizations in your area have career fairs or open houses. You can also find upcoming career fairs across the nation on websites such as nationalcareerfair.com.

Here are some suggestions for taking full advantage of job fairs:

- Dress as you would for an interview. If the event takes place at school and you will go directly from class in uniform, be sure it is clean and pressed.
- Prepare a list of questions in advance. It's easier to think of them beforehand than to remember them all in a noisy room. Good questions to ask include the following:
  1. What types of jobs does your facility offer?
  2. How can I get more information?
  3. What are the most important qualifications you look for when hiring employees?
  4. Can you give me a written job description?
  5. What is the application procedure?
  6. Who do I contact to set up an interview?
- Take copies of your resume. Carry them in a large envelope or folder to keep them clean and neat.
- Smile, make eye contact, and introduce yourself to recruiters. Your goal is to get information about the types of jobs they have and what they are looking for in applicants. Thank them for any information they give you. Leave graciously by telling them it was nice meeting them, you appreciate their help, and you look forward to speaking with them again.
- Take something in which you can collect brochures, job announcements, and business cards. A small notebook is helpful for taking notes.
- As soon as possible after the fair, organize what you collected and use your job lead log pages to record information about the people you met and what you learned. Prepare a list of follow-up activities, such as people to call and resumes to send.

Employer Meetings, Websites, and Telephone Job Lines

Some large facilities that do a lot of hiring have public meetings at which they explain their employment needs and application process. Contact personnel departments, watch the local newspaper, and visit employer Internet sites to find announcements. You may not have a chance to meet personally with the hiring staff, but it is still important that you make a professional impression by dressing and acting appropriately. Be prepared to take notes and ask questions.

Many employers, especially large organizations, have jobs listed on their websites. They also accept applications electronically. Read more about this in Chapter 11.

Some employers are still using job lines, taped announcements of current openings. These are accessed by telephone and provide information about how to apply for the jobs described. Some help wanted ads and job postings include telephone numbers. Try calling the personnel department at the facility in which you are interested to inquire whether they have this service.

EMPLOYMENT ADS

The help wanted section of the newspaper is one of the oldest and most traditional methods of locating openings. Although the Internet has become popular as a source of job leads, some newspapers still include employment ads that can be a good source of job leads. Writing a cover letter and mailing or faxing a resume is worth the time and expense it takes. Every action you take increases your chance of finding the right job.

In addition to the newspaper, many professional journals contain employment ads. These can be especially useful if you are willing to move to another area.

USING THE INTERNET

The Internet is the newest job-search tool. It greatly expands your job-search possibilities by being available 24 hours a day. It offers a wide range of how-to information, facts about specific occupations and employers, and job postings. So much information is available, in fact, that it's easy to get lost in cyberspace. You may suddenly realize that you've spent 3 hours moving from one interesting site to another without actually adding much to your job-search efforts!

Getting Started

An excellent place to start learning about using the Internet for the job search is the *Riley Guide* (www.rileyguide.com). Developed by a librarian and available both in print and online, it has provided free, updated career and employment information since 1994. The website serves as a gateway to hundreds of other websites on all phases of the job search. Other good sources that have been in business for some time are Quintessential Careers (www.quintcareers.com) and CareerBuilder (www.careerbuilder.com).

General Research

Studies have shown that only a small percentage of applicants are actually hired as the result of posting a resume on one of the large employment websites; there is simply too much competition. There are literally millions of resumes online at any one time. However, the Internet is a valuable job-search tool. It provides a vast and easily accessed source of information. You can read about health care trends, the general economy, and advances in medicine. You can scan job postings to see what characteristics employers mention most, get information about major facilities, and see samples of good resumes. To access general information, use the search engines discussed in Chapter 6 with key phrases such as "health care trends," "future of health care," "health care providers," and "health care employment." Government agencies such as the Department of Labor (www.dol.gov) and the Bureau of Labor Statistics (www.bls.gov) have information about the national job market, laws that affect employees, and resources for job seekers.

Other effective ways to take advantage of "the net" are discussed in the following sections.

Health Care Facility Websites

Many large health care facilities have websites that include photos, maps, information about the services they offer patients, and statements of their goals and overall mission. If you don't know the address, use a search engine such as Google (www.google.com) and enter the name of the company or facility. Many organizations now list their current job openings along with online applications. In fact, some facilities accept *only* electronic applications. (Chapter 11 contains information about submitting electronic resumes and completing online applications.)

Job-Posting Websites

Job openings are listed on hundreds, perhaps thousands, of websites. Although some websites are easier to use than others, most organize jobs by occupational fields, such as health care, and geographic location. Following are six general employment websites that have been operating for several years and are rated well by users:

1. www.indeed.com
2. www.careerbuilder.com
3. www.hotjobs.yahoo.com
4. www.jobbankinfo.org
5. www.jobcentral.com
6. www.monster.com

You can view the job listings on these sites without registering. If you wish to post your resume, however, you must register by supplying information such as your name, address, and telephone number. You then select a username and password to access your account each time you visit the website. A feature available to those who register on these sites is the assistance of a "search scout," an automated search that matches jobs to your resume and e-mails the results to you.

The general websites listed previously include health care categories and job postings. At the same time, there are employment websites specific to health care, such as the following:

1. www.healthjobsusa.com
2. www.healthcaresource.com
3. www.medzilla.com

In addition to these general health care sites, there are dozens of specialty websites that feature jobs in one career area, such as dental assisting. Links are available at www.quintcareers.com/healthcare_jobs.html.

Most professional organizations maintain websites, and some offer placement assistance for members. For example, the American Health Information Management Association (AHIMA) maintains job postings online for members. See Appendix A for a list of professional organizations and their contact information.

Keep in mind that new websites are continually being developed and old ones are merging, being deleted, or being moved to a different "address." Some of the addresses given in this book and in others may have changed by the time you try them. And it is certain that new websites will have been created.

Networking

The Internet provides opportunities for sharing information and ideas with others through mailing lists and newsgroups. **Mailing lists** (also known as *Listservs* and *e-mail discussion groups*) operate through e-mail. Each list is devoted to a specific topic: occupations, hobbies, health conditions, and so on. Once you have subscribed, you receive e-mail messages to which you can respond. Your e-mail is then sent to all other subscribers. Mailing lists offer a way to learn what other job seekers are doing and what's happening in your field around the country. Comprehensive directories of the thousands of mailing lists are available from CataList (www.lsoft.com/lists/listref.html) and Topica, Inc. (http://lists.topica.com). Another source of mailing list groups is available from Yahoo! at http://groups.yahoo.com.

Newsgroups offer another way to network online. A newsgroup is basically an online discussion group for a specific topic. Anyone can join and participate by reading and posting messages. Messages that address the same topic are called a "thread," and each time a different topic is introduced, a new thread is started. Most Web browsers have a search capacity called a "newsreader" that organizes the many newsgroups and enables you to post a message.

If you decide to use either mailing lists or newsgroups, it is important to learn the proper "netiquette" for participating. Experts suggest that you read a group's messages for at least 2 weeks before submitting anything. That way, you'll know the type and quality of material that is expected. It is also recommended that you check the "Frequently Asked Questions" (FAQ) section, if available, to avoid asking something that has already been covered. This is because all subscribers, not just you, receive the answer to your question and may find it annoying to receive information they already know and that is available elsewhere. When you do send messages, keep them short and to the point.

Web forums are another form of online discussion group offered through a variety of websites. You only need an e-mail address and Web browser to participate. You can ask questions, such as "How's the job climate in San Antonio?" and someone from that area is likely to answer. Lists of discussion groups are available on the Internet. Using a browser, enter the keyword "forum" and a topic of interest to get a list of ongoing forums.

One important rule is to never send advertising or use these groups to ask for a job. You may, however, find someone in the group whom you can contact personally via e-mail for possible assistance, just as you would other professional contacts. Good people to write to are those who have posted messages demonstrating that they have knowledge of or work in the occupational area you wish to enter. In your e-mail to that person, identify yourself and the interests you have that seem related to what this person has said in his or her electronic messages to the group. Do *not* ask the person for a job. The purpose of this contact is to ask for—or better yet, share—information about something you have in common. Once a relationship is developed online, and this person seems to have useful knowledge and is willing to share it, it is appropriate to ask for information and career advice.

Success Tips for Using the Internet

- **Learn more.** If you are not already proficient at using the Internet, take a class, find online help (see To Learn More at the end of this chapter), or get a copy of one of the many books on how to use it. If your school does not offer instruction, look for adult education classes in your community. Many are offered free of charge.
- **Be patient.** The Internet is a developing technology and still has a few bugs. You may get bumped offline just as you find what you are looking for.

  A promising-sounding website may have disappeared. But the wealth of information available is worth the time it takes to search.
- **Monitor where you are.** It's easy to get lost in a maze of links that takes you far from the original site. When you access a major site, write down its name and address so you can find it again.
- **Mark favorite sites.** Most Internet-access software allows you to create personalized lists of useful sites so you can find them later. Also, for any online

groups you join, save information in your job-search notebook about how to unsubscribe and the name and e-mail address of the person who manages the list.

- **Watch the time.** Using the Internet can be addictive. You can wander for hours linking and looking and actually accomplishing very little. If you find sites that look interesting but are unrelated to the task at hand, write down or mark their addresses and return to them later.
- **Beware of scams.** Take care when posting your resume or sending private information. If a website makes claims about jobs that seem too good to be true, it may simply be a means of getting personal information about you. Stick with major employment websites and the websites of employers whose existence you can verify in other ways.
- **Don't exceed 25%.** Remember, the Internet is only one tool for your job search. Use it wisely as a supplement to other methods. Some experts even recommend spending no more than 10% of your job-search time using the Internet.
- **Be careful what you post.** If you have pages on websites such as MySpace and Facebook, be *very* careful about what you post. Photos of yourself that may be amusing but that don't show you at your best may damage your chances for employment. Many employers reportedly search potential employees on the Internet, and some admit not hiring based on what they find.[1] You might consider using the Internet to your advantage. For example, if you have volunteered for a community fundraiser or serve meals at a community center, include photos of yourself participating in these activities.

Internet Tracking Form

If you use the Internet to find information, post your resume, and/or participate in groups, take a little time to record your activities. Use the Internet tracking form that follows to track the job opportunities you find online. Make copies of the form, or set up one of your own to keep in your job-search notebook or on your computer.

RESPONDING TO JOB POSTINGS AND ADS

Regardless of the source—Internet, professional journal, or newspaper—look under every category that might contain jobs for which you are prepared. For example, while "nursing assistants" are likely to appear under "nursing," they may also be listed under "medical" or "health care." If your training has prepared you for a variety of positions, be sure to check all possible job titles. For example, graduates of health information programs may be qualified for the following positions: coding specialist, health information technician, medical records coordinator or supervisor, and patient records technician. New job titles are constantly being created to describe the many activities performed in the modern health care facility. Use the skill inventories you created for yourself to help you identify all the jobs for which you might apply. Don't be discouraged if you find only a few postings or ads—or none—for your occupation. This may actually mean that there is such a shortage of applicants that employers have given up placing expensive ads.

When you respond in writing to a job opening, point out how you meet the employer's needs. You can do this in the cover letter, which will be discussed more fully in Chapter 11. For now, let's look at a couple of sample ads and see how to encourage the employer to read your resume and call you for an interview. Even very short ads contain information you can use.

There is not one best way to write an effective response to an employer. Highlight your qualifications with a format that best suits the stated requirements. It isn't necessary—or even desirable—to repeat what's in your resume. A few quick highlights about how you meet the specific requirements are sufficient, along with a fuller description of why you, in particular, can help this employer.

To Learn More

Bolles RN: *What color is your parachute? A practical manual for job-hunters and job-changers*, Berkeley, 2009, Ten Speed Press.
www.thejobhuntersbible.com
Bolles's book has become a classic job-search manual. The ideas are original, well researched, and reportedly very effective. The companion website is also packed with useful ideas, including hints on effectively using the Internet in the job search.

Career Builder
www.careerbuilder.com
Website includes job-search tools, career advice, list of career fairs around the country, and a salary calculator.

Dickel MR, Roehm, F: Guide to Internet job searching 2008-2009,
Columbus, Ohio, 2008, McGraw-Hill.

Nemko M, Edwards P, Edwards S: *Cool careers for dummies*, ed 2, Indianapolis, 2001, Wiley Publishing.
This book provides reader-friendly and effective information—even for "smarties."

Riley Guide
http://rileyguide.com
Margaret Dickel is a librarian who has been tracking the Internet as a job-search resource for many years. Her book is excellent, or you can access lots of information from her website.

Quintessential Careers

General job-search and career information: www.quintcareers.com
Health care jobs: www.quintcareers.com/healthcare_jobs.html
This website contains information on every phase of the job search and career development in the form of articles, resources, and tutorials.

U.S. Department of Labor, Bureau of Labor Statistics
www.bls.gov
The BLS website contains information about economic conditions, wages, and unemployment rates. By clicking on "jobseekers," you will find a list of links to other government websites covering industries, including health care, and specific occupations.

REFERENCE

1. Kate Lorenz, Warning: social networking can be hazardous to your job search. www.careerbuilder.com/Article/CB-533-Job-Search-Warning-Social-Networking-Can-Be-Hazardous-to-Your-Job-Search/?ArticleID=533&cbRecursionCnt=1&cbsid=920e95b94af84818bfb7a8e12af99ffd-288916701-R3-4 (Accessed 2/25/09.)

PRESCRIPTION FOR SUCCESS 10-1 INVENTORY OF TECHNICAL SKILLS

1. Refer to the Resume Building Block #3: Professional Skills and Knowledge form in Chapter 11, in which you began to list the skills you were learning in school. If necessary, gather additional sources of information to help you complete your inventory: lab checklists, course objectives, clinical performance evaluations, textbooks, and class handouts.
2. Create categories, such as the following, that are appropriate for your occupational area. List your specific skills under each heading:
   Equipment I Can Use
   Lab Procedures I Can Perform
   Tests I Can Perform
   Patient Procedures I Can Perform
   Administrative Procedures
   Computer Skills and Applications
   Medical Records
   Documentation and Charting
   Medical Insurance
   Billing
   Communication Skills
      Oral
      Written
3. Think of examples that demonstrate your mastery of each skill, such as your performance in the laboratory or classroom, completion of special projects, or work you did during your clinical experience. Are there areas in which you demonstrated particular expertise? You can use these examples to better present your qualifications to potential employers on both your resume and at job interviews.

PRESCRIPTION FOR SUCCESS 10-2 WHAT DO I WANT? AN UPDATE

Review Prescription for Success 1-8, and record any changes you have made.

1. Type of facility: large, small, urban, suburban, rural, inpatient, outpatient

____

2. Type of population served: economic status, age range, gender, ethnic groups

____

3. Work schedule: steady employment, per diem, flexible hours, fixed hours, overtime, days only, evenings and weekends

____

4. *Specialty area*

____

5. *Type of supervision*

____

6. Work pace: fast, moderate

____

7. *Amount of interaction with others* (All health care professionals are part of a team, although some work more independently than others.)

____

8. Range of duties: wide variety, concentrate on a few

____

PRESCRIPTION FOR SUCCESS 10-3 MY SUPPORT SYSTEM

Think about the people in your life who are qualified to help your job-search efforts. Who can you ask to help you with each of the following?

1. Proofreading your resume and other written materials

____

____

2. Interview practice

____

____

3. Postinterview evaluations

____

____

4. Encouragement

____

____

____

PRESCRIPTION FOR SUCCESS 10-4 | WHAT'S GOING ON?

Use your research skills to find answers to the following questions:

1. What is the unemployment rate in your area? ____________________
2. Who are the major health care employers?

   ____

   ____

   ____
3. What are the current hiring trends in health care?

   ____

   ____

   ____
4. How might these conditions affect your occupation?

   ____

   ____

   ____
5. How might they influence your job-search strategies?

   ____

   ____

   ____

PRESCRIPTION FOR SUCCESS 10-5 | CREATE A TARGETED RESPONSE

Find an employment ad, either printed or on the Internet. Identify the employer's requirements and write a response that demonstrates how you meet these requirements. (Attach copy of ad or computer printout.)

Your Response

____

____

____

____

____

____

CHAPTER 11

Writing Your Resume

PRODUCTION: THE SECOND "P" OF MARKETING

"You have to take life as it happens, but you should try to make it happen the way you want to take it."
—Old German Proverb

In Chapter 1, you read about the first step in the marketing process, planning. The second of the "5 Ps of Marketing" is production: using the information gathered from market research to design and put together a product that meets the needs of the customer. Your market research was finding out what patients and employers want and need from health care professionals.

Human beings have the unique ability to create their own lives. They can generate ideas, form mental images, and plan ways to achieve what they imagine. You have already generated the idea of becoming a health care professional and have completed the first step toward achieving that goal by enrolling in school. Whether you graduate and find satisfactory employment will depend, to a great extent, on your belief in your ability to succeed and your willingness to take the necessary actions to achieve your goals.

Henry Ford, who not only created fame and riches for himself but changed the history of transportation, is quoted as saying, "Whether you think that you can, or you can't, you are right." The tendency for people to get what they expect is known as the self-fulfilling prophecy. Our beliefs about ourselves—about what we can achieve—are more important than any other factor. Many prominent Americans, such as Abraham Lincoln and Thomas Edison, experienced many failures before finally achieving great success. Lincoln had business failures and lost elections before becoming one of our most famous presidents. And Edison conducted thousands of experiments before perfecting the electric light bulb, an invention that dramatically changed the world.

You can apply the principle of expecting success as you begin your career journey. All achievements begin as ideas, and what you picture mentally can become your reality. Positive images of you succeeding as a student act as powerful motivators. In addition to visual suggestions, your self-talk influences your success—or lack of it. We are continually holding conversations with ourselves that either give us encouragement ("I know I can pass this test.") or put us down ("I'll never be able to get this report finished."). By taking control of the pictures and words in your mind, you can apply their power to help you create the life you want.

A related and very powerful concept you can apply to your life is to act as if you already are what you hope to become. You can increase your chances of becoming a successful health care professional if you start approaching life as if you already were that person. Practice behaviors now that you know will be expected on the job. For example, because accuracy and efficiency are important characteristics for the health care professional, complete all class assignments as if the well-being of others depended on your accuracy. Working effectively with others as part of a team will be required in your work, so start using every opportunity to develop your teamwork skills. Cooperate with your classmates and instructors. Be proactive and look for opportunities to increase your personal and professional growth. Turn mistakes into lessons and learn from them. Approach personal difficulties as opportunities to learn and to grow. By the time you graduate, you will have become the health care professional you aspire to be.

PACKAGING: THE THIRD "P" OF MARKETING

Even an excellent product may not sell if it is poorly packaged. Companies know this and invest a lot of time and money to make their products visually appealing to customers. Appearance can make the difference between a product selling or collecting dust on the shelf. Most of us package ourselves to impress others or to fit into a specific social group. Americans spend billions of dollars annually on clothing, cosmetics, accessories, and hair care in an effort to create what we believe to be a pleasing appearance.

Appearance is especially important in the health care field because many patients form their opinions about the competence of health care professionals based on their appearance. Your effectiveness in meeting patient needs can be influenced by your appearance because patient satisfaction increases when health care professionals "look like they know what they are doing."

What is expected of the health care professional? How do you look competent? There are several ways. The first is to be fairly conservative in dress and grooming. It is best to avoid fashion trends such as brightly colored hair, tattoos, and body piercing. At the same time, it is true that employers are becoming more accepting of these trends. The problem is that some patients may interpret them as signs of rebellion, immaturity, and lack of common sense. Others are offended or even frightened by this type of appearance.

Even clothing that is not extreme may be inappropriate for work. Dressing for work is different from dressing casually for recreation or for social functions. What is perfect for a party may be totally out of place for a job interview or for the job itself.

A second consideration is to strive for an appearance that radiates good health. An important responsibility of the health care professional is to promote good health, and this is partly achieved by example. If you smoke or are overweight, putting you at risk for serious health problems, this would be a good time to adopt new healthy living habits. Other conditions such as teeth that need dental work, badly bitten fingernails, and dandruff indicate a lack of self-care, and this is inappropriate in a profession that encourages the practice of good personal health habits. The way you present yourself reflects your approach to life and your opinion of yourself. Failure to care for yourself can project a lack of self-confidence and can undermine patient faith in your effectiveness.

Third, the issues of cleanliness and hygiene are vitally important for professionals whose work requires them to touch others. Patients literally put themselves in the hands of health care professionals and must feel assured that they will benefit from, and not be harmed by, any procedures performed. It is natural to want the professional to look clean and neat and be free of unpleasant odors. For example, although the hands of the dental assistant may be clean and gloved, dirty uniforms or shoes (or even shoelaces!) give an unfavorable impression to the patient, who may wonder whether proper attention was given to sterilizing the equipment and cleaning the work area.

Finally, professionals must consider the safety and comfort of both patients and themselves. Perfumes and scented personal products cannot be tolerated by many patients. Long fingernails, flowing hair, and large dangling earrings may be attractive and appropriate for a social event, but in a health care setting they can scratch patients, contaminate samples, get caught in equipment, or be grabbed by young patients. Safety on the job cannot be compromised to accommodate fashion trends. Some clothing customs are determined by one's culture, such as head coverings and flowing skirts. These customs may also have to be modified to ensure the safety of both you and the patient.

PERSONAL REFLECTION

1. Is there anything about my appearance I want to improve in preparation for work in the health care setting?

   ____

   ____

   ____

   a. Fashion trends

   ____

   ____

   b. Health habits

   ____

   ____

   c. Cleanliness and hygiene

   ____

   ____

   d. Safety issues

   ____

   ____

2. How am I willing to change the way I dress, at least during working hours?

   ____

   ____

   ____

3. What can I do now to create a professional appearance?

   ____

   ____

   ____

Note: If you are not sure about any aspects of your appearance or grooming, speak privately with your instructor or someone else you trust. Dealing with these issues now will give you time to take care of them before you begin your job search.

PRESENTATION: THE FOURTH "P" OF MARKETING

Your resume, a written outline of your qualifications for work, is an important tool for presenting yourself and what you have to offer to prospective employers. The main purpose of a resume is to convince an employer to give you an interview, and later in this chapter you will learn how to write and organize an effective resume. The focus of the rest of this chapter is on learning about the content of the resume and how you can use it as a guideline to create your professional self. Starting to plan your resume now will help you do the following:

1. Recognize what you already have to offer an employer
2. Build self-confidence
3. Motivate yourself to learn both the technical and nontechnical skills that contribute to employment success
4. Identify anything you might want to improve about yourself
5. Know ahead of time what kinds of experiences will enhance your employability
6. Get a head start gathering information and collecting examples to demonstrate your value and skills

Your Resume as a Guide to Success

"Begin with the end in mind."

—*Stephen Covey*

Thinking about your resume at the beginning instead of waiting until the end of your educational program turns your resume into a checklist of "To Dos" for creating a product—your professional self—that you'll be able to offer with confidence to prospective customers: health care employers. The various components of a resume are explained in this chapter, along with suggestions on how to make them work for you while you are still in school.

Building Block 1: Career Objective. The career objective is a brief description, often only one sentence long, of the position or job title you are seeking. In addition to describing the job you are seeking, you may create a brief statement of what you can offer the employer:

- Obtain a position as an administrative and clinical medical assistant where I can contribute by applying up-to-date skills
- Occupational therapy assistant in a pediatric facility

As discussed earlier, it is wise to have reasonable expectations for your first employment position. Set positive long-term goals, but be realistic when starting out. Your first job is your chance to work with real people who have real problems. The wider the range of jobs you are willing to accept when first entering the field, the better your chances of obtaining employment.

As you go through your training, learn as much as possible about the various jobs for which you might qualify. You may be unaware of jobs that closely match your interests. It is not uncommon to rewrite objectives more than once before beginning the actual job search. Use the Resume Building Block #1: Career Objective form, on page 147, to begin defining the kind of job you want.

Building Block 2: Education. The education section contains a list of all your education and training, with emphasis on health care training.

Start your list with the school you attended most recently. Include grade point average and class standing (not all schools rank their students by grades) if they are above average. Use the Resume Building Block #2: Education form, on page 148, as a motivator to do your best academically.

Building Block 3: Professional Skills and Knowledge. *Professional skills and knowledge* refers to the skills and knowledge that contribute to successful job performance.

The way you organize this section when you actually write your resume depends on your educational program and the number and variety of skills acquired. You can list them individually if there are not too many (such as "Take vital signs") or as clusters of related skills (such as "Perform clinical duties").

Listing individual skills or clusters of skills is a good idea if your previous work experience is limited and you want to emphasize the recent acquisition of health care skills as your primary qualification. It is also helpful if you have trained for one of the newer positions in health care that is not familiar to all employers. For example, "patient care technician" is a relatively new type of multi-skilled worker who can be employed in a variety of health care settings. Even if you decide not to include a skills list on your resume, starting a list now will keep you aware of what you know and have to offer an employer. Employers report that many recent graduates do not realize just how much they really know, and therefore they fail to sell themselves at job interviews.

Find out if your school provides lists of program and course objectives and/or the competencies you will master. Some instructors give their students checklists to monitor the completion of assignments and demonstration of competencies. Other sources of information include handouts from your instructor, such as syllabi and course outlines; the objectives listed in your textbooks; and lab skill sheets. Develop your own inventory of what you have learned, using the Resume Building Block #3: Professional Skills and Knowledge form, on page 149, to begin a personal inventory of your skills. An additional benefit of tracking your progress is the sense of accomplishment you gain as you see the results of your hard work. You will be amazed by how much you are learning!

Building Block 4: Work History. The work history is a list of your previous jobs, including the name and location of the employer, your job title and duties, and the dates of employment.

You can benefit from this section of your resume even if you have no previous experience in health care. There are three ways to do this. The first is to review the duties and responsibilities you had in each of your past jobs. Which ones can be applied to health care work? Skills that are common to many jobs are called transferable skills. Take another look at the general skills listed in the SCANS report. Do you see any that you have used? Here are a few examples of both general and more technical skills common to many jobs:

- Work well with people from a variety of backgrounds
- Create efficient schedules that reduce employee overtime
- Purchase supplies in appropriate quantities and at competitive prices
- Resolve customer complaints satisfactorily
- Perform word processing duties
- Manage accounts receivable
- Provide customer service
- Provide appropriate care for infants and toddlers

Identifying transferable skills is especially important when you are entering a new field in which you have little or no experience. There is actually a type of resume that emphasizes skills and abilities rather than specific job titles held. It is called a "functional resume," and the format is described later in this chapter. At this time, start compiling a list of possible transferable skills.

The second way to maximize the value of the work history section of your resume is to state what you achieved in each job. In a phrase or two, describe how you contributed to the success of your employer. When possible, state these achievements in measurable terms. If you can't express them with numbers, use active verbs that tell what you did. Here are some examples:

- Increased sales by 20%
- Designed a more efficient way to track supplies
- Worked on a committee to write an effective employee procedure manual that is still in use
- Trained five employees to use office equipment correctly

A third way to add value to this section is to include your clinical experience. Although you must clearly indicate that this was a part of your training and not paid employment, it still serves as evidence of your ability to apply what you learned in school to practical situations. For many new graduates, this is their only real-world experience in health care. Students sometimes make the mistake of viewing their clinical experience as simply an add-on to their program—just one more thing to get through. They fail to realize the impact their performance can have on their career. Remember that clinical supervisors represent future employers. (In some cases they *are* future employers because some students are hired by their clinical sites.) Their opinion of you can help successfully launch your self-marketing efforts or cause them to fizzle, so commit to doing your best during your clinical experience. The inclusion of a successful clinical experience on your resume increases your chances of getting the job you want.

Use the Resume Building Block #4: Work History form, on page 150, to start compiling your work history.

Note: Do *not* be concerned if your work experience is limited or you can't think of any achievements. You may have finished high school recently or perhaps you spent several years working as a homemaker. Employers understand that everyone starts with a first job and you are receiving training to qualify you for work. And homemakers, as well as mothers and others who care for family members, gain experiences that are valuable to employers. Examples include caring for others, practicing time management, and handling family finances.

Building Block 5: Licenses and Certifications. Some professions require you to be licensed or have specific types of approval before you are allowed to work. Nursing is one example. Others include physical and occupational therapy and dental hygiene. Some professions have voluntary certifications and registrations, such as those earned by medical assistants. The kind of approvals needed vary by state and profession. Most licenses and certifications require certain types of training and/or the passing of a standardized exam. It is important that you clearly understand any professional requirements necessary or highly recommended for your profession.

Learn as much as you can now about the requirements for the occupation you have chosen. It is not advisable to wait until the end of your studies to start thinking about preparing for required exams. Ask your instructors about review classes, books, and computerized material. Check with your professional organization. (See the contact list in Appendix A) Become familiar with the topics on the exams, and plan your studies accordingly. Knowing the format of the questions (multiple choice, true-false, etc.) is also helpful. Increase your chances for success by preparing over time, the proven way to do well on exams. (Taking exams is covered in detail in Chapter 7.) Use the Resume Building Block #5: Licenses and Certifications form, on page 150 to start gathering information about certifications for your occupation.

Building Block 6: Honors and Awards. The section on honors and awards is an optional resume section. Your school may offer recognition for student achievements and special contributions. Community and professional organizations to which you belong may also give awards. Acknowledgments received for volunteer work can also be included in this section.

Investigate what you might be eligible for and use these rewards as incentives for excellent performance. Keep this in perspective, however. Awards should serve as motivators, not indicators of your value. They are nice to have but certainly not essential for getting a good job.

Use the Resume Building Block #6: Honors and Awards form, on page 151, to find out about the availability of and requirements for awards for which you might qualify.

Building Block 7: Special Skills. Special skills are those that don't fit into other sections but do add to your value as a prospective employee. Examples include proficiency in desktop publishing and the ability to use American Sign Language.

Research the needs of employers in your geographic area. Do you already have special skills that meet these needs? Would it substantially increase your chances for employment if you were to acquire skills outside the scope of your program—for example, becoming more proficient on the computer? If (and only if!) time permits, you might decide to attend workshops in addition to your regular program courses, do extra reading, or take a course on the Internet. Use the Resume Building Block #7: Special Skills form, on page 152, to record any skills that might supplement your qualifications.

Building Block 8: Volunteer Activities. Volunteer activities can be included on your resume if they relate to your targeted occupation or demonstrate desired qualities such as being responsible and having concern for others. If you are already involved in these types of activities, think about what you are learning or practicing that can help you on the job. If you aren't, consider becoming involved if you have a sincere interest and adequate time. Adult students face many responsibilities outside of class, and the additional activities mentioned in this chapter should be taken as suggestions, not must-dos. Mastering your program content should be your first priority. If applicable, use the Resume Building Block #8: Volunteer Activities form, on page 152, to investigate opportunities and record your service.

Building Block 9: Professional and Civic Organizations. Professional organizations provide excellent opportunities to network, learn more about your field, and practice leadership skills. Participation in civic organizations, groups that work for the good of the community, promotes personal growth and demonstrates your willingness to get involved in your community. Consider joining and participating actively in a professional or civic organization while you are in school. See whether your school or community has a local chapter. Use the Resume Building Block #9: Professional and Civic Organizations form, on page 153, to record your participation.

Building Block 10: Languages Spoken. In our multicultural society, the ability to communicate in a language other than English is commonly included on the resume. Find out whether many patients speak a language other than English in the area where you plan to work. Consider acquiring at least some conversational ability or a few phrases to use to reassure patients. Appendix B contains a list of useful Spanish phrases for the medical professional. If your school offers these languages as elective courses, they would be good choices. A patient benefits greatly, during the stress of illness or injury, when health care professionals know at least a few phrases of the patient's native language. Even speaking just a few basic phrases can increase your value to employers. Also consider learning about the customs, especially the ones related to health practices, of ethnic groups in your community. (Cultural differences are discussed in Chapter 4.) Use the Resume Building Block #10: Languages Spoken form, on page 153, if you have or plan to acquire knowledge of another language.

Portfolios

Although resumes are the principal method for job seekers to present their qualifications to potential employers, portfolios are being used to supplement the resume. A portfolio is an organized collection of items that document your capabilities and qualifications for work. A portfolio can give you a competitive edge at job interviews.

Starting to plan your portfolio now can cast your class assignments in a new light. More than work you turn in to your instructor, they can serve as demonstrations of your abilities to an employer. Strive to perform consistently at your highest level, producing work that will represent you well.

As you complete each course, save assignments that might be suitable for your portfolio. Store them in a folder or large envelope so they stay in good condition. In addition to written assignments, there are nontraditional ways to showcase your abilities. The items you collect need not be limited to evidence of your technical skills. For example, it is appropriate to include documentation of other activities, such as organizing an event for charity. No standard list of items to put in your portfolio exists, although your school may have prepared a list for students. In any case, only accurate and neat work should be included. How to finalize the contents and assemble your portfolio for presentation is covered later in this chapter.

PROMOTION: THE FIFTH "P" OF MARKETING

Think about how companies use promotional campaigns to give new products maximum exposure. They advertise—sometimes endlessly, it seems!—on television, in magazines and newspapers, and on the Internet to spread the word to as many consumers as possible about how the product will fulfill their needs. You will conduct a similar campaign when you conduct your job search. As with your resume and portfolio, you can begin to prepare now. Networking, references, and the job interview are the three main ways to promote yourself during the job search.

Networking

Networking, as we are using the word here, refers to meeting and establishing relationships with people who work in health care. It is an effective way to learn more about your chosen career. At the same time, it gets the word out about you and your employment goals. Examples of networking opportunities include professional meetings, career fairs, class field trips to health care facilities, and guest speakers who come to your school.

There are many ways to begin networking: at a professional meeting, introduce yourself to other members; after hearing a guest speaker in class, ask questions; at a career fair, ask a local employer for advice about what to emphasize in your studies. Be sure to follow up with a phone call or thank-you note to anyone who sends you information or makes a special effort to help you.

Another benefit of networking is building your self-confidence as you introduce yourself to people. You can improve your speaking ability and increase your ability to express yourself effectively. These are valuable skills you will use when attending job interviews. Start now to create a web of connections to help you develop professionally and assist you in your future job search and career.

REFERENCES

References are people who will confirm your qualifications, skills, abilities, and personal qualities. In other words, they endorse you as a product. Professional references are not the same as personal or character references. To be effective, professional references must be credible (believable) and have personal knowledge of your value to a prospective employer. Your best references have knowledge of both you and the health care field. Examples include your instructors, clinical experience supervisors, and other professionals who know the quality of your work. Previous supervisors, even in jobs outside of health care, also make good references.

Recall the discussion in this chapter about becoming a health care professional by conducting yourself as if you already were one. Start now to project a professional image to everyone you meet, including your instructors and other staff members at your school. Become the person whom others will be happy to recommend.

Job Interview

Job interviews provide the best opportunities to promote yourself to prospective employers. Interviewers often ask for examples of how you solved a problem or handled a given situation. Start thinking now about your past experiences and begin to collect examples from your work as a student, especially from your clinical experience, that will demonstrate your capabilities. It is not too early to start preparing so you can approach your future interviews as opportunities to shine, at ease and confident that you are presenting yourself positively. Job interviews are discussed in detail in Chapter 12.

PULLING IT ALL TOGETHER

You are now ready to gather the information in your Resume Building Blocks to construct a finished product. Just like actual blocks, the content from your Prescriptions for Success 10-3 through 10-11 can be put together in a variety of ways. The steps described in this section will help you create a document that best highlights your qualifications.

You will see as you progress through this chapter that there is no one best way to write a resume. Everyone has different talents and experiences. Even students who complete the same program at the same time come from a variety of backgrounds that can be presented in different ways. For example, a young person who graduated from high school shortly before beginning a dental assisting program will most likely benefit from emphasizing different areas than a classmate who worked in sales for 20 years before entering the same program.

There are also local customs and employer preferences regarding resumes. Seek the advice of your instructors, school career service personnel, and professional contacts. They keep in touch with employers and can offer sound advice.

At this busy time in the job-search process, you may be tempted to use a standard resume format. Filling in the blanks on a "one-type-fits-all" resume may seem to be a fast and easy way to complete this task. However, the time spent customizing your resume can pay off in several ways. For example, you will do the following:

1. Better recognize and review your own qualifications
2. Respond to employers' specific needs
3. Be prepared to support your claims with examples
4. Demonstrate your organizational skills
5. Show your initiative and creativity

Note: Your school may require or recommend that you use a format it has developed. In this case, it is probably best to use what is provided.

An effective way to increase your efficiency when putting together your resume is to use word-processing software. This gives you several advantages because you can:

- Try different layouts and formats
- Change and reorganize content quickly and easily
- Check for (most) spelling errors
- Change your objective or skill clusters to address specific employer needs
- Use special features such as bolding and changing the size and style of the letters
- Send your resume as part of an e-mail and/or post it on the Internet (this will be discussed later in this chapter)

If you don't know how to use a word-process program, now is a good time to learn if you have a little time. Today's software is quite easy to learn and even nontypists can produce great-looking documents by learning a few basic commands. Spacing, bolding, underlining, moving text, and printing can be accomplished with the click or two of a button. If you can spend a few hours to learn the basics of a word-processing program now, it will be a good investment of your time. Not only will this skill support your job-search effort, it will provide you with a valuable workplace skill. Even health care professionals who dedicate most of their time to hands-on patient activities can benefit from knowing how to word process. Today, computer skills are considered essential for most health care jobs.

10 STEPS FOR ASSEMBLING YOUR RESUME

Whether you create your resume on a computer or not, following a step-by-step process can help you assemble a resume to fit your needs. Box 11-1 summarizes the steps that are explained in the following sections.

Step One: Prepare the Heading

It is not necessary to write the word "Resume." Instead, clearly label the top of the page with your name, address, and telephone number. Centering your name is good for both appearance and practicality. Placing it on the far left side makes it more difficult for the employer to find if it is placed in a stack of other resumes or in a file. (You might even put your heading justified right.) Capitalizing your name and/or using a slightly larger font (letter) size than the rest of the document helps it to stand out.

JAIME RAMIREZ
3650 Loma Alta Lane
San Diego, CA 92137
(619) 123-4567
jrnurse@aol.com

Capitalize and boldface your name and consider using a larger size font. Include your ZIP code and area code. Be sure all numbers are correct. Include your e-mail address if you have one.

The following format is an option if your resume is long and you are trying to conserve space:

JAIME RAMIREZ
3650 Loma Alta Lane, San Diego, CA 92137
(619) 123-4567 jrnurse@aol.com

BOX 11-1 A 10-Step Checklist for Assembling Your Resume

1. Prepare the heading.
2. Add the objective.
3. Select the best type of resume for you.
4. Decide if you want to include a Summary of Qualifications section.
5. Choose which Resume Building Blocks to include.
6. Plan the order of your Building Blocks.
7. Decide whether you want to add a personal statement.
8. But…leave out personal information.
9. Plan the layout.
10. Create an attractive and professional-looking document.

Step Two: Add the Objective

The objective, from Resume Building Block #1, should be near the beginning of the resume so prospective employers can quickly see whether there is a potential match between your goals and their needs. This part of the resume may change slightly, as discussed before, if you are trying to match your objective with the stated needs of each employer. Your objective will not change if you have specific requirements you are not willing to change, if you have written a very general objective that meets a number of job targets, or if your objective simply states a job title such as "surgical technologist."

Step Three: Select the Best Type of Resume for You

The three basic types of resumes are chronological, functional, and combination. They provide different ways to present your work history and professional qualifications. Your particular background determines which type you should choose.

Chronological Resume. The chronological resume emphasizes work history. It shows the progression of jobs you have held to show how you have gained increasing knowledge, experience, and/or responsibility relevant to the job you want now. This type of resume is recommended if you have:

- Held previous jobs in health care
- Had jobs in other areas in which you had increases in responsibility or a strong record of achievements

- Acquired many skills that apply to health care (transferable skills)

In the chronological resume, each job you've had in the past is listed, followed by the duties performed and your achievements. The Work section is well developed and likely to be longer than most other parts of your resume.

Functional Resume. The functional resume emphasizes skills and traits that relate to the targeted job but that weren't necessarily acquired through health-care employment. They can be pulled from both work and personal experiences. For example, if you cared for a sick relative for an extended period of time, this is an experience you might decide to include. Review Prescription for Success 1-4 and the transferable skills on Resume Building Block #4 for ideas. Once you have identified and listed qualifications that fit your target jobs, organize them into three or four clusters with descriptive headings.

Functional resumes are advantageous in the following situations:

- If you are entering the job market for the first time
- If you have held jobs unrelated to health care
- If you have personal experiences you can apply to health care work

The Work History section of a functional resume consists of a simple list of job titles with each employer's name, city and state, and your dates of employment. A functional resume may take more time to develop than a chronological one, but the extra effort can really pay off because it allows you to highlight the qualifications that are your strongest bid for employment.

Combination Resume. The combination resume, as its name implies, uses features of both the chronological and functional types. The details of the job(s) held in or closely related to health care are listed, along with clusters of qualifications or a list of supporting skills. This resume is appropriate in the following situations:

- If you have held jobs in health care *and*
- If you have related qualifications you gained through other, non–health care jobs and experiences *or*
- If you have held a number of jobs in health care for which you performed the same or very similar duties

Let's look at how a recent occupational therapy assistant graduate who worked for 2 years as a nursing assistant and for 3 years as a preschool aide creates a combination resume. She decides to do the following:

- Include a list of the duties she performed in the nursing assistant job
- Create clusters to highlight her teaching and interpersonal skills, both important in occupational therapy
- List skills from her teaching and other experiences under each cluster heading

Choosing the Best Resume for You. Review your skills and experiences and use the guidelines in this section to choose the best type of resume for you. If you decide to use a chronological presentation, copy what you prepared for your Work History in Building Block #3.

If a functional resume would serve you better, use the following guidelines to create the clusters:

1. Consider the current needs of employers. Check your local help-wanted ads and job announcements, the National Healthcare Foundation Standards, and the SCANS competencies for ideas.
2. Think about the skills and traits that will contribute to success in your occupation.
3. Look over your work history, clinical experience, personal experiences, volunteer activities, and participation in professional organizations.
4. Refer to your completed Prescriptions for Success 1-4 and 9-1 for skills and characteristics you can use in clusters.
5. Create three or four headings for clusters that support your job target and give you an opportunity to list your most significant qualifications. The following list contains examples of appropriate clusters for health care occupations:
   - Communication Skills
   - Organizational Skills
   - Teamwork Skills
   - Interpersonal Relations
   - Computer Skills
   - Clerical Skills
6. List appropriate specific skills under each heading.

Step Four: Summary of Qualifications

Decide whether to include a Summary of Qualifications Section. This is an optional section. Its purpose is to list skills that support you as a product but that don't fit well in other sections. It can also serve to highlight how you will benefit the employer and encourage the reader to look over the rest of your resume. In other words, it can serve as an appealing introduction to you and your resume.

You may have decided to use a chronological resume but have additional experiences that don't belong in the Work History section. Or maybe you have designed a functional resume but have single experiences worth mentioning that don't fit any of the headings, as in the following examples:

- Excellent time-management skills
- Work calmly under pressure
- Proven problem-solving ability
- Cost conscious
- Enthusiastic team player
- Work well without supervision
- Enjoy learning new skills

A Qualifications section can also serve as a summary of highlights to draw attention to your most significant features. Such a summary might look like this:

- Eight years' experience working in health care
- Up-to-date administrative and clinical medical assisting skills
- Current CPR certification
- Fluent in spoken Spanish
- Excellent communication skills

Review the same information sources recommended in Step Four for preparing functional clusters. The difference in preparing the Qualifications section is you can combine different kinds of characteristics. They don't have to fall into neat categories but only have to demonstrate capabilities, traits, and special skills that relate to the job you want.

Note: If you have created clusters and are using them in a functional or combination resume, you may not need a Qualifications section. The important thing is not to repeat information in your resume. Step Five talks more about deciding what to include.

Step Five: Choose Which Resume Building Blocks to Use

You want your resume to be comprehensive, but at the same time you don't want to repeat information. For example, if you are using a functional format and have listed a special skill in one of your clusters, don't repeat it under another heading. Group as much as fits well into each Resume Building Block instead of having many headings with just one item listed. Think about which items fit together. The following are the most appropriate to combine:

1. Licenses and certifications can be placed in their own section, can be listed in the Education section, or can be listed as a Professional Qualification.
2. Honors and awards earned in school can be listed under Education. If you have a variety of awards, it might be better to highlight them by listing them in their own section.
3. Memberships can go under Education if they are related to school groups or your health care professional organization. If you have been active in the organizations and want to state what you've done or are involved in several organizations, they might better go in their own section.
4. Clinical experience can be listed under either Education or Work History. Wherever you place it, include some information about the duties you performed. For career changers and recent graduates, this may be a significant part of work history. Be sure to indicate clearly, however, that the work was unpaid and part of an educational program.
5. Languages you speak other than English can be listed under Qualifications, Special Skills, or Languages Spoken.

Deciding which headings to use and where to place content depends on the amount of content, how directly it relates to the kind of job you want, and your own organizational preferences. Suppose you speak two languages other than English. If they are spoken by many people in your geographic area, they are likely to be valuable job qualifications and might be listed in a Summary of Qualifications. If they are not commonly spoken in your area, they might best be listed under Languages—skills you want to show but that may not be directly related to the job. Think about the relative importance of your content as you decide how best to organize and label it.

Step Six: Plan the Order of Your Building Blocks

Place the sections that contain your strongest qualifications first. For example, if you are changing careers and recent education is your primary qualification, list that section before Work History.

Step Seven: Decide If You Want to Add a Personal Statement

In their book *Career Planning*, Dave Ellis and coauthors suggest adding a positive personal statement at the bottom of your resume.[1] This gives you an opportunity to make a final impression and add an original touch. It is a way to say, "Here is something personal and interesting about me that might help you, the employer." If you decide to write a personal statement, be sure it is a sincere reflection of you and not simply something that sounds good.

And, as with the entire resume, be sure it relates to your job target. Here are a couple of examples:

- "I enjoy being a part of a team where I can make a positive contribution by using my ability to remain calm and work efficiently under stressful conditions."
- "I get great satisfaction working with people from a variety of backgrounds who need assistance in resolving their health care problems."

If you decide to include a personal statement, review your reasons for choosing a career in health care along with what you believe are your best potential contributions to prospective employers. It is also a good idea to have someone else, such as your instructor, review your statement.

Step Eight: Leave out Personal Information

Don't include personal information such as your age, marital status, number of children, and health status. And never include false statements about your education or experience. If these are discovered later, they can be grounds for dismissal from your job.

Although it is important to have a Reference Sheet (list of references) available for potential employers who request it, it is not necessary to write a statement such as "References Available upon Request."

Step Nine: Plan the Layout

Each section of your resume, except the heading at the top and personal statement (optional) at the end, should be labeled: Objective, Education, Work History, and so on. Headings can be flush (aligned) with the left margin, with the content set to the right, as follows:

OBJECTIVE ________________________

____

EDUCATION ________________________

____

Alternatively, you can center your headings and list the information beneath and flush left.

OBJECTIVE

____

____

EDUCATION

____

____

____

The information you list under the headings can be arranged in a variety of ways. The design should be based primarily on whether you need to use or save space on the page. The second consideration is personal preference. However you choose to lay out your resume, strive for a balanced, attractive look. Note the varied use of capitalization and boldface to draw attention to the job title in the following examples:

WORK HISTORY Medical Transcriptionist
2001-Present
Hopeful Medical Center
Better Health, NJ

OR

MEDICAL TRANSCRIPTIONIST
2001-Present
Hopeful Medical Center
Better Health, NJ

OR

Medical Transcriptionist
2001-Present
Hopeful Medical Center
Better Health, NJ

Step Ten: Create an Attractive and Professional-Looking Document

Selecting and organizing content takes time and effort, so don't waste your efforts by failing to attend to the details of appearance. A poor appearance can land a resume in the wastebasket without even a review. The following tips will help you achieve a professional look:

- Leave enough white space so the page doesn't look crowded. Double-space between the sections.
- It is recommended that you limit your resume to one page. It is better to use two pages, however, than to crowd too much information onto one page. If you do use two pages, write "More" or "Continued" at the bottom of the first page and your name and contact information and "Page 2" or "Page Two" at the top of the second.
- Capitalize headings.
- Use bullets to set off listed items.
- Try using boldface for emphasis.
- Make sure your spelling and grammar are perfect.
- Leave at least a 1-inch margin on all sides.
- Use good-quality paper in white, ivory, or very light tan or gray.

Whether printing from the computer or using a copy machine, make sure the print is dark and clear. If you don't have access to a computer printer or a good copy machine, consider paying to have your resume printed. Although this limits your flexibility in customizing the resume for various employers, it will provide professional-quality copies.

Your basic resume can serve you throughout your health care career. Think of it as a living document on which you continually record your experiences and new skills.

RUDY MARQUEZ
1909 Franklin Blvd.
Philadelphia, PA 19105
(610) 765-4321 MAmarquez@aol.com

OBJECTIVE Position as a clinical medical assistant in an urgent care setting

QUALIFICATIONS

- 13 years experience as a certified medical assistant
- Current certifications in CPR and Basic Life Support
- Proven ability to communicate with patients and staff
- Proactive employee who anticipates office and physicians' needs
- Fluent in Spanish and Italian

WORK HISTORY

Medical Assistant 2005-present
Founders Medical Clinic Philadelphia, PA
- Perform clinical and laboratory duties
- Assist physicians with exams, procedures, and surgeries
- Reorganized patient education program, including selection of updated brochures, videos
- Provide patient education and present healthy living workshops
- Train and supervise new medical assistants

Medical Assistant 1999-2005
North Side Clinic Pittsburgh, PA
- Performed clinical and laboratory duties
- Developed system for monitoring and ordering clinic supplies that resulted in annual savings of over $25,000
- Received commendation for providing outstanding patient service

Medical Assistant 1997-1999
Dr. Alan Fleming Erie, PA
- Assisted Dr. Fleming with procedures and minor office surgeries
- Prepared treatment and examining rooms
- Took vital signs and administered injections
- Performed routine laboratory tests
- Handled computerized recordkeeping tasks
- Assisted in researching and purchasing new office computer system

EDUCATION

Associate of Science in Medical Assisting 1997
Emerson College of Health Careers, Erie, PA

Recently Completed Workshops and Continuing Education Courses
- Health Care Beliefs of Minority Populations
- Medical Spanish
- New Requirements for Maintaining Patient Confidentiality

ORGANIZATIONS

American Association of Medical Assistants (AAMA)
Pennsylvania Association of Medical Assistants
Philadelphia Lions Club

FIGURE 11-1 Example of a Chronological Resume. This type of resume, which lists a detailed work history, is recommended for applicants who already have experience working in health care.

See Figures 11-1, 11-2, and 11-3 for examples of completed resumes. Yours will look different, of course, but these will give you some ideas.

DISTRIBUTING YOUR RESUME

Make the best use of your printed resume by distributing it to people who have may have job openings—employers—and people who might know about jobs. Following are some suggestions to get you started:

- Employers who place help-wanted ads or post job openings on the Internet or elsewhere
- Employers who have unadvertised openings you have heard about from other sources
- Your networking contacts

HEATHER DIETZ
10532 Cactus Road
Yuma, AZ 85360
(520) 321-7654 thedietz@linkup.com

OBJECTIVE Entry-level position in health information management in which I can apply up-to-date knowledge and skills. I especially enjoy applying my organizational skills and working on challenging tasks that must be complete and accurate.

EDUCATION Associate of Science in Health Information Technology 2009
Desert Medical College Yuma, AZ

COMPUTER SKILLS

- Created electronic spreadsheet to track fund raising for Sage Elementary School PTA
- Taught self to efficiently use leading brand software programs in the following areas: word processing, database, spreadsheets, and accounting
- Set up and managed electronic accounting system for family-owned construction business
- Teach computer classes at Girl Scout summer day camp

ORGANIZATIONAL SKILLS

- Created system to monitor all church collections and fund-raising projects
- Initiated and developed computer career awareness program for Girl Scouts
- Secretary for college HIT student organization
- Completed HIT associate degree program with perfect class attendance while working part-time and managing family life

CLERICAL/ADMINISTRATIVE SKILLS

- 7 years bookkeeping experience
- Keyboarding speed of 78 wpm
- Excellent written communication skills

WORK HISTORY

Unpaid Internship at St. John's Medical Center, Yuma, AZ 2009
Medical Records Department

Bookkeeper 2003-2007
Buildwell Construction Company, Yuma, AZ

Bookkeeper 1998-2003
Perfect-Fit Cabinetry, Yuma, AZ

Secretary 1995-1998
Caldwell Insurance Company, Yuma, AZ

ORGANIZATIONS

Desert Medical College Health Information Technology Student Organization, Secretary
Sage Elementary School PTA, Treasurer
Faith Community Church, Member of Social Service Committee

FIGURE 11-2 Example of a Functional Resume. This type of resume, which lists skills that support a health care job, is recommended for applicants who have not worked in health care.

- Friends and relatives
- Anyone who indicates that he or she knows someone who might be hiring
- Your school's career services department

Keep enough copies of your resume on hand to respond to unexpected opportunities. Take copies to interviews (even if you have sent a copy in advance), career fairs, and the human resource departments of health care facilities. Be sure to have plenty on hand if you decide to drop in on employers as described in Chapter 10. A well-prepared resume in many hands is an effective way to get the word out that you are a serious job candidate.

It is usually not recommended, however, that you send resumes to dozens of employers in the hope of locating one that has a job opening. One exception is when there are more job openings than applicants. This can occur when there is a shortage, such as the current nationwide shortage of registered nurses. When there is a shortage, you are more likely to

EMILY COLLINS
8215 Mile High Drive
Denver, CO 80201
(303) 987-6543

OBJECTIVE Position as an Occupational Therapy Assistant working with clients who have physical disabilities

EDUCATION

Associate of Science Occupational Therapy Assistant 2010
Salud College Denver, CO
Graduated with Honors
Passed national certification exam
Fieldwork completed at Central Rehabilitation Hospital

Certificate Nursing Assistant 2005
San Juan Medical Center Denver, CO

HEALTH CARE WORK EXPERIENCE

Nursing Assistant 2005-2008
GoodCare Nursing Home, Denver, CO
- Encouraged patients to achieve their maximum level of wellness, activity, and independence
- Demonstrated interest in the lives and well-being of patients
- Helped patients to perform prescribed physical exercises
- Organized and participated in activities with patients
- Assisted patients with basic hygiene and dressing

INTERPERSONAL SKILLS

- Provided daily care for parent with Alzheimer's disease for 18 months
- Answered telephone, directed calls, and took messages for busy sporting goods manufacturer
- Received Connor Memorial Award from Salud College for making positive contributions and assisting classmates

TEACHING SKILLS

- Teach swim classes to all ages at YMCA
- Conduct CPR instruction for the American Heart Association
- Organize holiday programs and outings for nursing home residents (volunteer)
- Planned and supervised craft and play activities for school-age children
- Tutored ESL students at Salud College

WORK HISTORY

Preschool Aide 2004-2005
Bright Light Preschool, Denver, CO

Swim Instructor (part-time) 2004-present
YMCA, Denver, CO

Receptionist 2000-2004
Sportrite Manufacturing Co., Denver, CO

ORGANIZATIONS

American Occupational Therapy Association
American Heart Association, Chair of Local Fundraising Committee

FIGURE 11-3 Example of a Combination Resume. This type of resume is recommended for applicants who have some experience working in health care but who also want to highlight other skills that support their target job.

receive responses when sending unsolicited resumes. A second exception is when you are moving to a new area. Sending a large number of resumes, along with a cover letter explaining that you are relocating, may be more economical and productive than calling many potential employers.

NEW DEVELOPMENTS IN RESUMES

The capacities of the computer to sort and organize data, along with the speed and convenience of the Internet, have resulted in new forms of resumes and ways for job searchers and employers to connect.

E-Resumes

You will need to modify your resume if you are sending it to an employer electronically, if it will be scanned, or if you are posting it on an Internet site. This is to ensure that it transmits and scans properly. You will note that some changes require you to do exactly the opposite of the directions given in the previous sections to create an attractive printed resume! But this doesn't mean destroying or not using your original version—it means creating an additional version.

Start by converting your resume to what is called "plain text." If you created your resume using MS Word (on either a PC or a Mac), use the "save as" command and choose the plain text format (the ending will be .txt). This format strips your document of all special formatting—things like bullets, boldface, and italics. The instructions embedded to create these "special effects" do not translate well electronically, and your resume can become scrambled or interspersed with odd-looking characters.

Once you have created a plain-text version, do the following[2]:

1. Proofread it for oddly wrapped lines, scrunched up words, and similar problems that can happen when text is converted.
2. Delete "continued" or "page 2" if these exist.
3. Use caps to emphasize words that otherwise would have been boldfaced or italicized—your name, for example.
4. Replace bullets with standard keyboard symbols such as *, +, –, or ~. (Bullets may have converted to little boxes or other odd characters.)
5. If you need to add spaces, use the space bar, not the tab key.
6. If you use quotation marks anywhere, these only convert if they are straight, not curly (curly quotation marks are also called "smart quotes"). Check your word-processing program to see how to do this.

Just as with the original version of your resume, it is critical that this version be free of errors. Once sent or posted online, it is there for potentially millions of people to view.

Posting Your Resume on the Internet

There are many types of websites on which you can post your resume. Some are general employment sites, such as Monster. Others are specific to health care. And still others are employer websites that allow—or even require—you to apply electronically for specific job openings. Deciding whether to place your resume on the Internet and which type of website to choose depends on your job target and the kind of employer you are seeking. Although many websites allow job searchers to post their resumes for free, they charge employers to place help-wanted ads online and to view the resumes in their databases. Therefore larger organizations are the ones most likely to pay for this service. A physician's office or small clinic may not be able to justify the expense for its relatively small number of hires. Organizations with many employees, such as Kaiser Permanente or even a single hospital, may have their own websites and online application capabilities.

Spend some time considering whether to post your resume on the Internet. Although posting on a large website makes your resume available to millions of viewers, you are also competing with millions of other job seekers. Experts suggest that posting your resume on a few carefully chosen sites is worth some of your time but is not as likely to help you find a job as methods such as networking and applying directly to specific employers. (This advice does not apply to employer websites with job postings and instructions for applying and sending your resume electronically.)

Deciding on which public websites to post your resume should receive careful consideration.

In general, experts recommend that you should not pay to have your resume distributed. Many of these "services" simply send out mass e-mails containing the resumes of anyone who pays them. The resumes may or may not match the jobs posted (if indeed, the targeted employers even have job openings), and it is reported that resumes are often sent without contact information, such as your name and telephone numbers, so employers cannot reach you even if they are interested in learning more about you. You must explore websites for yourself, but starting with the recommendations of well-known job-search experts will help you avoid unreliable websites. The following three sites are well-established and appear on all "recommended" lists:

1. Monster.com
2. HotJobs.com
3. CareerBuilder.com

In addition, check sites dedicated to health care or your particular occupation and the website of your professional organization. (See the information on health-specific websites in Chapter 10.)

The following suggestions can help you choose an appropriate website[3]:

- Do not use websites that won't allow you to review at least a sample of their job lists before you provide personal information or your resume.
- Read the privacy policy! Some websites sell or give your information to other businesses. Important: *Never* put your social security number on your resume.

- Check the wording. Do the lists provided include real jobs, or are they examples of what the website claims to be trying to fill?
- Check for currency. Are there dates on the jobs listed? Are they recent?
- Look for information about who sponsors the site. Do they have credentials and/or experience in the job-search industry?
- If you do not get any responses to your resume within 45 days, remove it and find another website on which to post it.

As a courtesy to those who are looking for applicants, remove your resume from all websites on which you have it posted once you become employed. Another consideration is that your new employer may see your resume online and wonder if you are still looking for a better deal.

INTRODUCING YOUR RESUME: COVER LETTERS

A cover letter should be sent along with your resume, whether it goes by conventional ("snail") mail or is sent electronically. The purpose of a cover letter is to provide a brief personal introduction. It should be short, informative, persuasive, and polite. The fact that you write a letter can be persuasive in itself. It shows that you took the time and made the effort to consider why and how you meet this particular employer's qualifications. You did more than simply put a resume in an envelope or send it electronically.

Cover letters can be customized for different circumstances. Before discussing the different types, let's look at a few how-tos common to all cover letters:

1. Use a proper business letter format. Figure 11-4 contains an example.
2. Be sure your spelling and grammar are error-free.
3. Direct your letter to a specific person whenever possible. Look for a name in the employment ad, ask your contact for the name of the appropriate person, or call the facility and ask. If you are writing in response to an unadvertised position, having a name on your correspondence is especially important. Letters without names can get misdirected or discarded. Busy facilities don't have time to determine to whom to direct your inquiry.
4. Write an introduction. State who you are, why you are writing, who referred you or what ad you are responding to, and what position you are applying for. Employers may have more than one position open, so don't assume they will know which job you are applying for.
5. Develop the body of the letter. Explain why the employer should interview you—that is, what you have to offer and how you can help him or her. Summarize your qualifications for the job. Do your best to match them with what you believe the employer is seeking. At the same time, don't simply repeat the same information that is on your resume.
6. Include a closing paragraph. Ask the employer to call you for an interview or state that you will call for an appointment.
7. If you are sending your cover letter electronically (in the body of an e-mail, for example), keep the format simple: don't use bolding, bullets, or other special features and avoid using tabs to indent text.

Letter for an Advertised Position

In Chapter 10, we discussed responding to employment ads in a way that demonstrates how you meet the employer's needs. Use language in your letter that mirrors the words used in the ad or job announcement.

Letter for an Unadvertised Opening

You may learn about unadvertised job openings through your school or from your networking contacts. Mention your source of information in the introduction of your cover letter. (Be sure to obtain permission from the contact person before using his or her name!) Before writing the letter, learn as much as possible about the job. Sources of information include the person who told you about it, the employer's website, or an inquiry call to the facility.

Letter of Inquiry

There may be a facility where you would like to work, but you don't know if it has any job openings. Perhaps you have a friend who is happily employed there and has recommended it as a great place to work. Or it may have a reputation for excellent working conditions and educational and promotional opportunities. When you are not responding to a specific job opening, state your general qualifications that meet the current needs in health care. Explain why you are interested in working at the facility. Learn as much as possible about the facility so you can emphasize specific contributions you can make (Figure 11-4).

APPLICATIONS

Applications are commonly requested of job applicants, even if they have submitted a resume. Applications provide the employer with complete, standardized sources of information. Once you have been hired, the application is placed in your personnel file and can serve as a legal document and record of information about you and your previous employment.

Some applications contain important statements you are required to read and sign. For example, employers

10752 Learning Lane
Silver Stream, NY 10559
July 22, 2010

Ms. Sandra Walters, Manager
Caring Clinic
7992 Oates Road
Greenville, NY 10772

Dear Ms. Walters:

I am writing to inquire about job openings at Caring Clinic. My husband and I are relocating to Greenville in September and I am looking for a position in which I can apply my up-to-date skills as a phlebotomy technician. Caring Clinic has a reputation for excellent service to the health needs of the Greenville community and I would be proud to be a contributing member of your team.

As a recent graduate of Top Skill Institute, I had the opportunity to perform my internship at Goodwell Laboratory Services, an affiliate of Caring Clinic. I understand the importance of combining technical excellence with attention to customer service. While at Goodwell, my technical skills were highly praised by my supervisor, Mr. Jaime Gutierrez. In addition, I consistently received top ratings on patient satisfaction surveys.

My resume is enclosed for your review. I will call you in early September to see if I can set an appointment to meet with you. Thank you for your consideration.

Respectfully,

Carla Martinez

Carla Martinez

FIGURE 11-4 Example of a cover letter used to inquire about possible job openings.

of home health care workers may protect themselves from liability if employees have an accident when they are driving to and from job assignments. Read all statements carefully before signing. Applications and employment contracts may contain legal language and unfamiliar words. Don't hesitate to ask for an explanation of anything you don't understand.

After the work of constructing a resume, filling out an application may seem easy. But don't take it for granted. Take time to read the instructions, and fill it out as accurately and neatly as possible. This is especially important when applying for health care positions because neatness and accuracy are job requirements. Use this opportunity to demonstrate that you meet these requirements.

Success Tips for Filling out Job Applications

- Read the entire application before you begin to fill it in.

- Fill out all sections completely. Do not leave blanks or write in "See resume."
- Use black or blue pen, never pencil.
- Print neatly.
- Go to interviews prepared to fill out an application. Take complete information with you, including the following:
    - Social security number
    - Education, including dates and locations
    - Work history, including names of employers and dates of employment
    - Military service
    - References
- Proofread what you have written before submitting it.
- Be honest when answering questions. Giving false information can be grounds for dismissal if you are hired.
- For questions that don't apply to you, write "N/A" instead of leaving them blank. This way it is clear that you saw the question and didn't accidentally skip over it.
- Many entry-level jobs have a set salary. If the one you are applying for does not, it is best to write "negotiable."
- Be sure to sign and date the application.

Electronic Applications

Many employers now have application forms on their websites. When applying electronically, it is especially important to follow the directions and check your entries carefully before pushing the "send" button. Once the application has been sent, it is difficult to change incorrect information. In some cases, the online application takes the place of sending a resume. As with traditional written materials, what you submit is a reflection of you as a professional. In fact, some employers use electronic applications to test the computer skills of potential employees.

Use the Internet tracking form provided in Chapter 10 to record to whom you have sent electronic applications, your password (if any), and the specific information you have sent (for example, some applications ask for your salary requirements). If possible, print out your completed application and place it behind the tracking form in your job-search notebook.

REFERENCE SHEETS

As we discussed earlier in this chapter, references are people who will vouch for your qualifications and character. Good references can be a key factor in tipping the hiring scales in your favor. Give careful consideration to whom you ask to be references. They must be considered believable. Take care not to ask people who may be competing for the same jobs. Friends and relatives are not generally accepted as good work references, but they are often acceptable if you are asked to provide character references. In addition to being credible, references must have the following characteristics:

- Have the time and willingness to speak on your behalf to potential employers
- Be able to speak positively about you
- Have the ability to speak clearly and in an organized way

As mentioned earlier, the following people are good candidates to be work references:

- Instructors
- Other school personnel
- Clinical, externship, internship, or fieldwork supervisor(s)
- Previous employers
- Supervisors at places where you have performed volunteer work
- Professionals with whom you have worked on committees or projects

Contact each person you want to serve as a reference. Do this before you begin your job search. Never give out a name and then ask the person for permission afterward. This can put the person on the spot and makes it difficult if he or she prefers not to be a reference. Inform your references about the types of jobs you are applying for and what qualifications are important. This will enable them to be prepared to answer the potential employer's questions.

Create a written list of at least three references. At a minimum, include their names, titles, telephone numbers, and e-mail addresses. You may also want to include their addresses. Ask them if they can be contacted at work. If not, provide recommended times to call. It is essential that the telephone numbers be current and accurate. If you list a work number and the person is no longer employed there, your credibility may be questioned. Potential employers don't have time to call you back or make numerous calls trying to locate your references. Make it easy for them. This makes it easier for them to hire you.

Organize your reference list in an easy-to-read format, and print it on the same kind of paper as your resume. Write "References for (your name)" at the top of the page. The reference sheet should not be mailed with your resume unless it is specifically requested. Take copies with you to interviews to give to potential employers who ask for it. If you are visiting a human resource department, take a copy with you, because many employment applications have a section for listing references.

Be sure to let your references know when you are hired. Thank them for their willingness to assist you.

Keep them posted about your career progress. In the future, you may be in a position to help them, and that is what true networking is all about—mutual career support.

LETTERS OF RECOMMENDATION

Another type of reference is provided through letters of recommendation. These letters are usually written by supervisors or people in authority, such as instructors, who write statements about your work record, skills, and personal qualities. It is a good idea to request reference letters from employers throughout your career because they can serve as a record of endorsements and achievements over the years. As you leave each job (on good terms, it is hoped!), ask for a letter of recommendation from your supervisor.

Make copies of your letters of recommendation to place in your portfolio and/or to give to potential employers who request them. It is appropriate at interviews to mention that you have them available.

As with other references, be considerate. Ask only those people who you believe can write a positive letter. Also, try to give people enough time to compose a letter. Avoid giving a day's notice. Finally, let your references know what kind of job you are seeking so they can phrase their letters appropriately.

THE PORTFOLIO: SUPPORTING WHAT YOU SAY

Look over the items you have been collecting to put in your portfolio. (Review the suggestions given earlier.) Choose the ones that represent your best work and support the qualifications needed for your target jobs. Think about others you can include. For example, you might add a list of the courses you have taken if your educational program included classes not commonly offered in your program of study.

Organize your materials in a logical order, grouping related items together in sections. Place them in a binder or presentation folder using plastic protection sheets. It is not necessary to go to a lot of expense, but the folder should be well made and in a plain, conservative color. Prepare a title page labeled "Professional Portfolio" and include your name, address, and telephone number. If you have a large number of items, number the pages and prepare a table of contents.

You need to make only one portfolio if it is rather large; if it consists of only a few pages, make a few copies in case a potential employer asks you to leave it after the interview. Portfolios are not generally sent with your resume but are taken to interviews. You may mention to the interviewer that you have a portfolio. Don't simply hand it to the employer and expect him or her to read it (unless you are asked for it, of course). It is to be used during the interview to demonstrate your capabilities. For example, if you are asked about your knowledge of coding, you could show assignments in which you accurately coded a variety of diagnoses and procedures. Chapter 12 contains a section on using your portfolio at interviews.

To Learn More

Career Builder
http://msn.careerbuilder.com
Click on the Career Builder's Resume Center for advice and examples of resumes.

Covey SR: *The 7 Habits of Highly Effective People*, New York, 1990, Fireside.
This popular book lists seven principles that help individuals live effective lives. Students may find it helpful to learn about the seven habits:

- Habit 1: Be Proactive: Principles of Personal Choice
- Habit 2: Begin with the End in Mind: Principles of Personal Vision
- Habit 3: Put First Things First: Principles of Integrity and Execution
- Habit 4: Think Win/Win: Principles of Mutual Benefit
- Habit 5: Seek First to Understand, Then to Be Understood: Principles of Mutual Understanding
- Habit 6: Synergize: Principles of Creative Cooperation
- Habit 7: Sharpen the Saw: Principles of Balanced Self-Renewal

Enelow W, Kursmark L: *Expert resumes for health care careers*, Indianapolis, 2004, JISTWorks.
Dozens of examples of resumes for health care positions.

Erupting Mind
www.eruptingmind.com
This website contains dozens of reader-friendly articles that offer self-improvement advice. The topics covered include self-esteem, success skills, and using mind power with affirmations and visualization.

Gawain S: *Creative visualization: use the power of your imagination to create what you want in your life*, Novato, Calif, 2002, New World Library.
This book, originally published in 1977, remains a classic in the use of visualization and affirmation to attain personal success. Creative visualization has been used in the fields of health, education, business, sports, and the arts. The author explains how to use mental imagery and affirmations to produce positive changes in one's life.

Key Career Networking Resources for Job Seekers
www.quintcareers.com/networking_resources.html
This website contains links to many articles and additional websites about career networking.

Marino K: *Resumes for the health care professional,* ed 2, New York, 2000, John Wiley and Sons.
Dozens of examples of resumes for health care positions.

Online Writing Lab—Purdue University
http://owl.english.purdue.edu/owl
A very comprehensive source of help for all types of writing, including resumes and cover letters.

Quintessential Careers: "Researching Key Words in Employment Ads"
http://www.quintcareers.com/researching_resume_keywords.html

Riley Guide
www.rileyguide.com
The *Guide* has links to dozens of online resume-writing resources. All have been reviewed and evaluated for content and quality.

University of Mississippi Medical Center
Hospital Administrative Policy and Procedure Manual: Professional Appearance
http://hosped.umc.edu/docs/policies/(HADM.P-14)ProfessionalAppearance.pdf
See this website for an example of real-world requirements for health care employees.

U.S. Department of Labor: Occupational Outlook Handbook
www.bls.gov/OCO
This is a source of detailed information about hundreds of careers, including typical job descriptions, educational requirements, and average salaries. It is updated every 2 years.

REFERENCES

1. Ellis D, Lankowitz S, Stupka E, Toft D: *Career planning*, ed 2, New York, 1997, Houghton Mifflin.
2. Ireland S: *How to format your resume for email:* http://susanireland.com/eresumeguide/email/index.html.
3. Dickel MR, Roehm F: *Guide to Internet job searching 2008-2009*, Columbus, Ohio, 2008, McGraw-Hill.

RESUME BUILDING BLOCK #1 | CAREER OBJECTIVE

Employers want to know what kind of job you are looking for. You need to know this, too! You may change your objective for your first job several times as you learn new subjects and get ideas from your lab and clinical experiences.

To Do Now

Write at least two sentences that describe your objective, as you see it now, for your first job in health care.

1. ______________________________

____

____

2. ______________________________

____

____

Add new ideas here:

- ______________________________
- ______________________________
- ______________________________
- ______________________________
- ______________________________

Writing Your Resume

Objective

____

____

____

____

____

____

____

RESUME BUILDING BLOCK #2 | EDUCATION

Your education is more than a list of schools you've attended. Take the steps to get all you can out of your training program.

To Do Now
List five things you can do to get the most from your education.

1. ______
2. ______
3. ______
4. ______
5. ______

Write three academic goals..

1. ______
2. ______
3. ______

Writing Your Resume
List the schools you have attended, starting with the most recent.

RESUME BUILDING BLOCK #3 | PROFESSIONAL SKILLS AND KNOWLEDGE

To Do Now

Track the skills you are learning by keeping an inventory for each of your subjects. Fill in this form as you progress through your program. Here are some examples of the kinds of skills to include:

- Set up dental trays for common procedures
- Accurately complete medical insurance claim forms
- Create presentations using PowerPoint
- Teach a patient to use different ambulatory devices

	Course Title	Skills Acquired
1.	______	______
2.	______	______
3.	______	______
4.	______	______
5.	______	______
6.	______	______
7.	______	______
8.	______	______
9.	______	______
10.	______	______

Writing Your Resume

You can organize your professional skills and knowledge into clusters or write a list of individual skills.

______

______

______

______

______

RESUME BUILDING BLOCK #4 | WORK HISTORY

To Do Now
List the jobs you've had in the past and start recording transferable skills and accomplishments.

Job Title	Transferable Skills	Accomplishments

Writing Your Resume
Remember that the different types of resumes (chronologic, functional, and combination) will influence what information you include in your work history section.

Work History

RESUME BUILDING BLOCK #5 | LICENSES AND CERTIFICATIONS

To Do Now
Describe the licensing and/or certification requirements for your occupation, if any.

Are there voluntary approvals for which you can test or apply?

Are computerized, written, and/or practical exams required? What range of content is covered? How are the questions formatted (e.g., multiple choice, true-false)?

Are content outlines, review books, software, and/or practice exams available?

Writing Your Resume
LICENSE/CERTIFICATION/REGISTRATION (CHOOSE APPROPRIATE HEADING)

RESUME BUILDING BLOCK #6 | HONORS AND AWARDS.

To Do Now

List school awards for which you might qualify.

Eligibility requirements:

List community awards for which you might qualify:

Eligibility requirements:

List other awards for which you might qualify:

Eligibility requirements:

Writing Your Resume

HONORS AND AWARDS

RESUME BUILDING BLOCK #7 | SPECIAL SKILLS

To Do Now

Start recording special skills you think may be applicable to a job in health care.

Skill	Method of Acquisition	Application to Health Care

Writing Your Resume

SPECIAL SKILLS

RESUME BUILDING BLOCK #8 | VOLUNTEER ACTIVITIES

To Do Now

List any volunteer activities you might use on your resume. Do you have time while you are in school for new or additional activities that are directly related to your career goals?

Activity	Skills Acquired	Personal Qualities Demonstrated

Writing Your Resume

VOLUNTEER WORK AND COMMUNITY SERVICE

RESUME BUILDING BLOCK #9 | PROFESSIONAL AND CIVIC ORGANIZATIONS

To Do Now

List any professional and/or civic activities you might use on your resume. Are there organizations you can join to gain experience and enrich your educational program?

Organization	Activities	Skills Acquired

Writing Your Resume

PROFESSIONAL AND CIVIC ORGANIZATIONS

RESUME BUILDING BLOCK #10 | LANGUAGES SPOKEN

To Do Now

Languages you speak other than English:

Languages spoken by patients in your geographic area:

Opportunities to learn another language (even a few phrases useful in the health care setting):

Writing Your Resume

LANGUAGES SPOKEN

PRESCRIPTION FOR SUCCESS 11-1 | PLANNING AHEAD

1. Who do you already know who would be a good professional reference?

2. What can you start doing now to ensure you have access to at least four positive recommendations when you begin your job search?

CHAPTER 12

Interviewing for Jobs

THE INTERVIEW—YOUR SALES OPPORTUNITY

"You don't have to be perfect. Just be the best for the job."

—*Rick Baird*

Finally! The words you have been hoping to hear: "When can you come in for an interview?" Your job-search efforts are paying off. But wait a minute! You begin to worry: "What if I can't think of anything to say?" "What if I don't have the skills they are looking for?" "What if they ask me about . . . ?"

The purpose of this chapter is to help you put the "what ifs" to rest and see the interviewing process as an opportunity to present yourself at your best. In Chapter 3 we discussed the power of attitude and how, with practice, you can choose your reaction to any situation. Many applicants view interviews as opportunities to be rejected. But you have another choice. You can view an interview as an opportunity to determine an employer's needs and to show how you can meet them.

Think about it. Employers are busy people who don't have time to conduct interviews with people who are unlikely job candidates. You obviously meet the minimum qualifications. The interviewer wants to see whether you are a person who can back up your qualifications, communicate well, and contribute to the organization.

By learning what will be expected of you at an interview and practicing your presentation skills, you can attend each interview with confidence. A common reason for not being hired is lack of preparation for the interview. And this is a factor over which you, not the interviewer, has control.

The Customer's Needs

Good sales presentations are based on showing customers—employers—how they can benefit by buying a product—in this case, by hiring you. Recall from Chapter 1 that identifying the customer's needs is an important step for students who are beginning a program of career preparation. As we pointed out, it doesn't make sense to create a product that no one needs.

In the same way, if you attend an interview without knowing anything about what the employer is looking for, you put yourself at a disadvantage. This is because in order to be at your best during the interview, the following preparations must be completed in advance:

- Identify possible needs of the employer.
- Think of ways you might meet those needs as an employee.
- Anticipate what types of questions might be asked.
- Practice answering them.
- Create examples to demonstrate your qualifications.
- Prepare appropriate questions to ask.

All employers have general qualities they look for in applicants such as the ones identified in the SCANS report. And health care employers have expressed their needs through the National Healthcare Foundation Standards discussed in Chapter 1. In addition, individual employers have more specific requirements based on factors such as patient population, services offered, size of facility, budgets, and so on. It is important for you to learn as much as possible before attending the interview. Here is a checklist of possible sources of information:

- Direct contact by phone or in person: ask questions, request a job description, observe the facility
- Brochures produced by the organization
- People who work there, such as friends, classmates, or networking contacts
- The local newspaper: large facilities are sometimes the subject of news articles
- The employer's website
- Your school's career services department
- The Chamber of Commerce and other organizations that have information about large employers
- The local chapter of your professional organization

- Information gathered at career fairs and employer orientation meetings
- Employment ad if the position was advertised

If the facility is small, such as a one-physician office, you should know, at a minimum, the type of specialty practiced and the patient population served. When you are unable to learn very much before the interview, it is especially important that you listen carefully to the employer and ask good questions. How to do this is discussed later in this chapter.

The Interviewer Is Human, Too

"Research into interviewing shows that the person conducting the interview is often more stressed than the candidate."

—Allan-James Associates

In addition to knowing the employment needs of the employer, consider the personal situation of the interviewer. Many applicants view the interviewer as a person of great confidence who has all the power in the hiring process. Applicants mistakenly see themselves as the underdogs in a game they have little chance of winning. In reality, interviewers may be experiencing a number of pressures:

- Concern about finding the right candidate who can perform the job as needed
- An extremely busy schedule
- Lack of interviewing skills
- A demanding supervisor who will hold them responsible for the performance of the person who is hired
- Concern about finding the time and resources to orient and train a new employee

Understanding the interviewer's point of view requires empathy—attempting to see the world through the eyes of others (see Chapter 4). This may not seem easy in a job interview when you are nervous and concentrating on presenting yourself well. But it is this very shift of focus—from yourself to the interviewer—that leads to a more successful interviewing experience. It is through this attempt to understand and then show how you can help solve the employer's problems that you best present yourself as the candidate for the job.

HEADS UP! KNOWING WHAT TO EXPECT

Some interviews are highly structured, meaning that each candidate is asked the same set of prepared questions. Others are more like a conversation, with topics and questions generated freely. Most interviews fall somewhere between these patterns, with interviewers preparing at least a few questions in advance. The style of the interview and types of questions most likely depends on the size of the organization. Large health care systems, hospitals, and clinics usually have dedicated personnel to conduct initial interviews. As human resource professionals, they have the time and expertise to study the latest hiring practices and develop their interviewing skills. They are most likely to conduct behavioral interviews, described later in this chapter. A physician who has a single practice is more likely to focus on what skills you have acquired through your education and experience—specific skills he needs, for example, in a clinical medical assistant or receptionist.

In any case, always base your answers on the needs of the health care industry in general and the specific needs of the employer. Your purpose is to demonstrate how *you* can contribute to *their* success.

Traditional Interview Questions

There are many "golden oldie" questions that interviewers have been using for years. Here are a few examples:

1. How would you describe yourself?
2. What are your long-range career objectives?
3. Why did you choose this career?
4. What makes you qualified for this position?
5. How well do you work with people?
6. What motivates you to go the extra mile on a job?
7. How do you define success?
8. Why should I hire you?

You can see that these questions are very open-ended. You can answer them in many ways, which actually can present a problem if your answers are too vague or not related to the job under consideration. In each case, what employers want to know is how your answer applies to *them*. For example, in explaining why you chose a career in health care, focus on what it is about you that relates to the job you are applying for. Be specific. Saying, "I've always been a people person" doesn't give much information. Saying, "I've been interested in health care since I was 11, when I spent time playing chess with my grandfather after he had his stroke. I noticed how he really perked up when he played, and I became fascinated by how the brain works better when stimulated with an enjoyable activity. This led me to explore a career in occupational therapy" is more specific and gives the interviewer more insight into who you are and what this means in terms of health care employment. When answering, "Why should I hire you?" mention specific skills and personal and professional qualities that will make a positive contribution to the physician's practice, the department's success, patient satisfaction, and so on.

Prepare for traditional interview questions by reviewing your inventories of skills and qualities, along with specific supporting examples, and then thinking about how you can incorporate them into your answers.

Behavioral Interview Questions

Behavioral interviews have been part of the hiring process in many large organizations since the 1970s and are being increasingly used in the health care industry. In this type of interview, applicants are asked questions about their past performance—how they handled specific situations. Behavioral interviews are based on the premise that past performance is a good indicator of future performance.

Interviewers prepare in advance by listing the key qualifications for the jobs they post. Then they develop questions to help determine whether applicants possess the desired characteristics. Here is an example: suppose that getting along with others is very important. A question might be, "Describe a time when you had to work with someone with whom you found it difficult to get along." As you tell your story, the interviewer follows up with additional questions, such as "In what ways was this person difficult?" "What was it you needed to do together?" "What did you say to this person?" "Did you get the job done in spite of the difficulties?" "How did you feel about this situation?" "What did you learn from this?" There may be additional probing questions from the interviewer to get more detail as you tell your story and verify that this is an experience you really had. In the case of the difficult person, these might be, "How did these difficulties affect others, such as co-workers and customers?" "Did your supervisor become involved?" Table 12-1 contains examples of behavioral interview questions.

It has been shown that this kind of questioning about real events is more difficult for applicants to answer because they must be supported by facts. For this reason, behavioral interviewing has been found to be 55% predictive of future behavior on the job as compared with traditional interviewing, which is 10% predictive.[1]

Preparing to answer behavioral questions generally takes more preparation than for traditional questions. However, if you have been collecting examples of your skills and qualifications, as was first suggested in Chapter 11, you are already getting ready. The key is to anticipate the kinds of qualifications an employer wants and then search your inventory—and memory—for experiences you've had that illustrate that qualification. Examples can come from any area of your life. You may never have worked in health care. In fact, you may have limited work experience of any kind. But perhaps you have

TABLE 12-1 Behavioral Interview Questions

Qualifications	Sample Questions
Interpersonal skills	Tell me about a time when someone disagreed with you about a major decision. What did you say or do? How was the decision ultimately made? Describe a situation in which you were able to use persuasion to successfully convince someone to consider your ideas.
Flexibility	Describe a situation in which you were required to conform to a work policy you really didn't agree with. What was the policy? Why didn't you agree? How did you feel about the situation? Give me an example of a job in which your working conditions frequently changed. How did you adapt to these changes? Tell me about a time when you had to reorganize your schedule in order to help a co-worker meet a deadline. How did you help? What was the result?
Communication	Give me a specific example that shows how you typically deal with conflict. Describe a time when you had to communicate something difficult to your supervisor. What was the situation? How did you plan your communication? What did you say? What was the result? Describe a situation in which you felt you didn't communicate well. How did you follow up? What did you learn?
Customer service skills	Tell me about a time when you had to deal with a very upset customer or patient. How did you handle the situation? What was the result? Give me a few examples of what you have said to customers or patients who have approached you for help. How did you decide the appropriate way to work with each one? Describe something you did to help an employer improve customer service.
Stress management	Describe a stressful situation in which you applied your coping skills. What specifically caused the stress? How were you feeling at the time? What techniques did you use? How was the situation resolved?
Problem solving	Describe a time when you anticipated a potential problem and developed preventive measures. How did you identify the problem? What were the signs? How did you determine ways to prevent it? How did others feel about your actions? What was the final result? Describe a time when you were asked or assigned to do a task you didn't feel qualified to handle. What did you do?
Integrity	Describe an incident in which you made a serious mistake. How did you handle this with your supervisor and/or co-workers? Tell me about a time when you had to make an unpopular decision. What were the circumstances? Why were others unhappy with the decision? Why did you believe you were making the right decision?

raised children. That experience may help you answer questions about making an unpopular decision. These were likely based on good judgment, your values, even ethics and morality. Employers want to know you can make decisions that are guided by what is right rather than by what is popular. In addition to family life, there are other experiences you can draw from, such as the following:

- Clinical experience
- Previous work experience
- School: classes, labs, extra activities
- Community and service work

In a behavioral interview, it is essential to *listen carefully*. Not only must you understand the question, you need to understand *what it is the interviewer wants to know*—that is, what qualification is obviously important for this job, and how you can demonstrate that you have that qualification. Don't hesitate to ask for clarification if you don't understand the question.

It is totally acceptable to take a few moments to think about an answer. You undoubtedly have many experiences to draw from. However, if the question asks for an example you simply don't have—for example, "Tell me about a time when you had to fire a friend," and this has never happened to you—say so rather than trying to make up a story.

Many job-search experts recommend using the **STAR** approach when answering a behavioral question. It helps you organize your response and goes like this:

1. **S and T:** Choose and describe a Situation or Task that enables you to best demonstrate you have the qualification.
2. **A:** Explain the Actions you took in dealing with the situation. Give enough detail to show your skills, but take care not to ramble or give unnecessary information.
3. **R:** Describe the Results. Explain what happened, what you learned, and how the results made a difference. Give numbers and percentages when possible.

Being prepared in advance is especially important for behavioral interviews. Try to anticipate the qualifications the interviewer might be interested in. Some will probably be general, such as those listed in the SCANS skills. Others may be specific to the hiring facility or the job. It's a good idea to write your examples out in the form of stories so you'll have the details in mind if you need them. Some questions may ask you to describe failures and how you've handled them, so you might think of some examples. Reflect on what you learned from experiences that didn't turn out as you hoped they would.

Although it is advisable to have examples in mind and practice telling your "stories," take care not to try to memorize what to say. You need to think about what you are saying during the interview and not give a canned response that may not exactly apply.

BOX 12-1 Examples of Situational Questions

What would you do?

- You see a co-worker who does not have the authority to administer medications taking some from a locked cabinet.
- You disagree with your supervisor about how to handle a problem.
- You hear a co-worker discussing confidential patient information with her friend, who is not involved in the patient's care.
- You aren't sure how to prioritize your work, and no one is available to discuss it with you.
- You are working with an angry patient who insists on seeing the physician—who is not available—immediately.
- You have a problem to solve. What steps would you take?
- You offer ideas at staff meetings, but no one seems to take them seriously.

Situational Questions

Situational questions present situations and problems you might encounter on the job. You are asked to explain how you would respond and/or handle the problem. (See Box 12-1 for examples.) As with behavioral questions, you need to do some advance planning to be prepared to answer them:

- Learn as much as possible about the organization and the specific job. If possible, read the mission statement and goals of the organization.
- Recall your own values and mission statement. These may provide guidelines in answering questions that don't have easy answers but can be based on your sense of right and wrong.
- Review your personal inventory of skills and qualifications.

Occupation-Specific Questions

Questions in this category explore your specific knowledge, skill mastery, willingness to learn new procedures, and the general content of your training.

The type of question will vary, as in the following examples:

- Describe how to perform a specific procedure.
- Explain how to operate certain equipment.
- Describe appropriate action to take in a given situation that directly relates to this job.
- Suggest how to solve a health care problem.
- Explain how you plan to keep your skills updated.
- What do you know about...? (a theory, new procedure, etc.)

- Why do you want to work in pediatrics (dermatology, children's dentistry, etc.)?

Some employers give practical skill tests or ask you to physically demonstrate your knowledge. Examples of these tests include a keyboarding speed test, filing or record-keeping exercise, spelling test, calculation of drug dosages, or demonstration of a procedure. If you are asked to perform a practical test that is appropriate for your level of training, do so willingly. Use the request to show that you have confidence in your abilities and can handle stress. If the task is something you have not been trained to do but is required for the job, tell the interviewer you would welcome the opportunity to learn.

Work Preference Questions

You may be asked about your job preferences. Review your answers to Prescription for Success 9-2, "What Do I Want?" In addition, be prepared to answer questions such as the following:

- Do you want full-time or part-time work?
- What hours you are willing to work?
- What length of shift you prefer?
- What days and time of day you can work?

Remember to be realistic when applying for jobs. Don't waste employers' time—or your own—interviewing for jobs with conditions you already know are absolutely impossible for you to meet.

Personality Tests

In today's employment world, you may be asked to take a personality test as part of the interviewing process. Personality assessment tests are increasingly being used, especially in larger organizations. As many as 30% of all companies now use personality tests.[2] These tests consist of answering a series of questions on paper or on the computer and measure such qualities as persistence and whether a person is an extrovert or introvert (highly social or more private). Studies claim that better matches are found when applicants take these tests. This is because certain jobs require specific characteristics, and these are more reliably determined by tests than by interviews. Another claim is that individuals hired tend to be happier with their jobs because of this matching process.

The best advice for taking a personality test is to answer the questions honestly. The tests contain a variety of questions to assess each trait. If you answer as you think you should or if you randomly select answers, this can show up negatively. If you do not "pass" such a test, it is very possible you would not have enjoyed either the work or the setting. This has been one of the reported benefits of personality assessments: less turnover among employees who, with traditional hiring methods, end up deciding the job just isn't for them.

Computerized Job Interviews

Yes, believe it or not, some employers are conducting interviews with the help of a computer. The advantage for the employer, in addition to saving time, is that every applicant is asked a prepared set of questions, often as many as 100. Most interview programs consist of answers to be checked. This enables the comparison of "apples with apples" when deciding who to interview in person. The advantage for you, the applicant, is you have more time to think about your answers and can, through the type of questions asked, learn a little about the organization before coming face-to-face with a human interviewer.

Answer the questions carefully and honestly. Computers are able to notice inconsistencies in your answers. Studies have shown that people are more likely to "tell" a computer information they would never reveal to another person.[3] If you are ever faced with a computerized interview, take care not to give unnecessary information that may harm your chance of getting hired. Also, be aware that most computer-assisted interviews must be completed in a certain length of time, so be sure you know how much time you have and keep track of it as you move through the questions.

Other uses of the computer in the hiring process include scenarios in which applicants explain what they would do in a given situation, skill tests, integrity tests, and personality tests. Some organizations administer computerized interviews and tests on their own computers at their facility; others make them available on the Internet and give applicants a password to gain access to testing websites.

PRACTICE: YOUR KEY TO SUCCESS

"Successful interviews usually depend on good preparation."

—John D. Drake

Of course you cannot anticipate the exact questions that interviewers will ask. What you can do is prepare yourself to answer a variety of questions. There are some things you can practice to improve your interviewing skills:

- Listening carefully
- Asking for clarification when necessary
- Thinking through your "inventory" of capabilities and characteristics that apply when answering questions
- Thinking of examples to back up your answers
- Projecting self-confidence

Preparation means practice—actually answering questions, aloud, under conditions as close to those of an actual interview as possible. The best way to practice is to role-play with someone who acts as the interviewer. This can be an instructor, classmate, mentor, networking contact, friend, or family member. Many schools require mock (pretend) interviews as part of professional development classes. Take advantage of these opportunities, and do your best to conduct yourself as if you were at a real interview. Videotaping or having an observer take notes can be helpful, even if it's a little nerve-wracking. It's better to make a few mistakes now so you can avoid them at interviews.

If you believe that you might be asked to demonstrate skills or react to a scenario, include them in your practice sessions. The career services personnel at your school may be familiar with the interviewing practices of facilities in your area and can give you additional information about what to expect and how to best prepare.

The goal of interview rehearsals is not to memorize answers you can repeat. It is to develop a level of comfort about the interviewing process and have facts fresh in your mind so you can call on them as needed and respond to questions intelligently and confidently.

BE PREPARED: WHAT TO TAKE ALONG

Having everything you might need at the interview will help you feel organized and confident. It also demonstrates to employers that you are organized and think ahead, valuable qualities for health care professionals. Although your own list will be different, here are some suggestions for what to take along:

- Extra copies of your resume
- Your portfolio
- Copies of licenses, certifications, and other documentation
- Proof of immunizations and results of health tests
- Reference sheet
- Any documentation of skills and experience not included in your portfolio (or if you have chosen not to create a portfolio)
- Pens
- Small notepad
- Your list of questions (discussed later in this chapter)
- All information needed to fill out an application (see Chapter 11)
- Appointment calendar, planner, or electronic organizer
- Anything you have been requested to bring
- For your eyes only: extra pantyhose, breath mints, other "emergency supplies"

A small case or large handbag is a convenient way to carry your papers and supplies. It can be inexpensive, but it should be a conservative color, in good repair, and neatly organized so you can quickly find what you need.

FIRST IMPRESSIONS: MAKE THEM COUNT!

"The way in which we think of ourselves has everything to do with how our world sees us."

—Arlene Raven

Just 30 seconds! That's how long you have to make a lasting impression. The average person forms a strong opinion of another in less than 1 minute. This is why so much emphasis is placed on professional appearance both during the job search and later, on the job. Although it is possible to eventually reverse a negative first impression, it's a lot easier to make a good one in the first place. Employers are basing their opinions on this first meeting. They will be thinking, "If this is the best this person can do, what might I expect from them on the job?"

In Chapter 11 we discussed the messages that dress and grooming communicate. When you are applying for a job in health care, appropriate appearance can let the interviewer know that you:

- Understand the impact of your appearance on others (patients, other professionals)
- Know what is appropriate for the job
- Apply the principles of good hygiene
- Respect both yourself and the interviewer
- Take the interview seriously

There is no universal agreement about the proper clothing to wear when applying for health care jobs. Some schools encourage their students to wear a clean, pressed uniform. Other schools advise them to wear neat, everyday clothing that is not too casual. It is important to pay attention to the professional advice of the staff at your school. The best choices for clothing are generally conservative colors and simple styles.

There are a few don'ts that apply wherever you live. Never wear jeans or clothing that is revealing or intended for sports and outdoor activities. Don't wear a hat or sunglasses during the interview. If you're not sure about what to wear, ask your instructor or someone in your school's career services department for help. If extra money for interview clothes is a problem, ask if your school has a clothes-lending program. Many cities have excellent thrift shops that sell nice clothes at reasonable prices. Some even specialize in helping people dress for job interviews.

You may arrive at an interview and discover that most people at the facility are dressed very casually. Don't worry. It is far better to be overdressed in this situation than underdressed. You can adjust your style later, after you get the job.

There are some additional guidelines that apply to all health care job applicants:

- Be squeaky clean. Take a bath or shower, wash your hair, scrub your fingernails, and use a deodorant or antiperspirant.
- Save the fashion trends for later. Hair and nails should be natural colors, tattoos covered up, and visible rings and studs from piercings removed. Limit earrings to one set. Women should apply makeup lightly for a natural, not painted, look.
- Show that you know what is acceptable for the health care professional. Avoid long fingernails, free-flowing hair, and dangling accessories that can be grabbed by patients or caught in machinery. Wear closed-toe shoes. Strive to be odor-free. For example, don't smoke on the way to the interview. Even the fragrances in perfumes and other personal products, intended to be pleasant, should not be worn because many patients find them disagreeable or have allergic reactions.
- Men who wear facial hair should groom it neatly.

Your appearance may be perfect, but if you arrive late for an interview, it may not matter. Being late is a sure way to make a poor impression. Time management is an essential health care job skill, and you will have failed your first opportunity to demonstrate that you have mastered it. In addition, arriving late is a sign of rudeness and inconsideration for the interviewer's time. Making a few advance preparations will help to ensure that this doesn't happen to you:

- Write down the date and exact time of the appointment.
- Verify the address and ask for directions, if necessary.
- If the office is in a large building or complex, get additional instructions about how to find it.
- Inquire about parking, bus stops, or subway stops.
- If you are unsure of the location and it is not too far away, go there a couple of days before the interview to be sure you can find it.
- Allow extra time to arrive, and plan to be there about 10 minutes before the appointed time.
- If there is an emergency that can't be avoided (a flat tire or unexpected snow storm), call as soon as possible to offer an explanation and reschedule the interview.

Many job applicants don't realize that the interview actually starts before they sit down with the person asking the questions. That's right. From the first contact you made to inquire about a job opening or set the appointment, you have been making an impression. If you arrive for the interview and are rude to the receptionist, you may have already failed in your bid for the job. You cannot know what information is shared with the hiring authority. (Keep in mind, too, that these may be your future co-workers!)

Learn the name of the person who will be conducting the interview. Be sure you have the correct spelling for the thank-you note and pronunciation. When you are introduced, the following actions express both courtesy and self-confidence:

1. Make and maintain eye contact.
2. Give a healthy (not limp or hesitant) handshake.
3. Express how glad you are to meet him or her and how much you appreciate the opportunity to be interviewed.
4. Don't sit down until you are offered a chair or the other person is seated.

COURTESY DURING THE INTERVIEW

Maintaining eye contact (without staring, of course) while the other person is speaking indicates that you are interested in what he or she is saying. When you are speaking, it is natural to look away occasionally. Most of the time, however, you should look at the listener. This is a sign of openness and sincerity. (Review the guidelines for respectful communication in Chapter 4.) The following is a summary of behaviors to definitely avoid (even if the interviewer engages in them):

- Interrupting
- Cursing
- Using poor grammar (such as the word "ain't") or slang
- Gossiping, such as commenting on the weaknesses of other facilities, professionals, or your previous employer
- Telling off-color jokes
- Putting yourself down
- Chewing gum
- Appearing to snoop by looking at papers or other materials on the interviewer's desk, shelves, and so on
- Discussing personal problems

You don't want to come across as stiff or stuffy, but you do want to come across as professional. Try to be at ease and act natural while maintaining your best "company manners."

APPLY YOUR COMMUNICATION SKILLS

A successful job interview depends on the effective use of communication. An interview is essentially a conversation between two people who are trying to determine whether they fit each other's employment needs. As a job applicant, you must take responsibility for making sure that you understand the employer's needs, questions, and comments. At the same time, you have to express yourself clearly so that the interviewer understands you.

Active Listening

Understanding begins by listening actively. The importance of carefully listening to the interviewer cannot be overemphasized. So many times we become so caught up in thinking about what we're going to say next that we fail to fully hear, let alone actively listen, to the other person. This is especially true in an interview when we are nervous and worried about whether we will say the right thing. But this is the very situation in which we can most benefit from listening carefully so we can base what we say on what we hear.

Recall from Chapter 6 that active listening consists of paying attention, focusing on the speaker's words, and thinking about the meaning of what is said. This takes practice. When you participate in the mock interviews suggested earlier, do not look at the questions the person role-playing the interviewer is going to ask. Instead, focus on listening carefully to the questions and then formulating an appropriate response. Pausing to think and compose a good answer will be appreciated by interviewers. You are more likely to be evaluated on the quality of your answer, not on how quickly you gave it.

Mirroring

An effective communication technique for interviews is known as mirroring. This means you observe the communication style of the interviewer and then match it as closely as possible. This does not mean mimicking or appearing to make fun of the other person. It does mean adapting a style that will be most comfortable for the interviewer and help to build trust.

Feedback

Whatever the style of the interviewer, use feedback when necessary to ensure that you understand the message. Feedback, as you recall from Chapter 4, is a communication technique used to check your understanding of the speaker's intended message. It is not necessary—or even desirable—to repeat everything the speaker says. It is annoying tospeakers to have everything they say repeated, and you don't want to sound like a parrot. Using feedback unnecessarily will use up time better spent learning about the job and presenting your qualifications. Used when needed, however, feedback can help you understand the other person so you can respond appropriately and intelligently.

Organization

When speaking, do your best to present your ideas in an organized manner so they are easy for the listener to follow. This can be difficult when you are nervous, so take your time to think before you speak. Recall the STAR technique described earlier in this chapter. Sometimes we are uncomfortable with silence and feel that we have to talk to avoid it. But taking a few moments to consider what you are going to say will result in better answers. Saying something meaningful after a pause is more important than simply responding quickly.

Nonverbal Communication: It Can Make You or Break You

"If you want a quality, act as if you already have it."
—William James

You can speak smoothly and answer questions correctly and yet fail in your communication efforts. What has gone wrong? Your actions have betrayed you. That's right: what you do communicates as much as—or even more than—what you say. As we discussed in Chapter 4, our movements, posture, gestures, and facial expressions usually reveal our true feelings. You can enthusiastically claim that you would love the challenge of working in a fast-paced, think-on-your-feet clinical environment. But if your face and body language reflect fear, anxiety, or subtle expressions of "yuck!," your verbal message will not ring true. Remember that more than half of the meaning of our messages is communicated nonverbally. This is why videotaping yourself is very helpful when practicing interviewing skills. You can observe your nonverbal language and catch inappropriate facial expressions and other behaviors that might betray your words.

The point is not to suggest that you should try to mask your true feelings and put on an act to impress interviewers. Rather, the purpose of this discussion is to encourage you to be aware of how important your actions are and what they say about you. If there are aspects of a job you know you can't or don't want to perform, this is the time to find out. Keep in mind that one of your goals in an interview is to learn about the job and the organization so you can decide whether this is the place for you.

Developing a positive attitude about the interviewing process and having confidence in your own abilities will help ensure that your body language communicates appropriate positive messages. At the same time, developing the body language of a positive, confident person will help you become that person.

USING YOUR PORTFOLIO WISELY

Portfolios are gaining popularity among job seekers, including those in the health care field. They can be a very effective way to support your claims of competence by providing evidence of your accomplishments and qualifications.

Not all employers are familiar with portfolios. Announcing at the beginning of interviews that you have brought one and asking interviewers if they would like to see it is not the most effective way of using it to your advantage. Remember that one of your main goals at the interview is to show how you meet the employer's needs. You won't know enough about these needs until you spend a little time listening. Then you may be able to use your portfolio constructively. The following interviewer questions and statements might be answered with material in your portfolio:

1. Asks a question about your skills and abilities
   "Can you . . . ?"
   "Have you had experience . . . ?"
2. States what skills are needed or provides a job description
   "This job requires . . ."
   "We need someone who can use medical terminology correctly and chart accurately."
3. Shares a problem or concern
   "One of our problems has been with ensuring accurate documentation . . ."
   "We have difficulties with . . ."
4. Isn't familiar with the contents of your training program
   "Did your program include . . . ?"
   "What skills did you learn . . . ?"
5. "Asks for verification of licenses, certifications, and so on
   "Have you passed the ________________ exam?"
   "Are you a certified medical assistant?"
   "Are you licensed in this state?"

It isn't necessary—or even a good idea—to try to back up everything you say with your portfolio. In fact, if overused, a portfolio loses its effectiveness. And many questions are better answered with an oral explanation and/or example.

Become very familiar with your portfolio's contents so you can find items quickly. If necessary, create an easy-to-read table of contents. Frantically flipping through pages to find something will make you look (and feel) unprepared and disorganized. You will also waste valuable time, a very limited resource in most interviews.

Use your portfolio to give a brief summary presentation if you are given an opportunity at the end of the interview. For example, the interviewer might say, "Tell me why I should hire you," or ask, "What else should I know about you?" Use this presentation to quickly review your qualifications or to point out those that haven't been mentioned.

You may attend interviews where you don't use your portfolio at all. This is okay. It is always better—both during the job search and on the job—to be overprepared. This prevents you from missing opportunities when they do present themselves.

HANDLING STICKY INTERVIEW SITUATIONS

In spite of your best efforts, some interviews can be a little rocky. Remember, not every employer is skilled at interviewing. Consider this: you may have prepared and practiced more than the person conducting the interview! Table 12-2 contains difficult situations and suggestions for handling them gracefully. Keep in mind that the questions reveal something about the interviewer and possibly about the organization, so consider them when deciding if this is a place you want to work.

Dealing with Illegal Questions

It is illegal for employers to discriminate against an applicant on the basis of any of the following factors:

- Age (as long as the applicant is old enough to work legally)
- Arrests (without a conviction—being proven guilty)
- Ethnic background
- Financial status
- Marital status and children
- Physical condition (as long as the applicant can perform the job tasks)
- Race
- Religion
- Sexual orientation

Questions that require the applicant to reveal information about these factors are illegal. They are sometimes asked anyway. Some employers are ignorant of the laws. Or the interview becomes friendly and conversational, and personal information is shared. ("Oh, I went to Grady High School, too. What year did you graduate?") Employers may take the chance that applicants won't know the questions are illegal. And a few will ask because they know that most applicants will not take the time to report them for discrimination. It may not be obvious from the questions that answering them will, in fact, reveal information that cannot be considered when hiring. Take a look at the following examples:

Question	What It Can Reveal
What part of town do you live in?	Financial status
Do you own your home?	Financial status
Where are your parents from?	Ethnic background
Which holidays do you celebrate?	Religion
When did you graduate from high school?	Age

Illegal questions put you in a difficult situation, and there are no easy formulas for handling them. In deciding

TABLE 12-2 Handling Difficult Interview Situations

If the Interviewer	What You Can Do
Keeps you waiting a long time.	If you are interested in the job, do not show annoyance or anger. It is best not to schedule interviews when you have a very limited amount of time. Remember, this person may be overworked, and that's exactly why there is a potential position for you! Keep in mind that health care work does not always proceed at our convenience. A patient with an emergency, for example, will certainly have priority over an interviewee.
Allows constant interruptions with phone calls and/or people coming in.	Again, do not show that you are irritated. This person may be very busy, disorganized, or simply having a difficult day. (This could be another good sign that this employer really needs your help.)
Does most of the talking and doesn't give you an opportunity to say much about yourself.	Listen carefully, and try to determine how your qualifications relate to what you are hearing. Being a good listener in itself may be the most important quality you can demonstrate.
Seems to simply make conversation. Doesn't discuss the job or ask you questions.	Try to move the discussion to the job by asking questions: "Can you tell me about what you are looking for in a candidate?" "What are the principal duties that this person would perform?" It is possible that this is a test to see your reaction, so take care to be courteous.
Tries to engage you in gossip about school, etc.	Say you don't really know about the person or other professionals, facilities, or situation and cannot comment. Ask a question about the job to redirect the conversation.
Allows long periods of silence.	This may be a test to see how you react under pressure. Don't feel that you have to speak, and do your best to remain comfortable. (Say to yourself, "This is just a test, and I'm doing fine.") If it goes on too long, you can ask: "Is there something you'd like me to tell you more about? Discuss further?"
Doesn't seem to understand your training or qualifications.	Explain as clearly as possible. Use your portfolio, as appropriate, to illustrate your skills.
Makes inappropriate comments about your appearance, gender, ethnicity, etc.	Depending on the nature of the comment and your interpretation of the situation, it may be best to excuse yourself from the interview. For example, comments of a sexual nature or racial slurs should not be tolerated. You should discuss this situation with your instructor or career services department for advice on how to proceed.
Is very friendly, chatty, and complimentary about you.	Why in the world, you ask, is this a problem? It may not be. But be careful not to get so comfortable that you share personal problems and other information that may disqualify you for the job.

what to do, you need to ask yourself the following questions:

- Is the subject of the question of concern to me?
- Do I find the question offensive?
- Does the interviewer appear to be unaware that the question is illegal?
- What is my overall impression of the interviewer and the facility?
- Would I want to work here?
- How badly do I want this particular job?
- If this person is to be my immediate supervisor, is the question an indication that this is a person I don't really want to work with?
- What do I think the interviewer's real concern is? Is it valid?

Based on your answers, there are several ways you can respond to the interviewer.

1. Answer honestly.
2. Ask the interviewer to explain how the question relates to the job requirements.
3. Respond to the interviewer's apparent concern rather than to the question.
4. Ignore the question and talk about something else.
5. Refuse to answer.
6. Inform the interviewer that the question is illegal.
7. Excuse yourself from the interview and leave.
8. State that you plan to report the incident to the Civil Rights Commission or Equal Employment Opportunity Commission.

Employers do have the right—as well as the responsibility—to make sure that applicants can both physically and legally perform the job requirements. Sometimes there is only a small difference in wording between a legal and an illegal question, as in the following examples[4]:

Illegal	Legal
How old are you?	Are you over 18?
Where were you born?	Do you have the legal right to work in the United States?
What is your maiden name?	Would your work records be listed under another name?
Have you ever been arrested?	Have you ever been convicted of a crime?

Are you beginning to understand how employers can get confused and ask illegal questions? It is possible to be an excellent dentist or physical therapist but not an expert in the details of employment law. However you choose to respond to questions you believe are illegal, it is best to remain calm and courteous. You may decide you don't want to work there, but conduct yourself professionally at all times.

Many employment experts recommend that you respond to the employer's concerns rather than the questions. This requires that you determine what the concerns are.

One recommended strategy for handling common employer concerns is to bring them up before the interviewer does. This gives you the opportunity to present them in a positive light. Employers may be uncomfortable addressing certain issues and will simply drop you from the "possible hire" list. By taking the initiative, you gain the opportunity to defend your position and stay on the list. Table 12-3 contains suggestions for showing the employer the positive aspects of various employment "problems."

STAY FOCUSED ON THE POSITIVE

"Employers are hiring based on attitude: "Give me a 'C' student with an 'A' attitude."

—Melva Duran

Interviews are a time to do your best to stay positive. They are not the place to bring up problems or what you believe you can't do or don't want to do. Be positive and future-oriented, and prepared to emphasize the following:

- What you can do
- How you can help
- Ways you can apply what you've learned

As mentioned before, you should never criticize a previous employer, instructor, or anyone else. Potential employers realize they may someday be your previous employer and don't want to be the subject of your comments to others in the profession. It is also possible that the interviewer is a friend of the person you are criticizing!

Keep in mind that every interview is a sales presentation. A sales presentation is not the time to point out the product's faults. You want to emphasize the positive aspects of your skills and character, not your weaknesses. However, if you sincerely feel that you are not qualified for a job (and this is an important consideration in health care), you should never pretend that you are. Lacking needed skills is not a negative reflection on you as a person. It simply means that this job is not appropriate for you. Other jobs will be. In fact, there may be many reasons why jobs and applicants do not match. After all, that's the whole purpose of job interviews—for you and the employer to make that determination.

Discussion of personal problems should always be avoided. You are there to help solve the employer's problems, not find solutions to your own. Employers are looking for independent problem solvers. Bringing your own problems to the interview will not give them a good impression of your capabilities in this area. (There are exceptions. For example, if you are responsible for a disabled family member and need some consideration regarding your work schedule, it would be appropriate to mention this at the interview.)

Focusing on your own needs is negatively received by employers. Giving the impression that you are more concerned with what you can get from the job than what you can give is a sure way to get nothing at all. The following questions send the message "What's in it for me?" and should be avoided until you know you are actually being considered for the job:

TABLE 12-3 Point Out the Positives

The Problem	The Bright Side
You're very young, with little work experience.	You are energetic, eager to learn, "trainable," and looking for long-term employment. ("One of the advantages of being young is....")
You have a criminal record.*	You have learned from your mistakes and are eager to have an opportunity to serve others.
You're over age 40.	You are experienced, have good work habits, and are patient.
You've had many jobs, none for very long.	You have a variety of experiences, are flexible, can adjust to the working environment, and have now found a career to which you want to dedicate your efforts.

*Note: Some states do not allow individuals who have been convicted of specific crimes to work in certain health care occupations. In some cases, these individuals are not even allowed to take certification exams.

- How much does the job pay?
- What are the other benefits?
- How many paid holidays will I get?
- Is Friday a casual day?
- Can I leave early if I finish my work?
- When will I get a raise?

It is acceptable to inquire about the work schedule, duties, and other expectations. The time to negotiate specific conditions, including your salary, is after you have been offered the job.

IT'S YOUR INTERVIEW, TOO

Interviews are not only for the benefit of employers. You have the right, and the responsibility, to evaluate the opportunities presented by the jobs you are applying for. This may seem to contradict what we discussed in the previous section, but it doesn't. In fact, well-stated questions about the job communicate motivation and interest.

When you are in class, it is generally true that "there are no stupid questions." However, at a job interview, the quality of your questions does count. There is a difference between questions that should be avoided and ones that demonstrate that you:

- Have a sincere interest in the job
- Want to understand the employer's needs
- Understand the nature of health care work
- Have thought about your career goal
- Want information that will enable you to do your best

What you ask will depend on the job, the interviewer, and how much you already know about the job and the organization. It is a good idea to prepare in advance a list of general questions, along with a few that are specific to the job and the facility. This will help you remember what you want to ask. As we pointed out earlier, it is easy to forget when we feel under pressure, as may happen in the interview situation. Not everyone is skilled at "thinking in the seat," especially when it feels like the hot seat!

Here are a few suggested questions to get you started:

1. How could I best contribute to the success of this facility?
2. What are the most important qualities needed to succeed in this position?
3. What is the mission of this organization or facility?
4. What are the major problems faced by this organization or facility?
5. How is the organization structured? Who would I be reporting to?
6. What values are most important?
7. I want to continue learning and updating my skills. What opportunities would I have to do this?
8. How will I be evaluated and learn what I need to improve?
9. Are there opportunities for advancement for employees who work hard and perform well?

It is perfectly acceptable to ask questions throughout the interview where they fit in. This will be more natural and lead to a smoother interview than asking a long list at the end. You don't have to wait until you are invited to ask them.

In addition to asking questions, observe the facility and the people who work there. Does this "feel" like a place you would want to work? Is it clean? Organized? Does it appear that safety precautions are followed? What is the pace? Are the people who work there courteous and helpful? How do they interact with patients and with each other? If your interview is with the person who would be your supervisor, do you think you would get along? Do you believe you would fit in?

It may not be possible for you to see anything other than the interviewer's office. In fact, at a large facility your first interview may take place in the personnel office. You won't see the area where you would work. If this is the case, you will want to ask for a tour if you are offered a job.

LEAVING GRACIOUSLY

The end of the interview provides you an opportunity to make a final impression, so make it a good one. It is important to be sensitive to any signals the interviewer gives that it is time to wrap up. Failure to do so shows a lack of consideration for his or her time, and this is definitely not the parting message you want to leave. Some interviewers will make it obvious the interview is almost over by doing the following:

- Telling you directly
- Asking whether you have any "final" questions
- Telling you that everything has been covered

Less obvious signs include looking at his or her watch, clock, appointment book, or papers on the desk; pushing his or her chair back; or saying that the interviewer has "taken enough of your time." Show respect for the interviewer's time by moving along with the final steps of the interview:

1. Ask any final questions (limit these to a couple of the most important ones that haven't been answered).
2. Make a brief wrap-up statement.
3. Thank the interviewer for his or her time.
4. Inquire about what comes next.

If you are interested in the job, say so in the wrap-up statement. Tell the interviewer why you believe you can make a contribution; what impressed you about the organization; why you believe your qualifications fit the position; and so on. Express your enthusiasm about working there and state that you hope you are chosen for the position.

Whether you want the job or not, always thank the interviewer for his or her time. This applies even if the interview did not go well. Health care professionals and personnel staff are extremely busy. Let them know how much you appreciate being given the opportunity to present your qualifications.

Finally, if you aren't told about the next step in the application process, don't hesitate to ask. Inquire about when the hiring decision will be made. Find out if there is anything you need to send. If asked, give the interviewer your reference sheet. Be sure to get the interviewer's last name and correct title. An easy way to do this is to ask for his or her business card. And be sure that he or she has your telephone number and any other information needed to contact you. Then smile, give a firm handshake, and leave as confidently as you entered, regardless of how you believe the interview went.

COMPLETING AN IMPORTANT STEP

"You wouldn't be nervous if you didn't care."

—Robert Lock

You may be feeling a little—maybe very—overwhelmed at this point. "How can I remember all this and act natural and maintain eye contact and give good examples and . . . ?" It is a lot, and that's why it is so important to spend time learning about the interviewing process, preparing, and practicing. Take every opportunity to role-play. Make your practice sessions as realistic as possible. Figure 12-1 contains a summary list of positive interview behaviors.

When you inventoried your skills, were you surprised at how much you can do now that you would never have attempted before you started your educational program? You learned these skills by studying and practicing them—over and over. If you have been working on developing these skills, this is your chance to use them for job success. You are almost certainly more qualified for the job search than you realize. And using your skills to get a job will reinforce your ability to use them once you are on the job.

A final note: It's okay to be nervous. It can even be a good thing, because it means you are not taking this experience for granted. Interviewers know you are nervous, and it tells them that this job is important to you and that you care about the outcome. This is a positive message to communicate.

REWARD YOURSELF

"Celebrate all successes on the job search journey."

Attending an interview is a success, whether or not you are hired for a particular job. You have qualifications that were worthy of the interviewer's time, you prepared well, and you met the challenge of presenting yourself one-on-one to a potential employer. Take a moment to reward yourself for completing this important step.

MAXIMIZE THE INTERVIEW EXPERIENCE

"Nothing is a waste of time if you use the experience wisely."

—Auguste Rodin

Making the most of every interview means that you view each one as an experience that provides opportunities to improve your presentation skills and to learn more about the health care world. This knowledge can help you in future interviews and work-related situations such as performance evaluations. When you leave the interviewer's office, your reaction may be "Whew! That's over!" and the last thing you want to do is spend more time thinking about it. This is especially true if you feel the interview didn't go well. But this is precisely when you need to spend some time thinking about and evaluating the experience and your performance. Using an interview evaluation sheet will help you focus on the important factors that determine the success of an interview and create a plan for improvement. Make copies of the form provided in Prescription for Success 12-1, and keep a record of your interviews in your job-search notebook.

You might want to discuss your self-evaluation with someone you trust. Sometimes we are too hard on ourselves and need a second point of view to help us see the real situation. Review the interview with your instructor, career services personnel, or mentor. You may have friends and family members who can provide insight and support. Create an improvement plan and practice so you'll feel more confident at the next interview.

When seeking help or discussing interviews with others, it is best not to make negative remarks about the interviewer or the facility. This serves no purpose, unless you are seeking advice about whether to accept a job you have doubts about. A friend may have a friend who works there, and your words, said "in confidence," may be passed along to the wrong party.

You may believe you will receive a job offer. You very well might. But don't cancel or turn down other interviews until you are formally hired. You may have done a superb job and the facility plans to hire you. Then the next day, your soon-to-be supervisor is informed of a facility-wide hiring freeze. You don't want to be left out in the cold with no other options. You may even find something better before they make the offer. Stay actively involved in the search until you have a job.

THANK YOU LETTER

Whether the interview went like a dream or a nightmare, send a thank-you note. This courtesy is something many

At the Interview:
How To Show You've Got What It Takes

Employers want to hire someone who is:	How to show that you are that someone:
Qualified to perform the job	1. Be familiar with and able to document all your skills 2. Create a portfolio that contains evidence of your qualifications
Reliable	1. Arrive on time to the interview 2. Send any requested follow-up materials
Trustworthy	1. Have a good handshake 2. Maintain appropriate eye contact 3. Include only accurate information on your resume and job application 4. Do not lie during your interview 5. Avoid saying anything negative about a previous employer 6. Do not engage in any type of gossip
Professional	1. Dress appropriately 2. Be clean and well-groomed 3. Bring needed materials to interview
Motivated and willing to learn	1. Know something about the facility and why you want to work there 2. Ask questions about the job 3. Inquire about learning opportunities on the job 4. Have a plan for professional development
A good communicator and able to work well with others	1. Show consideration for everyone at the interview site 2. Introduce yourself 3. Behave courteously 4. Listen actively throughout the interview 5. Use feedback appropriately to check your understanding of the speaker's message 6. Answer all questions completely but concisely 7. Speak clearly and with proper expression
Likable	1. Smile 2. Be enthusiastic 3. Have a sense of humor 4. Show interest in job 5. Express interest in employer's needs 6. Be comfortable with yourself 7. Show respect for interviewer 8. Avoid showing impatience, annoyance
A problem-solver	1. Describe examples of problems solved in the past 2. Be prepared and willing to participate in any problem-solving exercises given 3. Suggest specific ways you can help the employer

FIGURE 12-1 The interview is your sales opportunity.

job seekers don't do. Yet it is a simple action that can set you apart from the others. Suppose the employer interviewed nine people in 2 days, in addition to carrying on a normal workload. Tired? Very likely. Able to remember each candidate clearly and recall who said what? Maybe. But why take the chance of being lost in the crowd?

If you know for sure that you don't want the job, send a thank-you note anyway. Keep it simple, say something positive about the interview, and express your appreciation for the time taken to meet with you. Do not say that you are not interested in the job. Figure 12-2 is an example of this kind of note.

Why, you might ask, would you write if you don't want to work there? There are at least three good reasons:

1. The employer may know someone else who is hiring. Impressed by your follow-up, he or she recommends you.

1642 Windhill Way
San Antonio, TX 78220
October 18, 2010

Nancy Henderson, Office Manager
Craigmore Pediatric Clinic
4979 Coffee Road
San Antonio, TX 78229

Dear Ms. Henderson:

Thank you so much for the time you spent with me yesterday. You have a busy schedule, and I appreciate the time you took to describe the opening for a medical assistant at Craigmore Pediatric. The Clinic enjoys a good reputation in San Antonio for the services it provides children in the community, and it was a pleasure to learn more about it.

Sincerely,

Karen Gonzalez

Karen Gonzalez

FIGURE 12-2 A simple thank-you letter.

2. An opening for a job that you do want becomes available at this facility. You are remembered for your thoughtfulness.
3. At this time, when courtesy and consideration for others are disappearing, it is the right thing to do.

Thank You–Plus Letter

If you want the job (see the next section for how-tos on making that decision), then take the time to write a thank-you–plus letter. The "plus" refers to a paragraph or two in which you do at least one of the following:

- Briefly summarize your qualifications in relation to the job as it was discussed in the interview
- Point out specifically how you can make a positive contribution—again, based on details you learned

Let the employer know you want the job and hope to be the candidate selected. Include your full name and telephone number.

Thank-you notes should be sent no later than the day after the interview. Consider keeping a box of cards in the car and writing the note immediately after you leave the interview. Interviewers will be impressed when they receive your note the very next day.

For some jobs, such as administrative positions, e-mailing a thank-you note may be acceptable because it demonstrates computer proficiency. Take the same care you would with a written letter: include a salutation, write complete sentences, use correct grammar, spell all words correctly, and use a proper closing.

ALERT YOUR REFERENCES

If you left a reference sheet with the interviewer, call your references as soon as possible to tell them they may receive a call. Of course, they already know that you have given their names out as references. (You did ask them, right?) Give them the job title, nature of the work, and type of facility. Add anything you learned about the type of candidate the employer is seeking. This gives your references an opportunity to stress those features that best support your bid for the job. Help them to help you by keeping them informed.

WHEN TO CALL BACK

Following up after an interview is a kind of balancing act: you don't want to be considered a pest by calling too soon and too frequently. On the other hand, you took the time to attend the interview and have a right to be informed when the hiring decision is made.

The best strategy is to wait until the day after you were told a decision would be made. Call and identify yourself and inquire about the decision. If none has been made, ask when you might expect to hear. Use your best telephone manners. This is still part of the interview, and courtesy counts. Never express impatience about a delay. You want to show interest, but you don't want to pressure the employer for a decision he or she is not ready to make. Sometimes the interviewer is deciding between two candidates and the decision may be influenced by your follow-up.

IS THIS THE JOB FOR YOU?

Jobs are usually not offered on the spot during the first interview. If this does happen to you, it is a good idea to ask when a decision is needed and say that you are very interested (if you are) but need a little time to make a decision. There are exceptions, of course. You may have performed your clinical work at this site and know for sure that this is the place for you. In this case, the interview may be a formality and it makes sense to accept the position immediately.

Interviewers will usually give you a time range during which a hiring decision will be made. You, too, need to make a decision: if this position is offered, will you accept it? Many factors will influence your decision. In Chapter 10, we discussed how the job market is affected by various economic and governmental conditions. When the unemployment rate is high, you probably can't be as choosy about the job you take. In fact, you may have very few choices, because there will be more candidates competing for a limited number of positions. You can be more selective when the unemployment rate is low. Of course, your location and specific occupation will influence the number of opportunities available to you. Some parts of the country are highly desirable places to live, and competition is intense. And some occupations will be in either high or low demand, depending on current health care trends.

Although you should consider these questions carefully, remember that the job that is "exactly what you want" probably doesn't exist. Finding the right job for you is a matter of finding a close match on the most important elements. You are starting a new career, and there are certain factors that will help your long-term success. Working with someone who is interested in teaching you, for example, may be a better choice than choosing a slightly higher-paying position that offers no opportunities for acquiring new skills. Many health care facilities make it a practice to promote from within. If there is a facility where you want to work, consider taking a job that gets you in the door.

DISCUSSING SALARY: WHEN AND HOW

Most career experts recommend that you not discuss salary with a potential employer until you have been offered the job. In many cases, this won't be an issue because salaries are predetermined and not negotiable. Some occupations, such as nursing, have labor unions, and the employer cannot change agreed-on salaries for specific positions.

Doing your research before you attend an interview may provide you with this information. If a range of salary is given for a position, the amount offered to you will most likely depend on the experience you bring to the job. Recent graduates tend to start at the low end of a range, earning more as they gain experience.

CONSIDERING AN OFFER

A job offer may be extended in a telephone call, at a second or even third interview, or in a letter. Even if you feel quite sure that this is the right job, you still need to be sure that you have all the information needed to make a final decision. It is essential that you understand the following:

- The exact duties you will be required to perform. If you haven't seen a written job description, ask for it now. If there is no written description, ask for a detailed oral explanation if this wasn't done in the interview.
- Start date. Be sure you are clear about the exact date and time you are to report for work.

- The days and hours you will work. Ask about the likelihood of required overtime and any change of hours or days that might take place in the future.
- Your salary. Earnings are expressed in various ways: hourly, weekly, biweekly, monthly, or annual rates. If you are quoted a rate that you aren't familiar with, you might want to convert it to one you know. For example, if you are accustomed to thinking in terms of amount per hour but are given a monthly salary, you may want to calculate the hourly equivalent.
- Orientation and/or training given. This is especially important for recent graduates. Learning the customs and practices of the facility can make a big difference in your success. Letting the employer know that you are interested in learning as much as possible about the facility and the job communicates the message that you are motivated and interested in being prepared to do your best.

You may have received all this information in the interview(s). Don't hesitate, however, to ask about anything you don't fully understand. It is far better to take the time now rather than to discover later that the job or working conditions were not what you expected. If you didn't have an opportunity to see any more than the interviewer's office, be sure to ask for a complete tour of the facility before deciding whether to accept the job.

UNDERSTANDING BENEFITS

Benefits can represent a significant portion of your compensation. Health insurance, for example, can cost hundreds of dollars per month for a family of four. If full family coverage is offered by the employer, this may be worth thousands of dollars each year. Find out if you must pay part of the cost of the premiums and what type of coverage is provided. Health insurance for individuals (or families) is often more expensive than the group rates available through an employer. And many individuals find it difficult to qualify on their own. Health insurance is becoming an increasingly important benefit to consider when choosing where to work. There are other types of insurance, too, that can add value to the benefits package, including dental, vision, life, and disability.

If you are planning to continue your education, tuition benefits might be important to you. Some employers cover all or part of educational expenses if the studies are related to your work and you receive a grade of C or better. Time off to take classes and workshops is an additional advantage. This benefit is especially helpful for health care professionals who are required to earn continuing education units on a regular basis. Related professional expenses that some employers cover are the dues for professional organizations and required uniforms.

Other benefits to consider when calculating your overall compensation include the number of paid vacation, holiday, and personal days offered and whether there is a retirement plan such as a 401(k) retirement plan. With this plan, you choose an amount to be deducted from your earnings each pay period. You pay no taxes on this money until you withdraw it anytime after you reach age 59½. The money is invested, often in mutual funds. Some employers match a certain percentage of the money you save, which is like giving you an additional, tax-free salary.

When considering the compensation offered by an employer, think in terms of the total package. One job may offer a higher hourly rate but require you to pay part of your health insurance premium. You may end up financially ahead by accepting the lower salary. On the other hand, if you are included on your spouse's group insurance plan, this might not be significant. Salary alone should not be the determining factor when deciding whether a job "pays enough."

Let's look at an example. Suppose you are offered Job A, which pays $24,000 and includes medical insurance, for which the employer pays $2700. The total value of this package, then, is $26,700. Another employer offers you Job B at $27,000 in salary with no insurance benefits. You need insurance and plan to pay for it yourself with the extra salary you will earn. Assuming that everything else about the two jobs is equal, with which one would you come out ahead financially? Almost certainly Job A. Let's see why.

1. You will pay taxes on wages of $24,000 rather than $27,000. (Health insurance benefits are not taxed.)
2. The $2700 for medical insurance is the cost for a member of a group plan. If you buy insurance as an individual, it may cost you even more. (And you may have to qualify medically, which makes it more difficult to get.)

Job A

$24,000 – $7200 (standard tax deduction and single exemption)	=	$16,800 (taxable income)
$16,800 × 15% tax rate	=	$2520 (taxes)
$24,000 – $2520	=	$21,480 (amount of money you keep)

Job B

$27,000 – $7200	=	$19,800 (taxable income)
$19,800 × 15%	=	$2970 (taxes)
$27,000 – $2970	=	$24,030
$24,030 – $2700 (amount spent on health insurance)	=	$21,330 (amount of money you keep)

The lesson here is to collect information and consider all aspects of the compensation plan. Although this was just an example, it shows how important it is to do the math. If you are unsure about how to do these calculations, ask for help. Your long-term financial health depends on it.

ACCEPTING AN OFFER

When you accept a job, express your appreciation and enthusiasm. In addition to responding orally, write a letter of acceptance. The letter should include a summary of what you understand to be the terms of employment.

When speaking with the employer, inquire about any necessary follow-up activities. It is also a good idea to disclose any future commitments or other factors that will affect your work. For example, if your son is scheduled for surgery next month and you know you will need to take several days off to take care of him, let the employer know this during the hiring process. It is a sign of integrity to make important disclosures before the hiring is completed. There may be little risk of losing the job by revealing reasonable, unavoidable future commitments. If the employer does refuse to accommodate you, it is better to learn now that this job lacks flexibility regarding family needs. You may want to reconsider your acceptance. (Be aware, however, that employers cannot grant repeated requests for days off because of family responsibilities. Their first responsibility must be to the patients they serve.)

You may want this job but need to negotiate some conditions. For example, suppose the work hours are 8:00 AM to 5:00 PM. You have a 3-year-old child who cannot be left at day care before 7:45 AM, and it takes at least 25 minutes to drive to work. It is better to ask if you can work from 8:30 AM to 5:30 PM than to take the position and arrive late every day. Many problems on the job can be avoided by discussing them openly in advance. (Again, you must also consider the employer's needs. Accommodations like this are not always possible if they disrupt the facility's schedule and patient flow.) And sometimes, having a "Plan B" will save the day—in this case, having someone reliable who can take your child to day care.

WHAT TO EXPECT

Once you are hired, employers can ask questions that were unacceptable during the hiring process. Information that cannot be used to make hiring decisions is often necessary to complete personnel requirements. Examples include the following[1]:

1. Provide proof of your age (to ensure you are of legal age to work).
2. Provide verification that you can legally work in the United States.
3. Identify your race (for affirmative action statistics, if applicable in your state).
4. Supply a photograph (for identification).
5. State your marital status and number and ages of your children (for insurance).
6. Give the name and address of a relative (for notification in case of emergency).
7. Provide your Social Security number (for tax purposes).

There may be mandatory health tests and immunizations. In addition, some employers require drug tests and background checks for all employees.

If you are asked to sign an employment contract, read it carefully first. As with all other employment issues, ask about anything you don't understand. Also, be sure to ask for a copy of anything you sign.

TURNING DOWN A JOB OFFER

After careful consideration, you may decide not to accept a job offer. It is not necessary to explain your reasons to the employer. Do express your appreciation and thanks for the opportunity, and do send a thank-you note. In addition to being an expression of courtesy, this leaves a positive impression on all employers. You may want to work at this facility in the future.

IF YOU DON'T GET THE JOB

"Failure is a delay, but not a defeat. It is a temporary detour, not a dead-end street."

—*William Arthur Ward*

It can be difficult when you are not selected for a job you really want. There are many reasons why applicants don't get hired. Some you can't change and must simply accept, such as the following:

- There was another applicant with more experience or skills that more closely met the employer's current needs.
- An employee in the organization decided to apply for the job.
- The employer believed that someone else was a better "match" for the organization in terms of work style, preferences, and so on.
- Budget cuts or other unexpected events prevented anyone from being hired at this time.

On the other hand, you may have lost this opportunity for reasons you can change. How do you know? First, do an honest review of your postinterview evaluation, school record, and resume. Are you presenting yourself in the best possible way? Second, look over the list in Box 12-2. Health care employers and career services personnel name these as major reasons why job applicants fail to get hired. Do you recognize anything that might apply to you?

You must be honest with yourself and commit to improving your attitude and/or job-search skills. If

BOX 12-2 Why Job Applicants Fail to Get Hired

1. Failure to sell themselves by clearly presenting their skills and qualifications
2. Too much interest in what's in it for them rather than what they can give
3. Unprofessional behavior or lack of courtesy
4. Lack of enthusiasm and interest in the job
5. Poor appearance
6. Poor communication skills
7. Unrealistic job expectations
8. Negative or critical attitude
9. Arrived late, brought children or the person who provided transportation, or other demonstrations of poor organizational skills

necessary, seek advice from your instructor, career services personnel, or mentor. Work on creating a winning attitude that will help you develop the interviewing skills it takes to get hired. Seek support from friends and family members if you are feeling down. They can help you keep your perspective and boost your self-confidence if it's a little low.

Although you may not feel enthusiastic about writing a note to an employer who chooses another applicant, consider this: you may have come in a close second. The next opening may be yours! So take a few moments and demonstrate your high level of professionalism by thanking the employer and letting him or her know that you are still interested in working for the organization.

If you don't get hired after attending an interview that you think went well, ask for assistance from an instructor or career services personnel. You may be able to get good feedback. Or perhaps this person can call the employer on your behalf to find out how you might improve your presentation or to see if you appeared to lack needed skills. Employers are sometimes more willing to share reasons with school personnel so they can better assist their students. Be willing to listen to any constructive criticism offered and to make any needed changes.

To Learn More

About.Com
http://jobsearch.about.com/od/interviewsnetworking/a/intfollowup.htm
"Job Interview Follow-Up"
http://jobsearch.about.com/cs/interviews/a/aceinterview.htm
Read about all aspects of interviewing, including behavioral interviews, proper interview behavior, and suggestions for dress.

Quintessential Careers
www.quintcareers.com/intvres.html
Gain access to dozens of articles and links to websites with information about interviewing, including examples of questions.
"Job Interview Follow-Up Do's and Don'ts"
www.quintcareers.com/interview_follow-up-dos-donts.html
"The Art of the Follow-Up after Job Interviews"
www.quintcareers.com/job_interview_follow-up.html
"Job Interview and Thank You Letters"
www.quintcareers.com/sample_thank-you_letters.html

REFERENCES

1. Lock RD: Job search, ed 3, Pacific Grove, Calif, 1996, Brooks/Cole.
2. Hansen K: Behavioral interviewing strategies for job-seekers. www.quintcareers.com/behavioral_interviewing.html (Accessed 2/27/09)
3. Cha AE: "Employers relying on personality tests to screen applicants." The Washington Post. March 27, 2005. Page A01. http://www.washingtonpost.com/ac2/wp-dyn/A4010-2005Mar26?language=printer (Accessed 3/1/09)
4. Graber S: The everything online job search book, Holbrook, Mass, 2000, Adams Media.
5. Lock RD: Job search: career planning guide, Book II, ed 3, Pacific Grove, Calif, 1996, Brooks/Cole.

CHAPTER

13

Code of Ethics and Standards of Practice

MASSAGE CODE OF ETHICS AND STANDARDS OF PRACTICE

Ethical Principles

The four basic principles that constitute the code of ethics for massage professionals are as follows:

- *Respect for the dignity of people*—Massage professionals will maintain respect for the interests, dignity, rights, and needs of all clients, staff, and colleagues.
- *Responsible caring*—Competent, quality client care will be provided at the highest standard possible.
- *Integrity in relationships*—At all times the professional will behave with integrity, honesty, and diligence in practice and duties.
- *Responsibility to society*—Massage professionals are responsible and accountable to society and shall conduct themselves in a manner that maintains high ethical standards.

Standards of Practice Based on Ethical Principles

In compliance with the principles of the code of ethics, massage professionals will perform the following:

1. Respect all clients, colleagues, and health professionals through nondiscrimination regardless of age, gender, race, national origin, sexual orientation, religion, socioeconomic status, body type, political affiliation, state of health, personal habits, and life-coping skills.
2. Perform only those services for which they are qualified and honestly represent their education, certification, professional affiliations, and other qualifications. The massage professional will apply treatment only when a reasonable expectation exists that it will be advantageous to the client's condition. The massage professional, in consultation with the client, will continually evaluate the effectiveness of treatment.
3. Respect the scope of practice of other health care and service professionals, including physicians, chiropractors, physical therapists, podiatrists, orthopedists, psychotherapists, counselors, acupuncturists, nurses, exercise physiologists, athletic trainers, nutritionists, spiritual advisors, and cosmetologists.
4. Respect all ethical health care practitioners and work with them to promote health and healing.
5. Acknowledge the limitations of their personal skills and, when necessary, refer clients to an appropriately qualified professional. The massage professional will require consultation with other knowledgeable professionals when:
   - A client requires diagnosis and opinion beyond a therapist's capabilities of assessment
   - A client's condition is beyond the scope of practice
   - A combined health care team is required

   If referral to another health care provider is necessary, it will be done with the informed consent of the client.
6. Refrain from working with any individual who has a specific disease process without supervision by a licensed medical professional.
7. Be adequately educated and understand the physiologic effects of the specific massage techniques used to determine if any application is contraindicated and to ensure that the most beneficial techniques are applied to a given individual.
8. Avoid false claims about the potential benefits of the techniques rendered and educate the public about the actual benefits of massage.
9. Acknowledge the importance and individuality of each person, including colleagues, peers, and clients.
10. Work only with the informed consent of a client and professionally disclose to the client any situation that may interfere with the massage professional's ability to provide the best care to serve the client's best interest.
11. Display respect for the client by honoring a client's process and following all recommendations by being present, listening, asking only pertinent questions, keeping agreements, being on time, draping properly, and customizing the massage to address the client's needs.

NOTE: Draping is covered in Chapter 8. The Ontario guidelines[2] specify these requirements for draping:

- It is the responsibility of the massage professional to ensure the privacy and dignity of the client and to determine whether the client feels comfortable, safe, and secure with the draping provided.
- The client may choose to be fully draped or clothed throughout the treatment.
- The female client's breasts are not undraped unless specified by referral from a qualified health care professional and the massage professional is working under the supervision of such a health care professional.
- The genitals, perineum, and anus are never undraped.

The client's consent is required for work on any part of the body, regardless of whether the client is fully clothed, fully draped, or partly draped.

12. Provide a safe, comfortable, and clean environment.
13. Maintain clear and honest communication with clients and keep client communications confidential. Confidentiality is of the utmost importance. The massage professional must inform the client that the referring physician may be eligible to review the client's records and that records may be subpoenaed by the courts.
14. Conduct business in a professional and ethical manner in relation to clientele, business associates, acquaintances, governmental bodies, and the public.
15. Follow city, county, state, national, and international requirements.
16. Charge a fair price for the session. Gratuities are appropriate if within reasonable limits. (Similar to percentages for other service providers, i.e., 10% to 20%.) A gift, gratuity, or benefit that is intended to influence a referral, decision, or treatment may not be accepted and must be returned to the giver immediately.
17. Keep accurate records and review the records with the client.
18. Never engage in any sexual conduct, sexual conversation, or any other sexual activities involving clients.
19. Avoid affiliation with any business that uses any form of sexual suggestiveness or explicit sexuality in advertising or promoting services or in the actual practice of service.
20. Practice honesty in advertising, promoting services ethically and in good taste and advertising only techniques for which the professional is certified or adequately trained.
21. Strive for professional excellence through regular assessment of personal strengths, limitations, and effectiveness and through continuing education and training.
22. Accept the responsibility to oneself, one's clients, and the profession to maintain physical, mental, and emotional well-being and to inform clients when the professional is not functioning at full capacity.
23. Refrain from using any mind-altering drugs, alcohol, or intoxicants before or during professional massage sessions.
24. Maintain a professional appearance and demeanor by practicing good hygiene and dressing in a professional, modest, and nonsexual manner.
25. Undergo periodic peer review.
26. Respect all pertinent reporting requirements outlined by legislation regarding abuse.
27. Report to the proper authorities any accurate knowledge and its supportive documentation regarding violations by massage professionals and other health or service professionals.
28. Avoid interests, activities, or influences that might conflict with the obligation to act in the best interest of clients and the massage therapy profession and safeguard professional integrity by recognizing potential conflicts of interest and avoiding them.

GOVERNMENTAL CREDENTIALS AND REGULATIONS

Licensing

- Requires a state or provincial board of examiners
- Requires all constituents who practice the profession to be licensed
- Legally defines and limits the scope of practice for a profession
- Requires specific educational courses or an examination
- Protects title usage (e.g., only those licensed can use the title of massage therapist)

Governmental Certification

- Administered by an independent board
- Voluntary but required for anyone using the protected title (e.g., massage therapist); others can provide the service but cannot call themselves massage therapists
- Requires specific educational courses and an examination

Governmental Registration

(Not to be confused with private registration processes)

- Administered by the state Department of Registry or other appropriate state agency

Voluntary Verification

- Does not necessarily require a specific education, such as a school diploma; often other forms of verification of professional standards, such as years in practice, are acceptable
- Does not provide title protection

Exemptions

- Means that a practitioner is not required to comply with an existing local or state regulation
- Excuses practitioners who meet specified educational requirements from meeting current regulatory requirements
- Does not provide title protection

STEPS FOR COMPLYING WITH LICENSING REQUIREMENTS

1. Find out whether your state or province requires licensing. Contact the Department of Licensing and Regulation, Occupational Licensing Division, for this information. If state licensing is required, find out what educational requirements must be met to take the examination.
2. If your state does not have licensing, contact the local government where you intend to work to inquire about local ordinances. Obtain a copy of the ordinances and read them carefully. Look especially for the educational, zoning, and facility requirements. Whether you live in a city, township, or similar government unit, the clerk's office is the department that usually has this information.

   NOTE: Even if there is no state or local regulation, attending only a licensed school or an approved training program is a good idea. Other states or local governments may require this type of education, and without it you cannot practice in their areas.
3. Shop carefully for your school of massage training. Contact the state Department of Education and confirm that the school is licensed and in compliance with state regulations.
4. Before renting, buying, or setting up your massage practice, contact the local government concerning zoning requirements and building codes. If you are considering a home office, check the zoning ordinances to make sure you will be in compliance. Again, your city or township officials (usually the clerk) are your best sources of information.

   Zoning permits require a public hearing. Your neighbors are notified by mail, and the hearing is advertised in the newspaper. Contact the zoning department to find out what action is required. Whether you are establishing your business in a home office or a business zone, contact the neighbors to explain your business and find out their response. Without their approval, or at least lack of opposition, you are unlikely to obtain a permit. Attend the hearing at all costs. Remember: *no permit = no business.* Zoning permits may require 6 to 8 weeks to complete. If you start your business without proper permits, you could be shut down at any time by government authorities.
5. Before you rent space or begin your business, contact the local government and apply for any necessary permits or business licenses. Make sure you meet all regulations. Fees can run anywhere from $25 to $500.

THE NATIONAL CERTIFICATION BOARD FOR THERAPEUTIC MASSAGE AND BODYWORK CODE OF ETHICS[1]

The Code of Ethics of the National Certification Board for Therapeutic Massage and Bodywork (NCBTMB) specifies professional standards that allow for the proper discharge of the massage therapist's and/or bodyworker's responsibilities to those served, that protect the integrity of the profession, and that safeguard the interest of individual clients.

Those practitioners nationally certified in therapeutic massage and bodywork in the exercise of professional accountability will conduct themselves as follows:

1. Have a sincere commitment to provide the highest quality of care to those who seek their professional services.
2. Represent their qualifications honestly, including education and professional affiliations, and provide only those services that they are qualified to perform.
3. Accurately inform clients, other health care practitioners, and the public of the scope and limitations of their discipline.
4. Acknowledge the limitations of and contraindications for massage therapy and bodywork, and refer clients to appropriate health professionals.
5. Provide treatment only when there is reasonable expectation that it will be advantageous to the client.
6. Consistently maintain and improve professional knowledge and competence, striving for professional excellence through regular assessment of personal and professional strengths and weaknesses and through continued educational training.
7. Conduct their business and professional activities with honesty and integrity, and respect the inherent worth of all people.
8. Refuse to unjustly discriminate against clients or other ethical health professionals.

9. Safeguard the confidentiality of all client information, unless disclosure is required by law, court order, or absolutely necessary for the protection of the public.
10. Respect the client's right to treatment with informed and voluntary consent. The NCTMB practitioner will obtain and record the informed consent of the client, or client's advocate, before providing treatment. This consent may be written or verbal.
11. Respect the client's right to refuse, modify, or terminate treatment regardless of prior consent given.
12. Provide draping and treatment in a way that ensures the safety, comfort, and privacy of the client.
13. Exercise the right to refuse to treat any person or part of the body for just and reasonable cause.
14. Refrain, under all circumstances, from initiating or engaging in any sexual conduct, sexual activities, or sexualizing behavior involving a client, even if the client attempts to sexualize the relationship.
15. Avoid any interest, activity, or influence that might be in conflict with the practitioner's obligation to act in the best interests of the client or the profession.
16. Respect the client's boundaries with regard to privacy, disclosure, exposure, emotional expression, beliefs, and the client's reasonable expectations of professional behavior. Practitioners will respect the client's autonomy.
17. Refuse any gifts or benefits that are intended to influence a referral, decision, or treatment and that are purely for personal gain and not for the good of the client.
18. Follow all policies, procedures, guidelines, regulations, codes, and requirements promulgated by the National Certification Board for Therapeutic Massage and Bodywork.

THE NATIONAL CERTIFICATION BOARD FOR THERAPEUTIC MASSAGE AND BODYWORK STANDARDS OF PRACTICE[2]

Standard I: Professionalism

The certificant must provide optimal levels of professional massage and bodywork services and demonstrate excellence in practice by promoting healing and well-being through responsible, compassionate, and respectful touch. In his or her professional role the certificant shall commit to the following:

1. Adhere to the NCBTMB Code of Ethics, Standards of Practice, policies, and procedures.
2. Comply with the peer review process conducted by the NCBTMB Ethics and Standards Committee regarding any alleged violations against the NCBTMB Code of Ethics and Standards of Practice.
3. Conduct themselves in a manner in all settings meriting the respect of the public and other professionals.
4. Treat each client with respect, dignity, and worth.
5. Use professional verbal, nonverbal, and written communications.
6. Provide an environment that is safe and comfortable for the client and which, at a minimum, meets all legal requirements for health and safety.
7. Use standard precautions to ensure professional hygienic practices and maintain a level of personal hygiene appropriate for practitioners in the therapeutic setting.
8. Wear clothing that is clean, modest, and professional.
9. Obtain voluntary and informed consent from the client before initiating the session.
10. If applicable, conduct an accurate needs assessment, develop a plan of care with the client, and update the plan as needed.
11. Use appropriate draping to protect the client's physical and emotional privacy.
12. Be knowledgeable of their scope of practice and practice only within these limitations.
13. Refer to other professionals when in the best interest of the client and/or practitioner.
14. Seek other professional advice when needed.
15. Respect the traditions and practices of other professionals and foster collegial relationships.
16. Not falsely impugn the reputation of any colleague.
17. Use the initials NCTMB to designate his or her professional ability and competency to practice therapeutic massage and bodywork only.
18. Remain in good standing with and maintain NCBTMB certification.
19. Understand that the NCBTMB certificate may be displayed prominently in the certificant's principal place of practice.
20. When using the NCBTMB logo and certification number on business cards, brochures, advertisements, and stationery, do so only in a manner that is within established NCBTMB guidelines.
21. Not duplicate the NCBTMB certificate for purposes other than verification of the practitioner's credentials.
22. Immediately return the certificate to NCBTMB if it is revoked or suspended.

Standard II: Legal and Ethical Requirements

The certificant must comply with all the legal requirements in applicable jurisdictions regulating the profession of massage therapy and bodywork. In his or her professional role the certificant shall commit to the following:

1. Obey all applicable local, state, and federal laws.
2. Refrain from any behavior that results in illegal, discriminatory, or unethical actions.
3. Accept responsibility for his or her own actions.
4. Report to the proper authorities any alleged violations of the law by other certificants.
5. Maintain accurate and truthful records.
6. Report to the NCBTMB any criminal convictions regarding himself or herself and other certificants.
7. Report to NCBTMB any pending litigation and resulting resolution related to his or her professional practice and the professional practice of other certificants.
8. Respect existing publishing rights and copyright laws.

Standard III: Confidentiality

The certificant shall respect the confidentiality of client information and safeguard all records. In his or her professional role the certificant shall commit to the following:

1. Protect the client's identity in social conversations, all advertisements, and any and all other manners unless requested by the client in writing, medically necessary, or required by law.
2. Protect the interests of clients who are minors or who are unable to give voluntary consent by securing permission from an appropriate third party or guardian.
3. Solicit only information that is relevant to the professional client/therapist relationship.
4. Share pertinent information about the client with third parties when required by law.
5. Maintain the client files for a minimum period of four years.
6. Store and dispose of client files in a secure manner.

Standard IV: Business Practices

The certificant shall practice with honesty, integrity, and lawfulness in the business of massage and bodywork. In his or her professional role the certificant shall commit to the following:

1. Provide a physical setting that is safe and meets all applicable legal requirements for health and safety.
2. Maintain adequate and customary liability insurance.
3. Maintain adequate progress notes for each client session, if applicable.
4. Accurately and truthfully inform the public of services provided.
5. Honestly represent all professional qualifications and affiliations.
6. Promote his or her business with integrity and avoid potential and actual conflicts of interest.
7. Advertise in a manner that is honest, dignified, and representative of services that can be delivered and remains consistent with the NCBTMB Code of Ethics.
8. Advertise in a manner that is not misleading to the public by, among other things, the use of sensational, sexual, or provocative language and/or pictures to promote business.
9. Comply with all laws regarding sexual harassment.
10. Not exploit the trust and dependency of others, including clients and employees or co-workers.
11. Display or discuss schedule of fees in advance of the session that are clearly understood by the client or potential client.
12. Make financial arrangements in advance that are clearly understood by and safeguard the best interests of the client or consumer.
13. Follow acceptable accounting practices.
14. File all applicable municipal, state and federal taxes.
15. Maintain accurate financial records, contracts and legal obligations, appointment records, tax reports, and receipts for at least 4 years.

Standard V: Roles and Boundaries

The certificant shall adhere to ethical boundaries and perform the professional roles designed to protect the client and practitioner and safeguard the therapeutic value of the relationship. In his or her professional role the certificant shall commit to the following:

1. Recognize his or her personal limitations and practice only within these limitations.
2. Recognize his or her influential position with the client and shall not exploit the relationship for personal or other gain.
3. Recognize and limit the impact of transference and countertransference between the client and the certificant.
4. Avoid dual or multidimensional relationships that could impair professional judgment or result in exploitation of the client or employees and/or co-workers.
5. Not engage in any sexual activity with a client.
6. Acknowledge and respect the client's freedom of choice in the therapeutic session.
7. Respect the client's right to refuse the therapeutic session.
8. Refrain from practicing under the influence of alcohol, drugs, or any illegal substances (with the exception of prescribed dosage of prescription medication, which does not significantly impair the certificant).
9. Have the right to refuse and/or terminate the service to a client who is abusive or under the influence of alcohol, drugs, or any illegal substance.

Standard VI: Prevention of Sexual Misconduct

The certificant shall refrain from any behavior that sexualizes, or appears to sexualize, the client/therapist relationship. The certificant recognizes that the intimacy of the therapeutic relationship may activate practitioner and/or client needs and/or desires that weaken objectivity and may lead to sexualizing the therapeutic relationship. In his or her professional role the certificant shall commit to the following:

1. Refrain from participating in a sexual relationship or sexual conduct with the client, whether consensual or otherwise, from the beginning of the client/therapist relationship and for a minimum of 6 months after the termination of the client/therapist relationship.
2. In the event that the client initiates sexual behavior, clarify the purpose of the therapeutic session, and if such conduct does not cease, terminate or refuse the session.
3. Recognize that sexual activity with clients, students, employees, supervisors, or trainees is prohibited even if consensual.
4. Not touch the genitalia.
5. Only perform therapeutic treatments beyond the normal narrowing of the ear canal and normal narrowing of the nasal passages as indicated in the plan of care and only after receiving informed voluntary written consent.
6. Only perform therapeutic treatments in the oropharynx as indicated in the plan of care and only after receiving informed voluntary consent.
7. Only perform therapeutic treatments into the anal canal as indicated in the plan of care and only after receiving informed voluntary written consent.
8. Only provide therapeutic breast massage as indicated in the plan of care and only after receiving informed voluntary consent from the client.

REFERENCES

1. From National Certification Board for Therapeutic Massage and Bodywork: Code of ethics (adopted 2/17/95), McLean, Va, The Board.
2. From National Certification Board for Therapeutic Massage and Bodywork: Code of ethics (adopted 2/17/95) and standards of practice (adopted 2/9/00), McLean, Va, The Board.

CHAPTER

14

Medical Terminology

TABLE 14-1 Common Root Words

Root (Combining Vowel)	Meaning	Root (Combining Vowel)	Meaning
abdomin (o)	Abdomen	neur (o)	Nerve
aden (o)	Gland	ocul (o) Eye	Eye
adren (o)	Adrenal gland	orth (o)	Straight, normal, correct
angi (o)	Vessel	oste (o)	Bone
arterio (o)	Artery	ot (o)	Ear
arthr (o)	Joint	ped (o)	Child, foot
broncho (o)	Bronchus, bronchi	pharyng (o)	Pharynx
card, cardi (o)	Heart	phleb (o)	Vein
cephal (o)	Head	pnea	Breathing, respiration
chondr (o)	Cartilage	pneum (o)	Lung, air, gas
col (o)	Colon	proct (o)	Rectum
cost (o)	Rib	psych (o)	Mind
crani (o)	Skull	pulm (o)	Lung
cyan (o)	Blue	py (o)	Pus
cyst (o)	Bladder, cyst	rect (o)	Rectum
cyt (o)	Cell	rhin (o)	Nose
derma	Skin	sten (o)	Narrow, constriction
duoden (o)	Duodenum	stern (o)	Sternum
encephal (o)	Brain	stomat (o)	Mouth
enter (o)	Intestines	therm (o)	Heat
fibro (o)	Fiber, fibrous	thorac (o)	Chest
gastr (o)	Stomach	thromb (o)	Clot, thrombus
gyn, gyne, gyneco	Female	thyr (o)	Thyroid
hem, hema, hemo, hemat (o)	Blood	toxic(o)	Poison, poisonous
hepat (o)	Liver	trache (o)	Trachea
hydr (o)	Water	ur (o)	Urine, urinary tract, urination
hyster (o)	Uterus	urethr (o)	Urethra
ile (o), ili (o)	Ileum	urin (o)	Urine
laryng (o)	Larynx	uter (o)	Uterus
mamm (o)	Breast, mammary gland	vas (o)	Blood vessel, vas deferens
my (o)	Muscle	ven (o)	Vein
myel (o)	Spinal cord, bone marrow	vertebr (o)	Spine, vertebrae
nephr (o)	Kidney		

TABLE 14-2 Common Prefixes

Prefix	Meaning	Prefix	Meaning
a-, an-	Without or not	intro-	Into, within
ab-	Away from	leuk-	White
ad-	Toward	macro-	Large
ante-	Before, forward	mal-	Bad, illness, disease
anti-	Against	mega-	Large
auto-	Self	micro-	Small
bi-	Double, two	mono-	One, single
circum-	Around	neo-	New
contra-	Against, opposite	non-	Not
de-	Down, from, away from, not	para-	Abnormal
dia-	Across, through, apart	per-	By, through
dis-	Separation, away from	peri-	Around
dys-	Bad, difficult, abnormal	poly-	Many, much
ecto-	Outer, outside	post-	After, behind
en-	In, into, within	pre-	Before, in front of, prior to
endo-	Inner, inside	pro-	Before, in front of
epi-	Over, on	re-	Again
eryth-	Red	retro-	Backward
ex-	Out, out of, from, away from	semi-	Half
hemi-	Half	sub-	Under
hyper-	Excessive, too much, high	super-	Above, over, excess
hypo-	Under, decreased, less than normal	supra-	Above, over
in-	In, into, within, not	trans-	Across
inter-	Between	uni-	One
intra-	Within		

TABLE 14-3 Common Suffixes

Suffix	Meaning	Suffix	Meaning
-algia	Pain	-megaly	Enlargement
-asis	Condition, usually abnormal	-oma	Tumor
-cele	Hernia, herniation, pouching	-osis	Condition
-cyte	Cell	-pathy	Disease
-ectasis	Dilation, stretching	-penia	Lack, deficiency
-ectomy	Excision, removal of	-phasia	Speaking
-emia	Blood condition	-phobia	Exaggerated fear
-genesis	Development, production, creation	-plasty	Surgical repair or reshaping
-genic	Producing, causing	-plegia	Paralysis
-gram	Record	-rrhage, -rrhagia	Excessive flow
-graph	Diagram, recording instrument	-rrhea	Profuse flow, discharge
-graphy	Making a recording	-scope	Examination instrument
-iasis	Condition of	-scopy	Examination using a scope
-ism	Condition	-stasis	Maintenance, maintaining a constant level
-itis	Inflammation	-stomy, -ostomy	Creation of an opening
-logy	Study of	-tomy, -otomy	Incision, cutting into
-lysis	Destruction of, decomposition	-uria	Condition of the urine

TABLE 14-4 Common Abbreviations

Abbreviation	Meaning	Abbreviation	Meaning
abd	Abdomen	IBW	Ideal body weight
ADL	Activities of daily living	ICT	Inflammation of connective tissue
ad lib	As desired	id	The same
alt dieb	Every other day	L	Left, length, lumbar
alt hor	Alternate hours	lig	Ligament
alt noct	Alternate nights	M	Muscle, meter, myopia
AM (AM, am)	Morning	meds	Midline
ama	Against medical advice	ML	Medications
ANS	Autonomic nervous system	n	Normal
approx	Approximately	NA	Nonapplicable
as tol	As tolerated	OB	Obstetrics
BM	Bowel movement	OTC	Over the counter
BP	Blood pressure	P	Pulse
Ca	Cancer	PA	Postural analysis
CC	Chief complaint	PM (PM, pm)	Afternoon
c/o	Complains of	PT	Physical therapy
CPR	Cardiopulmonary resuscitation	Px	Prognosis
CSF	Cerebrospinal fluid	R	Respiration, right
CVA	Cerebrovascular accident, stroke	R/O	Rule out
DM	Diabetes mellitus	ROM	Range of motion
DJD	Degenerative joint disease	Rx	Prescription
Dx	Diagnosis	SOB	Shortness of breath
ext	Extract	SP, spir	Spirit
ft	Foot or feet	Sym	Symmetric
fx	Fracture	T	Temperature
GI	Gastrointestinal	TLC	Tender loving care
GU	Genitourinary	Tx	Treatment
h (hr)	Hour	URI	Upper respiratory infection
H_2O	Water	WD	Well developed
Hx	History	WN	Well nourished

CHAPTER

15

Sanitation Practices

SANITATION PRACTICES FOR MASSAGE PROFESSIONALS[1]

The following sanitation requirements for practicing massage professionals have been developed from the Oregon model.

- The massage professional must clean and wash the hands and forearms or feet thoroughly with an antibacterial/antiviral agent before touching each client. Any professional known to be infected with any communicable disease or to be a carrier of such disease or who has an infected wound or open lesion on any exposed portions of the body is excluded from practicing massage until the communicable condition is alleviated.
- The professional must wear clean clothing. If at all possible, lockers or closets for personnel should be maintained apart from the massage room for the storage of personal clothing and effects.
- All doors and windows opening to the outside must be tight fitting and must ensure the exclusion of flies, insects, rodents, or other vermin. All floors, walks, and furniture must be kept clean, well maintained, and in good repair.
- All rooms in which massage is practiced must meet the following requirements: (1) heating must be adequate to maintain a room air temperature of 75° F; (2) ventilation must be sufficient to remove objectionable odors; and (3) lighting fixtures must be capable of producing a minimum of 5 foot-candles of light at floor level; this level of lighting should be used during cleaning.
- All sewage and liquid waste must be disposed of in a municipal sewage system or approved septic system. All interior water distribution piping should be installed and maintained in conformity with the state plumbing code. The water supply must be adequate, deemed safe by the health department, and sanitary. Drinking fountains of an approved type or individual paper drinking cups should be provided for the convenience of employees and patrons.
- Every massage business must have a sanitary toilet facility with an adequate supply of hot and cold water under pressure, and it must be conveniently located for use by employees and patrons. Bathroom doors must be tight fitting, and the rooms must be kept clean, in good repair, and free of flies, insects, and vermin. A supply of soap in a covered dispenser and single-use sanitary towels in a dispenser must be provided at each lavatory installation, as well as a covered waste receptacle for proper disposal; a supply of toilet paper on a dispenser must be available for each toilet.
- Lavatory and toilet rooms must be equipped with fly-tight containers for garbage and refuse. These containers should be easily cleanable, well maintained, and in good repair. Any refuse must be disposed of in a sanitary manner.
- Massage lubricants, including but not limited to oil, alcohol, powders, and lotions, should be dispensed from suitable containers, to be used and stored in such a manner as to prevent contamination. The bulk lubricant must not come in contact with the massage professional. It should be poured, squeezed, or shaken into a separate container or the massage professional's hand. Any unused lubricant that comes into contact with the client or massage professional must be discarded.
- The use of unclean linen is prohibited. Only freshly laundered sheets and linens should be used for massage. All single-service materials and clean linens should be stored at least 4 inches off the floor in shelves, compartments, or cabinets used for that purpose only. All soiled linens must be placed in a covered receptacle immediately and kept there until washed in detergent and an antiviral cleaning agent (e.g., a 10% bleach solution, or one part bleach to nine parts water) in a washing machine that provides a hot water temperature of at least 140° F.
- Massage tables must be covered with impervious material that is cleanable and must be kept clean and in good repair. Equipment that comes in contact with the client must be cleaned thoroughly with soap or

other suitable detergent and water, followed by adequate sanitation procedures before use with each individual client (a 10% bleach solution, made up daily, is recommended). All equipment must be clean, well maintained, and in good repair.

- When cleaning the massage area, observe the following rules:
  - Do not shake linen, and dust with a damp cloth to minimize the movement of dust.
  - Clean from the cleanest area to the dirtiest. This prevents soiling of a clean area.
  - Clean away from your body and uniform. If you dust, brush, or wipe toward yourself, microorganisms will be transmitted to your skin, hair, and uniform.
  - Store used linens in a closed bag or container while in the massage room or during transport.
- Floors are dirty; any object that falls on the floor should not be used on or for a client.

STANDARD PRECAUTIONS[2]

Standard precautions synthesize the major features of universal precautions (blood and body fluids), which are designed to reduce the risk of transmission of bloodborne pathogens, and body substance isolation, which is designed to reduce the risk of transmission of pathogens from moist body substances. Standard precautions apply to (1) blood; (2) all body fluids, secretions, and excretions, except sweat, regardless of whether they contain visible blood; (3) nonintact skin; and (4) mucous membranes. Standard precautions are designed to reduce the risk of transmission of microorganisms from both recognized and unrecognized sources of infection in hospitals.

Hand Washing and Gloving

Hand washing is considered by many to be the single most important measure for reducing the risk of transmitting organisms from one person to another or from one site to another on the same patient. Washing your hands as promptly and thoroughly as possible between clients is very important. In addition to hand washing, gloves play an important role in reducing the risk of transmission of microorganisms.

Gloves are worn for two important reasons: (1) to provide a protective barrier and (2) to reduce the likelihood that microorganisms on the massage practitioner's hands will be transmitted to clients. Wearing gloves does not replace the need for hand washing, because gloves may have small, unapparent defects or may be torn during use, and hands can become contaminated during the removal of gloves. Gloves must be changed and the old ones discarded after each use.

A mask provides protection against the spread of infectious, large-particle droplets that are transmitted by close contact and that generally travel only short distances (up to 3 feet) from infected patients who are coughing or sneezing. Massage professionals occasionally use masks.

Gowns and Protective Apparel

Various types of gowns and protective apparel are worn to provide barrier protection and to reduce the opportunity for transmission of microorganisms in medical settings.

Immunocompromised Clients

Standard precautions, or the equivalent, are used for the care of all clients.

Hand Washing

1. Wash the hands after touching blood, body fluids, secretions, excretions, and contaminated items, regardless of whether gloves are worn. Wash the hands immediately after removing gloves, between client contacts, and when otherwise indicated to avoid transfer of microorganisms to other clients or environments. It may be necessary to wash the hands between tasks and procedures on the same client to prevent cross-contamination of different body sites.
2. Use a plain (nonantimicrobial) soap for routine hand washing.
3. Use an antimicrobial agent or a waterless antiseptic agent if hand washing is not possible.

Gloves

1. Wear gloves (clean, nonsterile gloves are adequate) when touching blood, body fluids, secretions, excretions, and contaminated items. Put on clean gloves just before touching mucous membranes and nonintact skin.
2. Change gloves between tasks and procedures on the same client after contact with material that may contain a high concentration of microorganisms.
3. Remove gloves promptly after use, before touching uncontaminated items and environmental surfaces, and before going to another client, and wash hands immediately to avoid transferring microorganisms to other clients or environments.

Mask, Eye Protection, and Face Shield. Wear a mask and eye protection or a face shield to protect the mucous membranes of the eyes, nose, and mouth during procedures and client care activities that are likely to generate splashes or sprays of blood, body fluids, secretions, and excretions.

Gown. Wear a gown (a clean, nonsterile gown is adequate) to protect skin and to prevent soiling of clothing during procedures and client care activities that are likely to generate splashes or sprays of blood, body fluids, secretions, or excretions. Select a gown that is appropriate for the activity and the amount of fluid likely to be encountered. Remove a soiled gown as promptly as possible, and wash hands to avoid transfer of microorganisms to other clients or environments.

REFERENCES

1. Modified from Oregon Board of Massage Technicians: Sanitation requirements for the state of Oregon, Oregon Administrative Rules, November, 2006.
2. Modified from the Division of Healthcare Quality Promotion, National Center for Infectious Diseases, Centers for Disease Control and Prevention. http://www.cdc.gov/ncidod/dhqp/guidelines.html Accessed July 20, 2007.

CHAPTER 16

Preventing the Transmission of HIV, Hepatitis, and Tuberculosis

Using the information presented in this section, the student will be able to perform the following:

- Define AIDS in detail
- Identify behavior that could result in the transmission of HIV or HBV infection and other contagious conditions

A *syndrome* is a group of clinical symptoms that constitute a disease or abnormal condition. (*Clinical* means reported or observed symptoms not discovered by laboratory tests.) With syndromes, an individual need not have all the symptoms. Syndromes may be caused by many different things, but with AIDS, the cause is a dysfunction in the body's immune system, one of the body's primary defenses against disease.

The diseases of AIDS are caused by germs we encounter every day. In fact, some of these germs live permanently in small numbers inside the human body. When the immune system weakens, these germs are able to multiply freely, therefore the diseases they cause are called *opportunistic diseases.*

HIV, which seems to be responsible for AIDS, is a retrovirus. As a group, retroviruses can live in the host for a long time without causing any sign of illness. In most animals, retrovirus infections last for life. These viruses die when exposed to heat, they can be killed by many common disinfectants, and they usually do not survive well if the tissue or blood they are in dries up. However, retroviruses have a high mutation rate and consequently tend to evolve very quickly into new strains. HIV shares this and other traits with other known retroviruses.

HIV replicates (lives) in the group of white blood cells called *lymphocytes,* or *T cells.* Among the T cells, HIV's favorite target is the T4 cell. The T4 cell, also called the *helper/inducer T cell,* performs a vital job in the immune system. HIV infection of the T4 cells creates a defect in the body's immune system, which may eventually result in AIDS. Long-term infection with HIV without the development of AIDS is becoming more common. Improved treatment, a better understanding of the disease on the part of health care professionals, increased public education, and less stress from public stigma support this process.

THE MECHANICS OF TRANSMISSION

For transmission, HIV must travel from inside one person to the inside of another person. Because viruses are unable to enter the body through intact skin, they must enter through an open wound or one of a number of possible body openings (most of which contain mucous membranes). *Mucous membranes* are thin tissues that protect most openings and passages in the human body. These membranes secrete mucus, which contains antigerm chemicals and keeps the surrounding tissues moist. Mucous membranes can be found in the mouth, inside the eyelids, in the nose and air passages leading to the lungs, in the stomach, along the digestive tract, in the vagina, in the anus, and inside the eye and the opening of the penis. From the surface of a mucous membrane, many viruses can travel through the membrane and enter the tiny blood vessels inside. The mucous membranes of the eyes and mouth often are doorways for highly infectious viruses, such as the flu virus. The danger with HIV is very different. The major infection sites for this virus are the bloodstream and the central nervous system. HIV can be found in any body fluid or substance that contains lymphocytes.

The presence of HIV in a substance does not necessarily indicate that the substance is capable of transmitting the infection. In theory, all body fluids are capable of transmitting disease; in reality, however, the most dangerous substances seem to be blood, semen, and pre-ejaculate fluid; cervical and vaginal secretions; and perhaps feces. Despite much research, a clear-cut case of saliva causing transmission has not been found, although kissing theoretically could transmit the virus. The concentration of HIV (i.e., the number of viral particles per unit of volume) is very important in infectivity. If a substance has a high concentration of HIV, it is more likely to transmit the virus. A pregnant woman can transmit the virus to her unborn child. The concentration of HIV in mother's milk and in saliva, urine, and tears is low, but theoretically these are infectious substances that could transmit HIV infection. However, no cases have been reported to be caused by contact with these secretions. Sweat cannot transmit HIV.

HIV SURVIVAL OUTSIDE THE HOST

If HIV is present in a substance that leaves the body, the viral particles are capable of remaining infectious until the substance dries up. Depending on the circumstances, this could be a matter of minutes or hours. If the substance stays moist, the viral particles can survive much longer. For example, in water and blood solutions (10% blood, 90% saline), HIV can survive at room temperature for 2 weeks. In refrigerated blood, such as that used for transfusions, HIV can survive indefinitely.

The public has a widespread fear that AIDS can be contracted through casual contact, such as shaking hands, being in the same room with an individual infected with HIV, touching doorknobs, or sharing bathroom facilities. The fear is far, far greater than the risk. Diseases spread by casual contact invariably are spread through saliva or sputum, and they exist in the saliva or sputum in very high concentrations. The concentration of HIV in saliva and sputum is very low, if it exists in these substances at all. After 10 years of documentation of the AIDS epidemic, there are no known cases of AIDS or HIV infection being transmitted by casual social contact, not even among people living in the same household. In some cases household members have even shared toothbrushes with infected housemates without contracting the virus.

To date no medical or health care workers have contracted HIV from casual contact. The contact between the massage professional and the client falls under this classification. We touch only the skin, which is not a transmission route.

HEPATITIS

Hepatitis is an inflammatory process, an infection of the liver caused by a virus. It is classified as type A, B, C, D, E, or G. Hepatitis A, caused by the hepatitis A virus (HAV), is a less serious form and is usually transmitted by fecal contamination of food and water. Hepatitis B is a potentially fatal disease caused by the hepatitis B virus (HBV), which is transmitted through routes similar to those for HIV. HBV is 100 times more contagious than HIV, and it is estimated that more than 1 million people in the United States are carriers of HBV. Two types of vaccine are available for preventing the transmission of HBV. Hepatitis C accounts for 86% of new cases of hepatitis each year. The hepatitis D virus (HDV) infects only those who have hepatitis B, and its symptoms are more severe than other forms of hepatitis. Vaccines do not appear to be effective for HDV. Hepatitis E is transmitted through food and water contaminated by fecal material. Hepatitis G is a sexually transmitted virus.[5]

Standard precautions prevent the spread of hepatitis. It is important to be cautious of all behaviors in which body fluids are contacted or unsanitary conditions may be present that may allow the transmission of HIV and the hepatitis viruses.

TUBERCULOSIS

Tuberculosis (TB) is an infection caused by a bacterium that usually affects the lungs but may invade other body systems. It is estimated that approximately 1.86 billion people—more than one third of the world's population—are infected with TB. Transmission occurs via airborne droplets that are produced when an infected person coughs, sneezes, or talks. TB can also be spread through contaminated food.

In many infected individuals, tuberculosis is asymptomatic. In others, symptoms develop so gradually that they are not noticed until the disease is advanced. However, symptoms can appear in immunosuppressed individuals within weeks of exposure to the bacillus. Symptoms include fatigue, weight loss, lethargy, anorexia (loss of appetite), and a low-grade fever that usually occurs in the afternoon. A cough that produces purulent sputum develops slowly and becomes more frequent over several weeks or months. Night sweats and general anxiety often are present. Because these are common signs and symptoms of all chronic infections, referral is necessary for diagnosis. Dyspnea, chest pain, and hemoptysis may also occur as the disease progresses.

Tuberculosis is diagnosed by a positive tuberculin skin test (PPD), sputum culture, and chest x-ray. A positive tuberculin skin test indicates that an individual has been infected and has produced antibodies against the bacillus. By itself the positive skin test does not indicate the presence of an active disease. Treatment consists of antibiotic therapy to control active or dormant tuberculosis and to prevent transmission. Massage professionals should be tested yearly because of their contact with the public.

CHAPTER

17

Effects of Massage

Both mechanical and reflexive responses are linked to massage techniques that deliver moderate to deep pressure, which stimulates pressure receptors. This type of massage is often referred to as *Swedish massage* or *therapeutic massage*. Some of the benefits outlined in this chapter are related to touch, but most are linked to Swedish massage. One study in particular implemented deep Swedish massage or deep-tissue massage. In this study, massage using light pressure generally produced adverse results. In fact, the study was criticized because it stated that massage did not have any effect on circulation. However, after closer examination, the fact that only light pressure was used for the experimental (massaged) group was discovered.

In a study conducted by Daniel Cherkin and colleagues, speculation was offered to explain why massage was effective in treating low back pain. As you would expect, effects on soft tissues were noted. Other factors attributed to massage effectiveness were the client spending 1 hour in a relaxed environment, receiving ongoing attention from the therapist, being touched in a therapeutic context, and increased body awareness during and after the massage. Education about exercise and other positive lifestyle changes was another benefit clients received as part of their massage.

Do the effects of massage last? Most benefits cease shortly after the massage treatments are terminated, but this is also true of other health-related treatments such as diet, exercise, and meditation. The key to long-term effects is the education clients receive concerning lifestyle habits and changes. These changes can be a healthy diet, frequent walks, and increased fluid intake. Clients are also taught other methods of self-care such as how to breathe for relaxation, a basic self-massage routine, or the stretching of muscle groups. Massage does have long-lasting effects on some specific injuries or pathological conditions. These effects include reducing scar tissue formation, decreasing edema, loosening lung phlegm, and relieving constipation. Chronic conditions often require ongoing massage treatments.

Massage therapy and the response it creates within the body can affect the cardiovascular system, lymphatic and immune systems, skin and related structures, nervous and endocrine systems, muscles, connective tissues, respiratory system, digestive system, and urinary system. Also noted are miscellaneous effects and indications for specific conditions and individuals.

This next lengthy section includes a listing of the documented effects of massage. Although every effort has been made to cite reliable sources, varying degrees of the quality of the research can be found (see the previous section on Scientific Method). Literature on massage therapy tends to lack the rigorous application of empirical research methods and is many times anecdotal in nature. The reference section at the end of this book has a complete list of works cited. If you have any concerns about a particular claim, then obtain the actual research and peruse the study.

EFFECTS OF MASSAGE ON THE CARDIOVASCULAR SYSTEM

- **Dilates blood vessels.** Superficial blood vessels become dilated resulting from reflex action.
- **Improves blood circulation.** Deep stroking improves blood circulation by mechanically assisting venous blood flow back to the heart. The increase of blood flow is comparable to that associated with exercise. The fact that local circulation during a massage increases up to three times more than circulation at rest has been documented.
- **Decreases blood pressure.** Blood pressure is decreased by blood vessel dilation. Both diastolic and systolic readings decline and last approximately 40 minutes after the massage.
- **Creates hyperemia.** Increased blood flow creates a hyperemic effect, which is visible on some skin types.
- **Stimulates release of acetylcholine and histamine.** These two substances are released as a result of vasomotor activity, thereby helping prolong vasodilation.
- **Replenishes nutritive materials.** Increased circulation aids in the delivery of products such as nutrients and oxygen to cells and tissues.

- **Promotes removal of waste products.** Increased circulation also aids in the removal of metabolic wastes. The notion is often said that massage *dilutes the poisons*.
- **Reduces ischemia.** Massage reduces ischemia. Ischemia is linked to pain and trigger-point formation.
- **Reduces heart and pulse rates.** Massage decreases heart rate through activation of the relaxation response.
- **Increases stroke volume.** Stroke volume is the amount of blood ejected from the left ventricle during each contraction. As the heart rate decreases, more time exists for the heart's lower chambers (ventricles) to fill with blood. The result is a larger volume of blood pushed through the heart, thereby increasing stroke volume.
- **Increases red blood cell (RBC) count.** The number of RBCs and their oxygen-carrying capacity are increased. This effect is due to (1) promoting the spleen's discharge of RBCs, (2) recruiting blood from engorged internal organs into general circulation, and (3) stimulating stagnant capillary beds and returning this blood into general circulation.
- **Increases oxygen saturation in blood.** When RBC count rises, oxygen saturation of the blood increases.
- **Increases white blood cell (WBC) count.** The presence of WBCs increases after massage. The body may perceive massage as a mild stressor (an event to which the body must adapt) and recruits additional WBCs. The increase in WBC count enables the body to protect itself more effectively against disease.
- **Enhances the adhesion of migrating WBCs.** The surfaces of WBCs become increasingly sticky after a massage, thereby increasing their adhesive quality and therefore their effectiveness.
- **Increases platelet count.** Massage has been found to increase the number of blood platelets.

Mini-Lab

Obtain two uninflated balloons—a small one and another twice the size of the first. Place a cup of water in each balloon. Which balloon has the lesser amount of pressure, the smaller or the larger? The larger one has the lesser pressure. This illustrates how massage can lower blood pressure through reflex action and increasing the parasympathetic response. By increasing the diameter of the vessel, the pressure inside the vessel decreases.

EFFECTS OF MASSAGE ON THE LYMPHATIC AND THE IMMUNE SYSTEMS

- **Promotes lymph circulation.** Lymph circulation depends on pressure: from muscle contraction, pressure changes in the thorax and abdomen during breathing or applied pressure from a massage. Hence, massage promotes this circulation.
- **Reduces edema.** Massage reduces edema (swelling) by enhancing lymph circulation.
- **Decreases the circumference of an area affected with edema.** When an area swells, the diameter increases. When the swelling subsides, circumference decreases.
- **Decreases weight in patients with edema.** Fluid retention adds weight to an individual. When edema is addressed with massage, weight is consequently reduced.
- **Increases lymphocyte count.** Lymphocytes are types of WBCs. This effect indicates that massage supports immune functions.
- **Increases the number and function (or cytotoxicity) of natural killer cells, CD4 cells, and CD4/CD8 ratio.** All the aforementioned cells are types of WBCs. This increase further suggests that massage strengthens immune functions.

EFFECTS OF MASSAGE ON THE SKIN AND RELATED STRUCTURES

- **Increases skin temperature.** Warming of the skin indicates a reduction of stress.
- **Improves skin condition.** As circulation increases, added nutrients are made available to the skin, thereby improving its condition, texture, and tone. Clinical observations have determined that massage also improves the appearance (i.e., color and texture) of the skin.
- **Stimulates oil glands.** Stimulation of the oil (sebaceous) glands causes an increase in oil (sebum) production. This stimulation improves the skin's condition and reduces skin dryness.
- **Improves skin conditions.** Unless a condition contraindicates massage, skin conditions may improve by decreasing redness, reducing thickening or hardening of the skin, increasing healing of skin abrasions, and reducing itching.

EFFECTS OF MASSAGE ON THE NERVOUS AND THE ENDOCRINE SYSTEMS

- **Reduces stress.** Activating the relaxation response reduces stress.
- **Reduces anxiety.** Interestingly, a reduction in anxiety is noted in both the person who received the massage and the person who gave the massage.
- **Promotes relaxation.** General relaxation is promoted through activation of the relaxation response. Relaxation has a diminishing effect on pain.
- **Decreases beta wave activity.** Associated with relaxation, a decrease in beta brainwave activity occurred during and after the massage (confirmed by electroencephalogram [EEG]).

- **Increases delta wave activity.** Increases in delta brainwave activity, which occur during massage, are linked to sleep and to relaxation; both are promoted with massage (confirmed by EEG).
- **Increase in alpha waves.** An increase in alpha brainwaves during massage indicates relaxation (confirmed by EEG).
- **Increases dopamine levels.** Increased levels of dopamine are linked to decreased stress and reduced depression.
- **Increases serotonin levels.** Increased levels of serotonin suggest a reduction of both stress and depression. Theories suggest that serotonin inhibits pain signals, indicating that increased levels of serotonin also reduce pain.
- **Reduces cortisol levels.** Massage reduces cortisol levels by activating the relaxation response. Elevated levels of cortisol not only represent heightened stress but also inhibit immune functions.
- **Reduces norepinephrine levels.** Massage has been proved to reduce norepinephrine, a stress hormone.
- **Reduces epinephrine levels.** Epinephrine, another stress hormone, is reduced with massage.
- **Reduces feelings of depression.** Both chemical and electrophysiological changes from a negative to a positive mood were noted and may support the decrease in depression after massage therapy. Depression associated with chronic pain was also reduced.
- **Decreases pain.** Massage relieves local and referred pain, presumably by increasing circulation, thereby reducing ischemia. Massage also stimulates the release of endorphins (endogenous morphine), enkephalins, and other pain-reducing neurochemicals. General relaxation brought on by massage therapy also has a diminishing effect on pain. The pressure of a massage interferes with pain information entering the spinal cord by stimulating pressure receptors, further reducing pain. Massage interrupts the pain cycle by relieving muscular spasms, increasing circulation, and promoting rapid disposal of waste products. Massage also improves sleep patterns. During deep sleep, a substance called somatostatin is normally released. Without this substance, pain is experienced.
- **Reduces analgesic use.** Because pain is reduced with massage, the need for excessive use of pain medication is also reduced.
- **Activates sensory receptors.** Depending on factors such as stroke choice, direction, speed, and pressure, massage can stimulate different sensory receptors, affecting massage outcome. For example, cross-fiber tapotement stimulates muscle spindles, which activates muscular contraction, whereas a slow passive stretch and deep effleurage activate Golgi tendon organs, thereby inhibiting contraction. Activation of pressure receptors reduces pain (see Table Talk: The Gate Theory).
- **Faster and more elaborate development of the hippocampal region of the brain.** As part of the limbic system, development of the hippocampal region is related to superior memory performance.

Table Talk

The Gate Theory

In 1965 Ronald Wall and Patrick Melzack postulated the gate theory of pain relief, which explains why massage, ice, and heat are effective in the treatment of pain. The *gate theory* states that transmission of impulses into the spinal cord is *gated* (can be open or shut). Gating is affected by the degree of activity, or transmission, in sensory nerves. Multiple signals may be competing for the same gate—or entrance into the spinal cord. The one who hits the gate first wins. The gate then closes and prevents or inhibits other nerve impulses.

Nerve-transmission speed is affected by nerve diameter. Impulses traveling along larger nerve fibers are faster than those traveling along smaller nerves. Sensory nerves for pressure, temperature, and sharp acute pain lie close together in large concentrations near the body's surface. These sensory nerves are long and large in diameter and transmit impulses quickly, protecting the body from harm. Strong stimuli to these receptors generate a quick sensory input to the spinal cord. A reflex is generated to move the affected body part out of harm's way. Touching a needle or a hot pan elicits this type of immediate reflex response.

The sensory receptors for aching pain originate in the deeper tissues. These nerves are composed of short, thinner nerve fibers, which tend to transmit pain that has been present for some time (i.e., headache, dull pain) and requires no immediate protective action. These nerves transmit stimuli that are of lesser importance and lesser consequence to the body. The purpose of the deep, slower transmitting nerves is to make the conscious mind aware that a problem exists, which can be used to prevent overuse or dependence on an injured body part.

Suppose that a gymnast is having performance compromised by soreness in the right calf. This pain originates from the deeper, slower nerves. When a pressure stimulus such as massage is applied to the calf, the new sensory input travels along the faster, larger nerve network, entering the spinal cord first. The gate closes, excluding pain information from entering the cord. The body experiences the pressure of the massage stroke as an interruption of pain.

Massage therapists can use the gate mechanism when applying pressure, heat, and cold. All of these have the potential to interfere or interrupt pain signals.

EFFECTS OF MASSAGE ON MUSCLES

- **Relieves muscular tension.** Massage relieves muscular restrictions, tightness, stiffness, and spasms.

- **Relaxes muscles.** Muscles relax as massage reduces excitability in the sympathetic nervous system.
- **Reduces muscle soreness and fatigue.** Massage enhances blood circulation, thereby increasing the amount of oxygen and nutrients available to the muscles. Increased oxygen and nutrients reduce muscle fatigue and postexercise soreness. Massage promotes rapid disposal of waste products, further reducing muscle fatigue and soreness. Massage interrupts the pain cycle. A fatigued muscle recuperates 20% after 5 minutes of rest and 100% after 5 minutes of massage. A reduction in postexercise recovery time was indicated by a decline in pulse rate and an increase muscle work capacity.
- **Reduces trigger point formation.** Trigger point formation in both muscle and fascia is greatly reduced by massage.
- **Manually separates muscle fibers.** Compressive strokes and cross-fiber friction strokes separate muscle fibers, thereby reducing muscle spasms.
- **Increases range of motion.** When muscular tension is reduced, range of motion is improved. The freedom of the joints is dictated by the freedom of the muscles.
- **Improves performance (balance and posture).** Many postural distortions are removed when trigger points and muscle tension are reduced. Range of motion increases, gait becomes more efficient, the posture is more aligned and balanced, and performance is improved as the net result.
- **Lengthens muscles.** Massage mechanically stretches and broadens tissue, especially when combined with Swedish gymnastics (joint mobilization and stretches). These changes are detected by Golgi tendon organs, which inhibit contraction signals, further lengthening muscles. Massage retrains the tissue from a contracted state to an elongated state, thereby increasing resting length. This principle is one of the principles behind neuromuscular reeducation.
- **Increases flexibility.** By lengthening muscles and promoting relaxation, massage has also been shown to increase flexibility.
- **Tones weak muscles.** Muscle spindle activity is increased during massage strokes (e.g., tapotement, vibration). An increase in muscle spindle activity stimulates minute muscle contractions, thereby helping tone weak muscles. This effect is particularly beneficial in most cases of prolonged bed rest, flaccidity, and atrophy.
- **Reduces creatine kinase activity in the blood.** Creatine kinase is an enzyme that helps ensure that enough adenosine triphosphate (ATP) is available for muscle contraction. By reducing the activity of creatine kinase in the blood, massage indirectly helps decrease muscle spasm, which increases muscle relaxation.
- **Decreases electromyography (EMG) readings.** Decreased EMG readings signify a decrease in neuromuscular activity and reduction of neuromuscular complaints.

Mini-Lab

Sit in a chair with your feet flat on the floor. Moving only your head and neck, look over your left shoulder, and notice how far you can comfortably move. Do the same, looking to the right. With your right hand, grab the top of your right shoulder. As you apply pressure, slowly move the shoulder up and down 10 times. Maintain the pressure, and roll your shoulder back 10 times, then forward 10 times. Do this same movement with the left shoulder. Squeeze the back of your neck. Without releasing the pressure, turn your head (as if saying *no*), nod your head (as if saying *yes*), and move your nose in a circle clockwise and counterclockwise 10 times each. After the *squeeze and move* activity, look over your right and left shoulders again. Notice how much farther you can go. This increase is the result of self-administered massage.

EFFECTS OF MASSAGE ON CONNECTIVE TISSUES

- **Reduces keloid formation.** Massage applied to scar tissue helps reduce keloid formation in scar tissue beneath the site of massage application.
- **Reduces excessive scar formation.** Deep massage reduces excessive scar tissue formation, helping create an appropriate scar that is strong yet does not interfere with the muscle's ability to broaden as it contracts.
- **Decreases adhesion formation.** Deep, specifically applied massage helps decrease adhesions. This decrease, in turn, facilitates normal, pain-free motion of the affected muscles and joints.
- **Releases fascial restrictions.** Pressure and the heat it produces convert fascia from a gel state to a solid state (thixo-tropy), thereby reducing hyperplasia. Softening of the fascia surrounding muscles allows them to be stretched to their fullest resting length, thereby increasing joint range of motion and freeing the body of restricted movements.
- **Increases mineral retention in bone.** Massage increases the retention of nutrients such as sulfur and phosphorus in bones.
- **Promotes fracture healing.** When a bone is fractured, the body forms a network of new blood vessels at the break site. Massage increases circulation around the fracture, thereby promoting fracture healing. Increased circulation around a fracture leads to increased deposition of callus to the bone. Callus is formed between and around the broken ends of a fractured bone during healing and is ultimately replaced by compact bone.
- **Improves connective tissue healing.** Occurring only with deep-pressure massage, proliferation and

activation of fibroblasts were noted. Fibroblasts generate a connective tissue matrix, which promotes tissue healing by increasing collagen production and increasing the tensile strength of healed tissue.

- **Reduces surface dimpling of cellulite.** Massage flattens out fat deposits located under the skin and makes the skin seem smoother. Cellulite (a type of fat) appears as groups of small dimples or depressions under the skin caused by an uneven separation of fat globules below the skin's surface, which are displaced by manual manipulation. Massage does not reduce the amount of cellulite below the skin; instead, it temporarily alters the shape and appearance of cellulite.

EFFECTS OF MASSAGE ON THE RESPIRATORY SYSTEM

- **Reduces respiration rate.** Massage slows down breathing because of activation of the relaxation response.
- **Strengthens respiratory muscles.** The muscles of respiration have a greater capacity to contract, thereby helping improve pulmonary functions.
- **Decreases the sensation of dyspnea.** Dyspnea (short or difficult breathing) is lessened as a result of massage.
- **Decreases asthma attacks.** Through increased relaxation and improved pulmonary functions, a person with asthma experiences fewer attacks after massage.
- **Reduces laryngeal tension.** Laryngeal tension may occur from excessive public speaking or singing. Massage reduces the stress on the larynx and tension on the muscles of the throat.
- **Increases fluid discharge from the lungs.** The mechanical loosening and discharge of phlegm increase with rhythmic alternating pressures. Tapotement (cupping) and vibration on the rib cage are often used to enhance this effect. Phlegm loosening and discharge are further enhanced when combined with postural drainage (promoting fluid drainage of the respiratory tract through certain body positions) and when the client is encouraged to cough.
- **Improves pulmonary functions.** Relaxation plays a significant role in how massage improves pulmonary function, but massage also loosens tight respiratory muscles and fascia. The affected pulmonary functions are as follows:
  - **Increased vital capacity.** This measurement is the amount of air that can be expelled at the normal rate of exhalation after a maximum inhalation, representing the greatest possible breathing capacity.
  - **Increased forced vital capacity.** This measurement is the amount of air that can be forcibly expelled after a forced inhalation.
  - **Increased forced expiratory volume.** This measurement is the volume of air that can be forcibly expelled after a full exhalation.
  - **Increased forced expiratory flow.** This measurement is the volume of air that can be forcibly expelled after a full inhalation.
  - **Improved peak expiratory flow.** This measurement is the greatest rate of airflow that can be achieved during forced expiration beginning with the lungs fully inflated.

EFFECTS OF MASSAGE ON THE DIGESTIVE SYSTEM

- **Promotes evacuation of the colon.** By increasing peristaltic activity in the colon through massage, movement of bowel contents toward the anus for elimination is aided.
- **Relieves constipation.** Because evacuation of the colon is promoted, constipation is relieved.
- **Relieves colic and intestinal gas.** Increased peristaltic activity also helps relieve colic and the expulsion of intestinal gas.
- **Stimulates digestion.** Massage also promotes activation of the relaxation response, which stimulates digestion.

EFFECTS OF MASSAGE ON THE URINARY SYSTEM

- **Increases urine output.** Massage activates dormant capillary beds and recovers lymphatic fluids for filtration by the kidney, which, in turn, increases the frequency of urination and amount of urine produced. Massage is also relaxing and thus stimulates the parasympathetic nervous system, which promotes general homeostasis, thereby increasing urine output.
- **Promotes the excretion of nitrogen, inorganic phosphorus, and sodium chloride in urine.** Levels of these metabolic waste products are elevated in urine after massage.

MISCELLANEOUS EFFECTS OF MASSAGE

- **Reduces fatigue and increases vigor.** Many clients experienced a sense of renewed energy after massage.
- **Improves sleep patterns.** When clients who have had massage therapy went to sleep, they reported a deeper sleep and felt more rested after waking.
- **Reduces job-related and posttraumatic stress.** Massage reduces many types of stress, including job-related and posttraumatic stress.
- **Improves mood.** The mental health status and mood improved after massage.

- **Decreases feelings of anger.** Clients reported a decrease in aggression and feelings of anger with massage.
- **Improves body image.** Massage improved body image in clients who stated having a poor body image before the massage.
- **Improves self-esteem.** Individuals who received and who gave massages reported enhanced self-esteem.
- **Promotes communication and expression.** Individuals who received and gave massages reported an increase in the quantity and quality of their social interactions. They talked more freely and openly and enjoyed themselves more during these interactions. Massage can also assist the ease of emotional expression with relaxation.
- **Improves lifestyle habits.** After massage, clients reported improved lifestyle habits such as increased activities of daily living (ADL), fewer cups of coffee, fewer physical symptoms, fewer visits to the physician, and increased levels of exercising (e.g., walking).
- **Increases physical well-being.** Massage enhances well-being through stress reduction and subsequent relaxation.
- **Reduces touch aversion and touch sensitivity.** Victims of rape and spousal abuse reported a reduction in touch aversion after massage. Hypersensitivity to touch was reduced in other individuals.
- **Increases academic performance.** A decrease in math computation time and an increase in accuracy were noted in massage studies.
- **Increases mental alertness.** Massage increases mental alertness by relaxing the body and mind and by removing stress.
- **Satisfies emotional needs.** Clients reported using the therapeutic relationship to satisfy their emotional needs for attention, acceptance, caring, and nurturing touch.

> *"There's an alternative. There's always a third way, and it's not a combination of the other two ways. It's a different way."*
>
> *David Carradine*

INDICATIONS OF MASSAGE FOR SPECIFIC CONDITIONS AND SPECIAL POPULATIONS

Most individuals can benefit from massage therapy. This section focuses on specific conditions that have been documented to benefit from massage. For further reading, please see the bibliography at the end of the chapter.

- **Alzheimer's disease.** Massage decreased physical expressions of agitation (e.g., pacing, wandering) and improved sleep patterns.
- **Anemia.** An increase in RBCs and an increase in oxygen saturation in the blood suggest that massage is beneficial for individuals with anemia.
- **Asthma.** Studies indicate that massage improved pulmo-nary functions and reduced the occurrence of asthma attacks.
- **Attention deficit hyperactivity disorder (ADHD).** Individuals diagnosed with ADHD who receive massage were observed to be less fidgety and hyperactive and spent more time completing assigned tasks. Students themselves reported an improved short-term mood state.
- **Burn victims.** Burn victims who were massaged experienced a decrease in pain and itching and reduced anxiety before débridement. Massage also reduced feelings of depression and anger.
- **Cancer.** Edema, pain, fatigue, anxiety, nausea, and feelings of anger and depression were reduced when patients with cancer had routine massages. Massage also increased lymphocyte and natural killer cell counts.
- **Cerebral palsy (CP).** Massage promotes circulation of blood and lymph and relieves muscular tension in individuals with CP. Increases in flexibility were also reported.
- **Chronic fatigue syndrome (CFS).** Clients with CFS experience reduced feelings of depression and anxiety and fewer symptoms such as fatigue. CFS affects muscle strength; improved grip strength was also documented.
- **Constipation.** Elimination problems were relieved through massage.
- **Diabetes.** Blood glucose levels, anxiety, and depression were reduced with massage. An increase in dietary compliance was also reported.
- **Eating disorders.** Patients with anorexia nervosa and bulimia stated a reduction of depression and anxiety. These individuals stated that they experienced an improvement in eating habits and an increase in positive body image.
- **Edema.** Swelling resulting from edema was reduced with massage, as long as the swelling was not a result of inflammation or disease.
- **Fibromyalgia.** Not only were stress, anxiety, and feelings of depression reduced, but decreases in pain, stiffness, fatigue, and insomnia were also documented in individuals with fibromyalgia. Massage was rated more effective than standard physical therapy or prescriptive drugs.
- **Headaches.** Most headaches (muscular, cluster, eye strain, mental fatigue, and sinus) were relieved with massage. People also reported a reduction in headache frequency and headache duration but not always in intensity. One study did report less analgesic use as a result of pain reduction.
- **High blood pressure.** Massage decreased blood pressure (both systolic and diastolic readings) and helped

promote healthy lifestyle habits in patients with high blood pressure (hypertension).

- **Individuals infected with the human immunodeficiency virus (HIV).** The number of natural killer cells, CD4 cells, and CD4/CD8 cell ratio increased after 1 month of massage therapy. These cells are important because they have been shown to provide protection against acquired immunodeficiency syndrome and opportunistic diseases. Massage also helped individuals infected with HIV to relax.
- **Hospitalized patients.** Massage increased relaxation, provided a sense of well-being, and produced a positive mood change for patients. Most (more than two thirds) attributed enhanced mobility, greater energy, increased participation in treatment, and faster recovery to massage therapy.
- **Hospice patients.** Hospice patients experienced reduced pain and had a decline in heart rate and blood pressure, indicating decreased stress and anxiety.
- **Infants.** Preterm, cocaine-exposed, HIV-exposed, and full-term infants experienced less colic, less repetitive crying, and improved feeding habits and gained more weight than infants in the same categories who were not massaged. Massage was found more effective than rocking for inducing infant sleep.
- **Injuries.** Massage speeds the healing of overuse injuries, sprains, and strains.
- **Insomnia.** Inducing relaxation alleviates insomnia.
- **Low back pain.** Addressing trigger points decreases low back pain. Medical costs were reduced by approximately 40% along with reduced analgesic use. Massage increased range of motion and promoted relaxation. Patients reported that massage made them feel cared for, happy, physically relaxed, less anxious, calm, and restful and gave them a feeling of closeness with the individuals who gave massages. Massage was rated more effective than standard physical therapy or prescriptive drugs.
- **Lung disease.** For clients with chronic obstructive pulmonary disease, massage strengthened respiratory muscles, reduced heart rate, increased oxygen saturation in blood, decreased shortness of breath, and improved pulmonary functions. Respiratory drainage is encouraged through cupping tapotement and vibration. Clients with cystic fibrosis further reported decreased anxiety and improved mood with massage treatments.
- **Multiple sclerosis (MS).** Individuals with MS who received massages experienced reduced anxiety and depression, improved self-esteem, and positive body image and implemented changes to their lifestyle that promoted health such as exercising and stretching.
- **Nerve entrapment.** Conditions of nerve entrapment, such as carpal tunnel syndrome, thoracic outlet syndrome, and sciatica, were relieved by release of the myofascial component.
- **Pervasive developmental disorder (PDD).** Massaged children with PDD or autism spent less time in solitary play and had an increase in attention to sounds and their social relatedness to their teachers. Behaviors such as touch aversion were reduced.
- **Poor circulation.** Massage improved blood circulation.
- **Pain (chronic).** Pain levels decreased, most often significantly. The depression and anxiety associated with individuals with chronic pain improved, as well as their quality of life.
- **Pregnancy and postpartum.** Massaged pregnant women reported fewer obstetrical and postpartum complications, reduced prematurity rates, shorter and less painful labors, improved psychological support, and fewer days in the hospital after labor and delivery. When nurses, midwives, or spouses massaged the pregnant or laboring women's perineal area, injury such as tearing during fetal delivery was reduced. Feelings of postpartum depression declined with massage. Depressed adolescent mothers reported less stress, anxiety, and depression.
- **Premenstrual syndrome (PMS).** Massage reduced swelling, pain, and anxiety and improved the mood of women experiencing PMS.
- **Psychiatric patients.** Child, adolescent, and adult psychiatric patients were observed to be better adapted to a group, and the medical staff reported better clinical progress with massage. A decrease in depression and anxiety was noted with reduced cortisol levels and norepinephrine blood levels and increased dopamine levels. In many individuals, a decreased self-destructive behavior was reported, and the mental health status improved in the people in the massaged group. A decrease in the episodes of dysfunctional behavior was found in patients with dementia.
- **Rheumatoid arthritis.** Massage reduced trigger point formation, provided relief from pain and anxiety, reduced morning stiffness and edema, and increased range of motion of the joints. Studies also revealed an increase tolerance of exercise and other educational approaches.
- **Stress and anxiety.** Stress and anxiety are reduced by activation of the relaxation response.
- **Temporomandibular joint (TMJ) dysfunction.** The muscular component of TMJ dysfunction was addressed with massage, and reduced pain and dysfunction was the result.

Once the benefits and indications of massage are known, an understanding of contraindications and endangerment sites becomes clear. For instance, by increasing lymph circulation, massage affects the tissue and fluids of the body; because massage increases the circulation of blood, thrombosis must be a contraindication.

"It's time again. Tear up the violets and plant something more difficult to grow."

James Schuyler

CONTRAINDICATIONS FOR MASSAGE THERAPY

During the assessment process, the therapist takes into consideration information obtained from the client. Some of this information comes through direct questioning, and some is obtained through observation and palpation. All information gathered culminates in a treatment plan that establishes goals and addresses modifications. In most instances, only slight adjustments are made, such as propping up a stiff shoulder so the client is comfortable lying on the table or using only light pressure over the abdomen because of a hernia. Some conditions warrant avoiding an area, such as the site of a recent burn or a client's feet because of a sebaceous cyst. Some conditions and symptoms may even preclude massage altogether. The presence of a disease or physical condition that makes treating a particular client in the usual manner impossible or undesirable is called a **contraindication.**

Ruling out the presence of any conditions in which massage may have harmful effects is the duty and obligation of the therapist.

The two categories of contraindications are *absolute* and *local.* Conditions in which massage is inappropriate, is not advised, and may be harmful to the client are known as **absolute contraindications.** Only rarely would a physician order massage under these conditions, but some exceptions occur, such as preeclampsia.

Many conditions or diseases are **local contraindications** in which massage can be administered while avoiding the infected area or the area in question.

Although massage is inappropriate in cases of absolute or local contraindications, the therapist may elect to use an energetic modality such as polarity that involves little or no physical contact. In other cases in which contraindications exist, advanced techniques such as lymphatic drainage may be appropriate. A well-trained, experienced therapist should possess the critical thinking skills involved in making these important decisions with the client. Record extensively in the client's records all discussions regarding his or her conditions and the type of treatment plan on which the two of you agree.

Much of the client intake and assessment involves screening clients for the appropriateness of massage. Some helpful guidelines follow.

If a client has a condition or disease that is indicated for massage, then treat as a cautious indication and follow several basic guidelines, which include:

- Tailor the massage to client's vitality and stamina (e.g., slower, gentler massage; a massage of shorter duration; assisting the client on and off the table).
- Position the client for comfort (e.g., side lying position for pregnant clients, seated position for paraplegics, extra bolstering for clients with spinal abnormalities, semireclining for clients with emphysema).
- Obtain physician clearance before the initial treatment to acquire more information regarding client's health status (e.g., arteriosclerosis, cerebral palsy). Make sure the client has signed a medical release form.

Obtaining a pathology book written specifically for massage therapists that lists each one of these conditions is highly recommended, such as our companion text: *Mosby's Pathology for Massage Therapists,* by Salvo and Anderson. This and similar texts define each pathological condition and details how to proceed (or not proceed) with massage.

"It is the heart that understands and the hand that soothes."

Martha Rogers

ENDANGERMENT SITES

Endangerment sites are areas of the body that contain superficial, delicate structures that are relatively unprotected and are therefore prone to injury. These sites merit caution during treatment. In most instances, the therapist simply adjusts pressure or avoids pointed or sustained pressure. Endangerment sites include structures such as nerves, blood vessels, organs, and small or prominent bony projections. These areas may be treated during a massage session, and they often are, but caution must be exercised, working slowly, lightly, and carefully when in or around these sites. Exceptions to this rule would be energy work and techniques with which little or no pressure is used, such as therapeutic touch.

This section examines types of endangerment sites and why caution is warranted. In the next section, areas of the body where most endangerment sites exist are identified.

- **Nerves.** When nerves are compressed during massage, the client may experience numbness, tingling, burning, or shooting pain. That massage will damage the nerve is doubtful, but these sensations may alarm your client or make him or her feel uncomfortable. If the pressure is prolonged, then the client may experience a temporary loss of motor control.
- **Blood vessels.** Pressure applied to superficial blood vessels may cause a temporary reduction in blood flow and may possibly affect blood pressure. When massaging an area where a superficial artery is present, apply light pressure and feel for a pulse. If a pulse is felt, then avoid prolonged pressure on the

specific pulse location. Caution areas for arteries also include the neighboring veins of the same name, with the exception of the aorta, the carotid artery, the great saphenous vein, and the jugular vein. Arteries and veins lie in proximity to each other, and caution of one vessel generally reflects caution of the other. Note that many of these endangerment sites are common pulse point locations.

- **Bony structures.** Compression of certain small, fragile, or prominent bony areas may cause pain and bruising.
- **Organs and glands.** Pressure or striking movements such as tapotement to the kidney or eye area may cause bruising, sharp pain, nausea, or temporary dysfunction. Swollen lymph nodes are also endangerment sites.

The following specific locations of each type of endangerment site can be located on the endangerment site map (Figure 17-1). All endangerment sites are bilaterally symmetrical with the exception of those located on the midline of the body. Remember, you can and should work these areas, but be mindful of the following structures:

- **Abdomen.** The structures of which to be aware regarding pressure in the abdomen include the abdominal and descending aorta, liver, linea alba (connective tissue band running down the abdominal wall, which can herniate), lumbar plexus, vagus nerve (deep pressure on psoas major may stimulate the vagus nerve and cause symptoms such as sweating and nausea), and xiphoid process (can fracture under heavy pressure).
- **Axilla.** The axilla contains several nerves and blood vessels that can become compressed during massage, such as the axillary and brachial arteries, as well as axillary, median, musculocutaneous, radial, and ulnar nerves, all branches of the brachial plexus.
- **Elbow.** The elbow is divided into a front (antecubital) and a back (cubital) area. Endangerment areas of the elbow include the brachial, radial, and ulnar arteries, as well as the median and the radial and ulnar nerves.

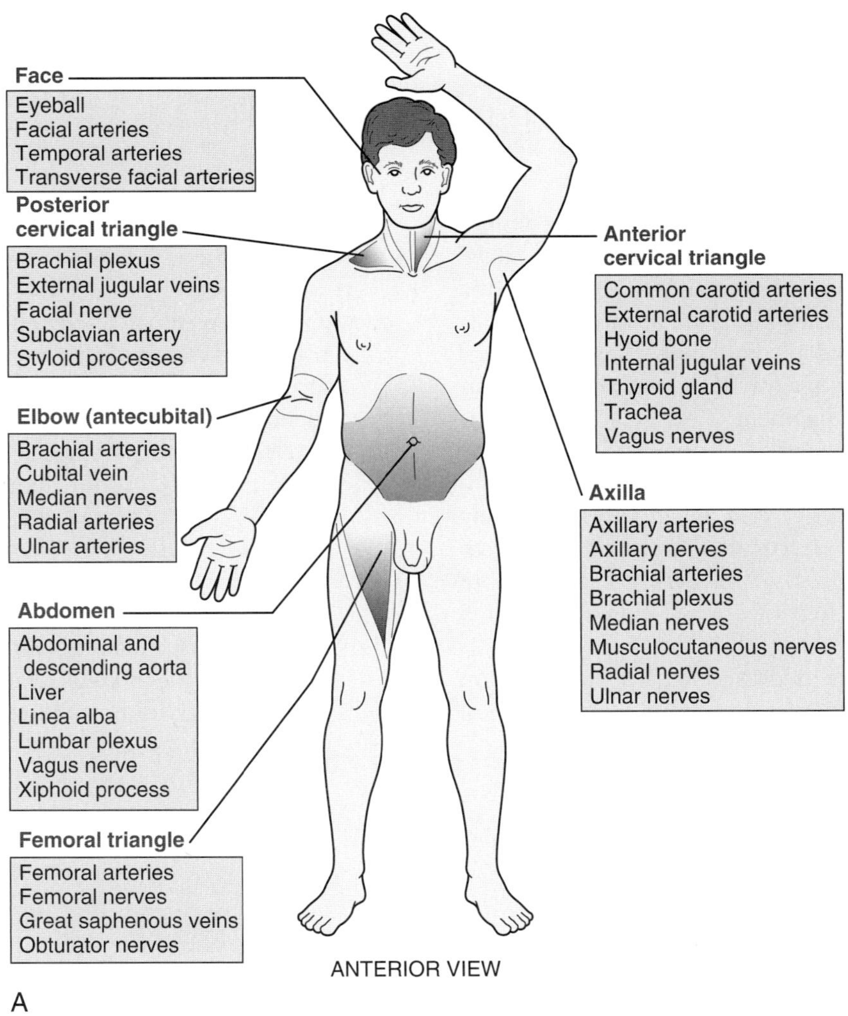

FIGURE 17-1 Endangerment site map. Massage therapists should exercise extreme caution when working these areas. **A**, Anterior view.

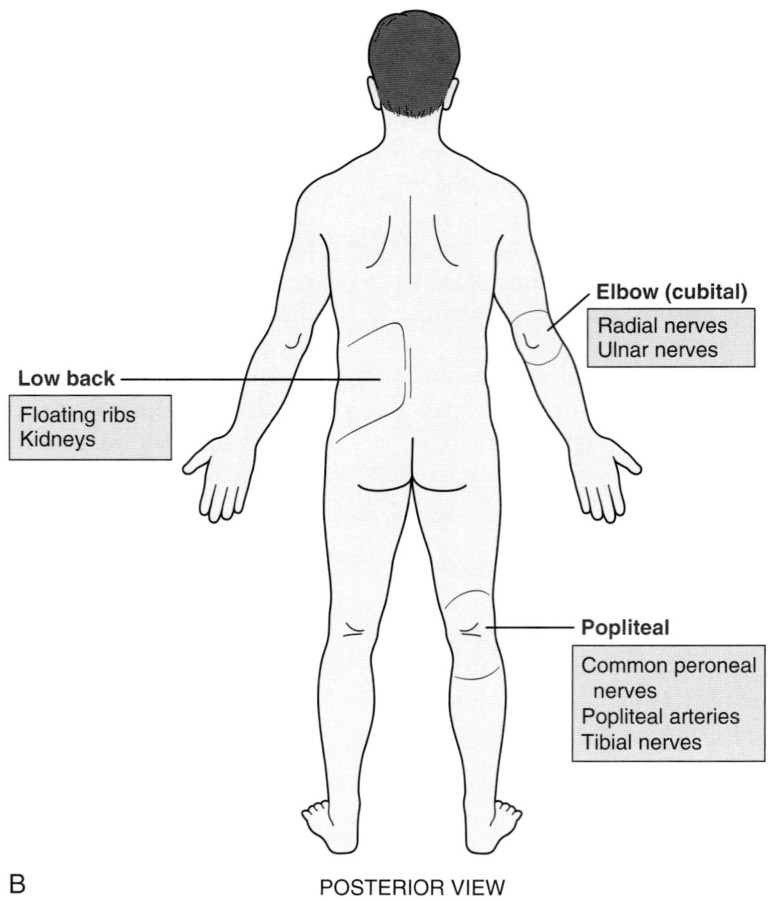

FIGURE 17-1, cont'd B, Posterior view.

- **Face.** Avoid direct pressure on the eyeball, temporal artery (runs vertically anterior to the ear), facial arteries (alongside the upper and lower jaw), and transverse facial arteries (anterior to the ear).
- **Femoral triangle and medial thigh.** The borders of the femoral triangle are the muscles gracilis and sartorius and inguinal ligament. This area contains the femoral arteries and nerves, great saphenous veins, and obturator nerves.
- **Low back.** Do not get carried away with the striking tapotement or the electrical massager on the low back. Two structures for which to watch out here are the floating ribs and kidneys (located retroperitoneally).
- **Popliteal.** Located behind the knee are the common peroneal and tibial nerves and the popliteal arteries.
- **Throat.** The throat region contains two triangular regions, the anterior and posterior cervical triangles.
  - *Anterior cervical triangle's* defining borders—the trachea, the base of the jaw (mandible), and muscle sternocleidomastoid—contains seven endangerment sites, which are the common carotid arteries, external carotid arteries, hyoid bone, internal jugular veins, thyroid gland, trachea, and vagus nerves.
  - *Posterior cervical triangle,* which uses the clavicle (collar bone) and the muscles sternocleidomastoid and trapezius, as its defining borders and presents the following endangerment sites: brachial plexus, external jugular veins, facial nerve, subclavian artery, and styloid processes of the temporal bone.

BOX 17-1 Pathologies and Massage Contraindications

Conditions That Require Physician Clearance
- Acromegaly
- Aneurysm
- Atherosclerosis
- Burns
- Cancer
- Cerebrovascular accident
- Chronic obstructive pulmonary disease
- Congestive heart failure
- Coronary artery disease
- Hemophilia
- Hodgkin's disease
- Kidney stones
- Leukemia
- Myasthenia gravis
- Nephrosis
- Peritonitis
- Polycystic kidney disease
- Shingles*
- Uremia

Conditions With Local Contraindications
- Abdominal diastasis (avoid abdomen)
- Abnormal lumps (avoid area)
- Acne vulgaris (avoid infected area)
- Athlete's foot (avoid infected area)
- Blister (avoid area)
- Bruise (avoid bruised area if less than 72 hours old)
- Carpal tunnel syndrome (avoid inflamed area)
- Colitis (avoid abdomen)
- Cretinism (avoid throat area)
- Crohn's disease (avoid abdomen)
- Cystitis (avoid abdomen)
- Decubitus ulcers (avoid ulcerated area)
- Diverticular diseases (avoid abdomen)
- Folliculitis (avoid infected area)
- Foreign objects embedded in the skin such as glass, pencil lead, and metal (avoid area)
- Furuncle/carbuncle (avoid infected area)
- Goiter (avoid throat area)
- Gouty arthritis (avoid infected area)
- Graves' disease (avoid throat region and any enlarged lymph nodes)
- Hernia such as hiatal, femoral, inguinal, and umbilical (avoid herniated area)
- Herpes simplex (avoid infected area)
- Hyperthyroidism (avoid throat area)
- Hypothyroidism (avoid throat area)
- Impetigo (avoid infected area)
- Irritable bowel syndrome (avoid abdomen)
- Local inflammation (avoid inflamed area)
- Onychomycosis (avoid infected area)
- Open wounds (avoid wounded area)
- Paronychia (avoid infected area)
- Phlebitis (lightly over affected area)
- Polyps (avoid abdomen)
- Poison ivy, poison oak, poison sumac (unless affected area is widespread, in which case this is an absolute contraindication)
- (Seborrheic keratosis (avoid infected area)
- Shingles (avoid infected area)*
- Spina bifida (avoid lumbosacral area)
- Swollen lymph glands (avoid swollen area)
- Thrombophlebitis (lightly over affected area; avoid inner thigh region)
- Ulcers (avoid abdomen)
- Unhealed burns and abrasions (avoid injured area)
- Urinary incontinence (avoid abdomen)
- Urinary tract infection (avoid abdomen)
- Varicose veins (lightly over affected area)
- Wart (avoid infected area)

Conditions With Absolute Contraindications
- Appendicitis
- Autoimmune diseases or acute inflammatory processes during exacerbation period (or flare-up)
- Cardiac arrest
- Chickenpox
- Cholecystitis (during flare-up)
- Cirrhosis of the liver (if due to viral agent)
- Contact dermatitis (if widespread area is involved)
- Diarrhea (if due to infection)
- Embolism
- Encephalitis
- Fever
- Gallstones (if during a gallbladder attack)
- German measles
- Gout (during acute phase)
- Hemorrhage
- Hepatitis (during acute phase)
- Hives (during acute phase)
- Hypertension (if not controlled by diet, exercise, and/or medication)
- Infectious diseases (many are contained in this list)
- Inflammation
- Influenza
- Intestinal obstruction
- Jaundice
- Laryngitis (if caused by infectious agent)
- Lice
- Lupus (during a flare-up)
- Measles
- Meningitis
- Migraine headache (during the migraine headache episode)
- Mononucleosis
- Multiple sclerosis (during flare-up)
- Mumps
- Pancreatitis (if acute pancreatitis)
- Pericarditis
- Pharyngitis (if due to infection)
- Pleurisy (if caused by infectious agent)
- Pneumonia (during acute phase)
- Preeclampsia
- Psychiatric diagnoses of manic depressive psychosis, schizophrenic psychosis, and paranoid conditions
- Pulmonary embolism
- Pyelonephritis
- Rabies
- Recent injury (wait 72 hours or until medical clearance is given)
- Recent surgery (until medical clearance is given)
- Respiratory distress syndrome
- Rheumatoid arthritis (during flare-up)
- Ringworm
- Scabies
- Scarlet fever
- Scleroderma (during flare-up)
- Severe, acute pain
- Sickle cell disease (during flare-up)
- Tonsillitis
- Tuberculosis

*If you, the therapist, have not had the chicken pox, do not massage; it is a contraindication for you.

CHAPTER 18

Anatomy and Physiology

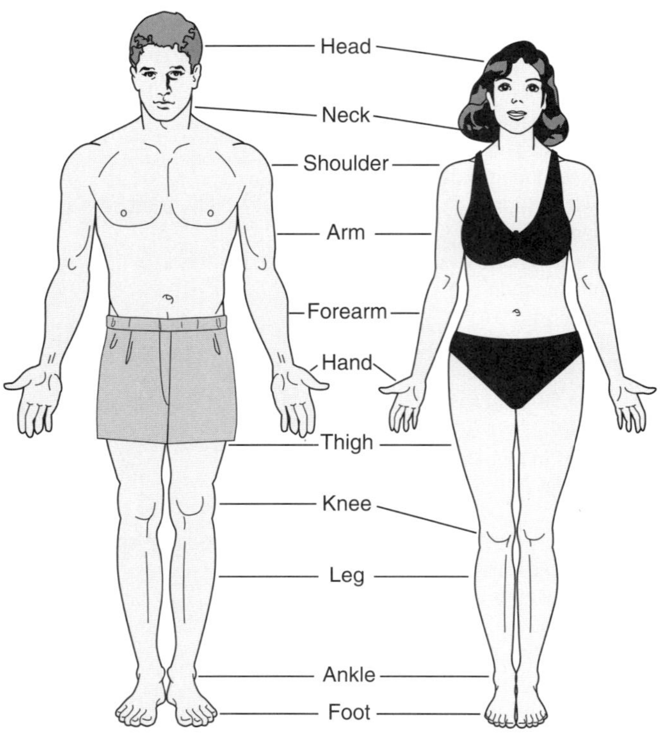

FIGURE 18-1 Anatomic position. The person is standing upright, facing forward, feet slightly separated, arms hanging at the sides with palms facing forward. Structures are named and their positions are described using this standard position.

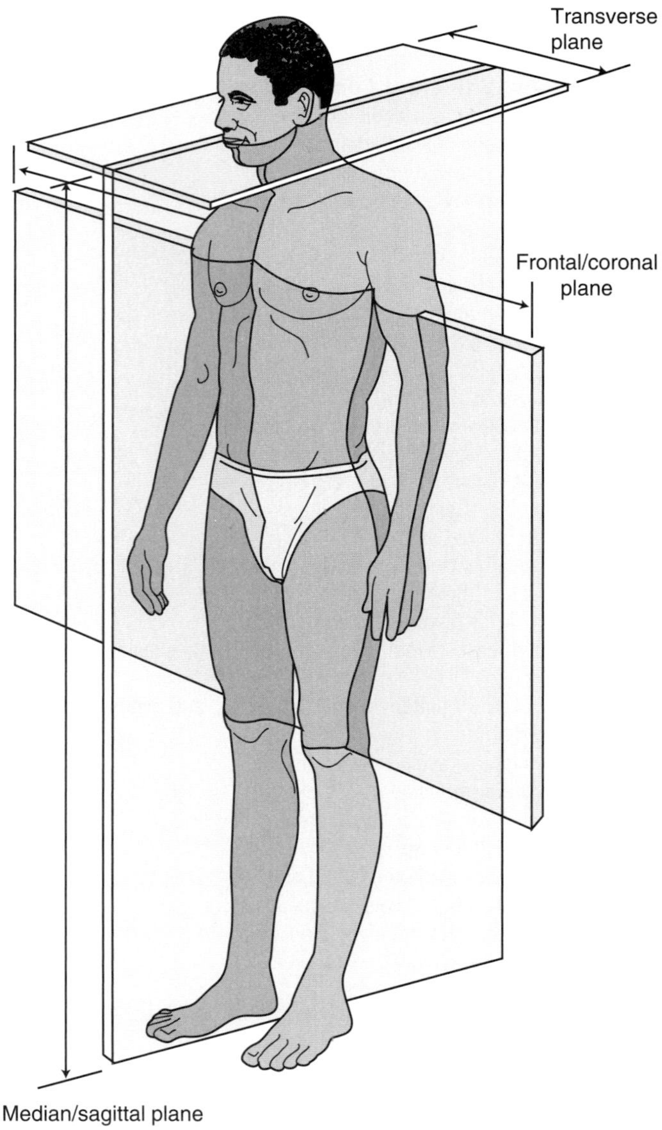

FIGURE 18-2 Anatomic planes.

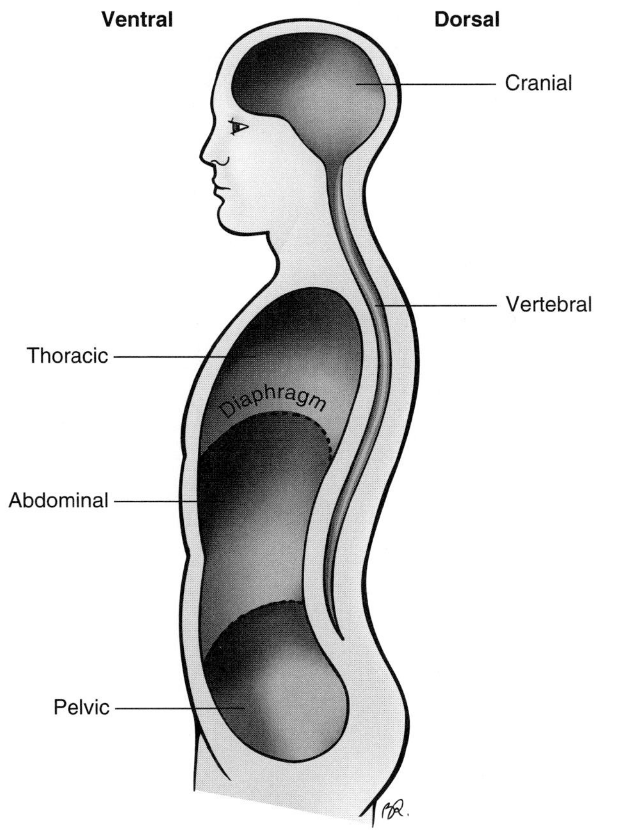

FIGURE 18-3 Body cavities. *(From Fritz S:* Mosby's fundamentals of therapeutic massage, *ed 4, St Louis, 2009, Mosby.)*

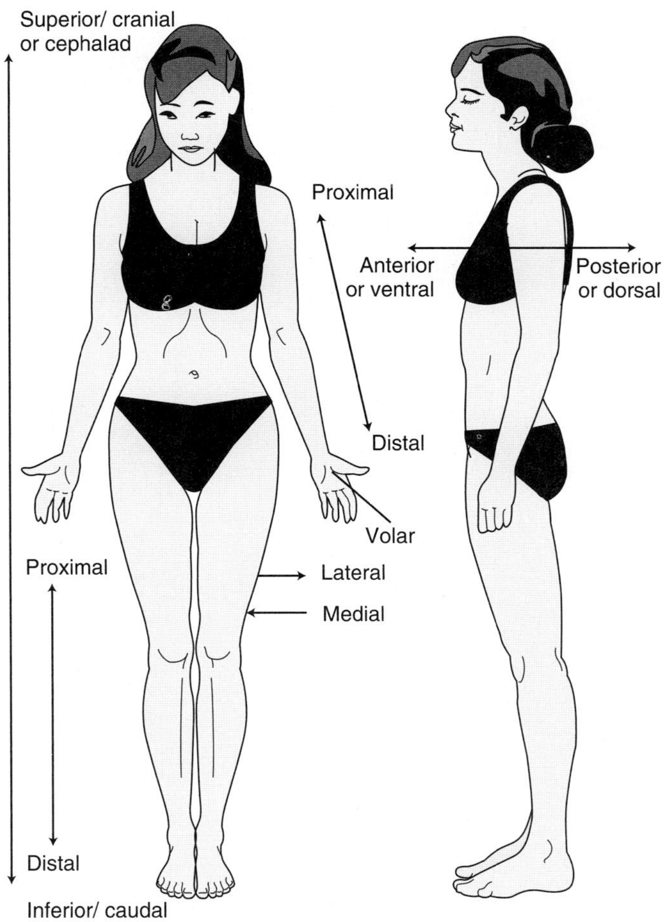

FIGURE 18-4 Directional terms.

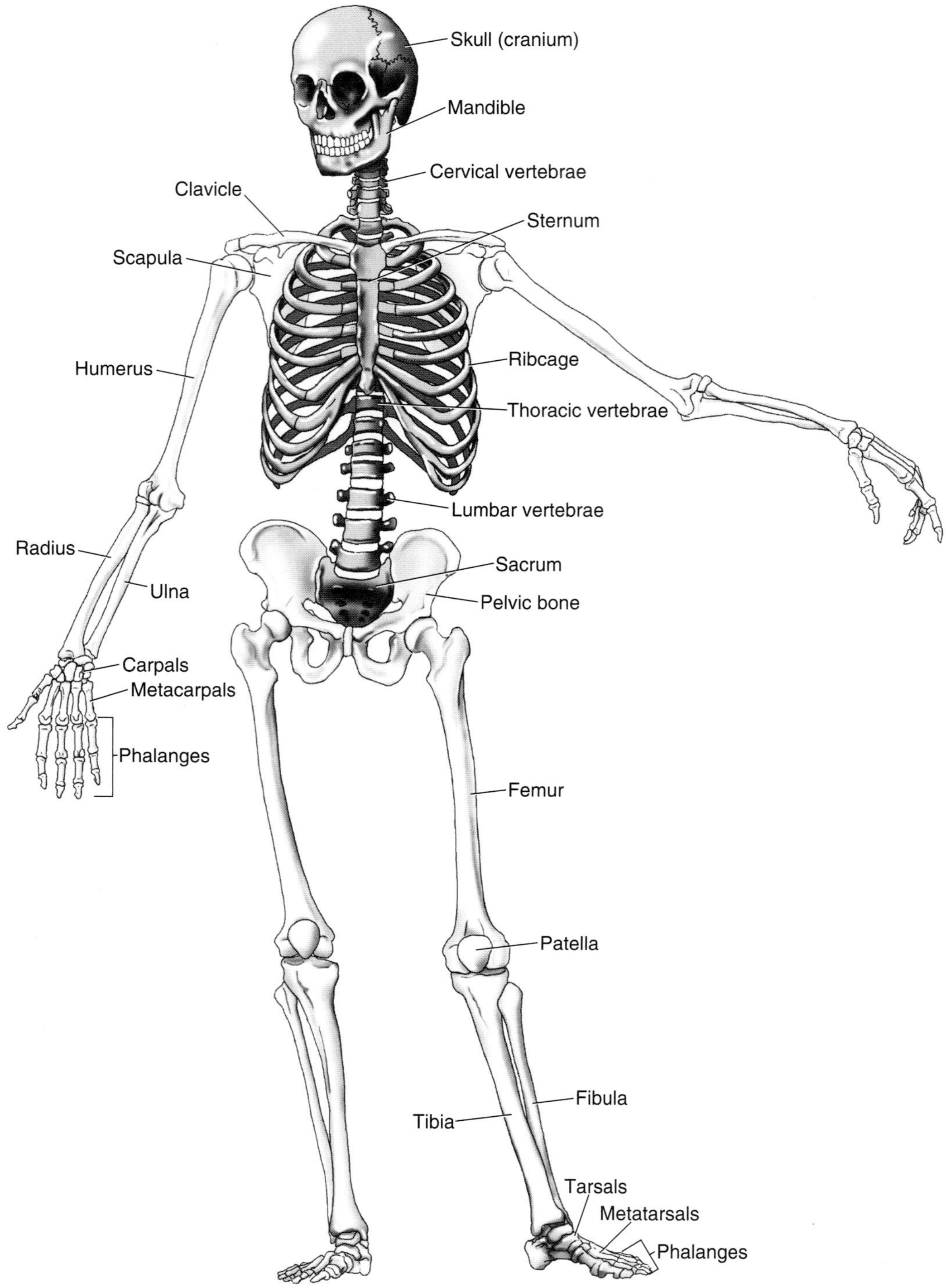

FIGURE 18-5 Skeleton. The *dark gray* bones are the axial skeleton; the *light gray* bones are the appendicular skeleton. **A,** Anterior view.

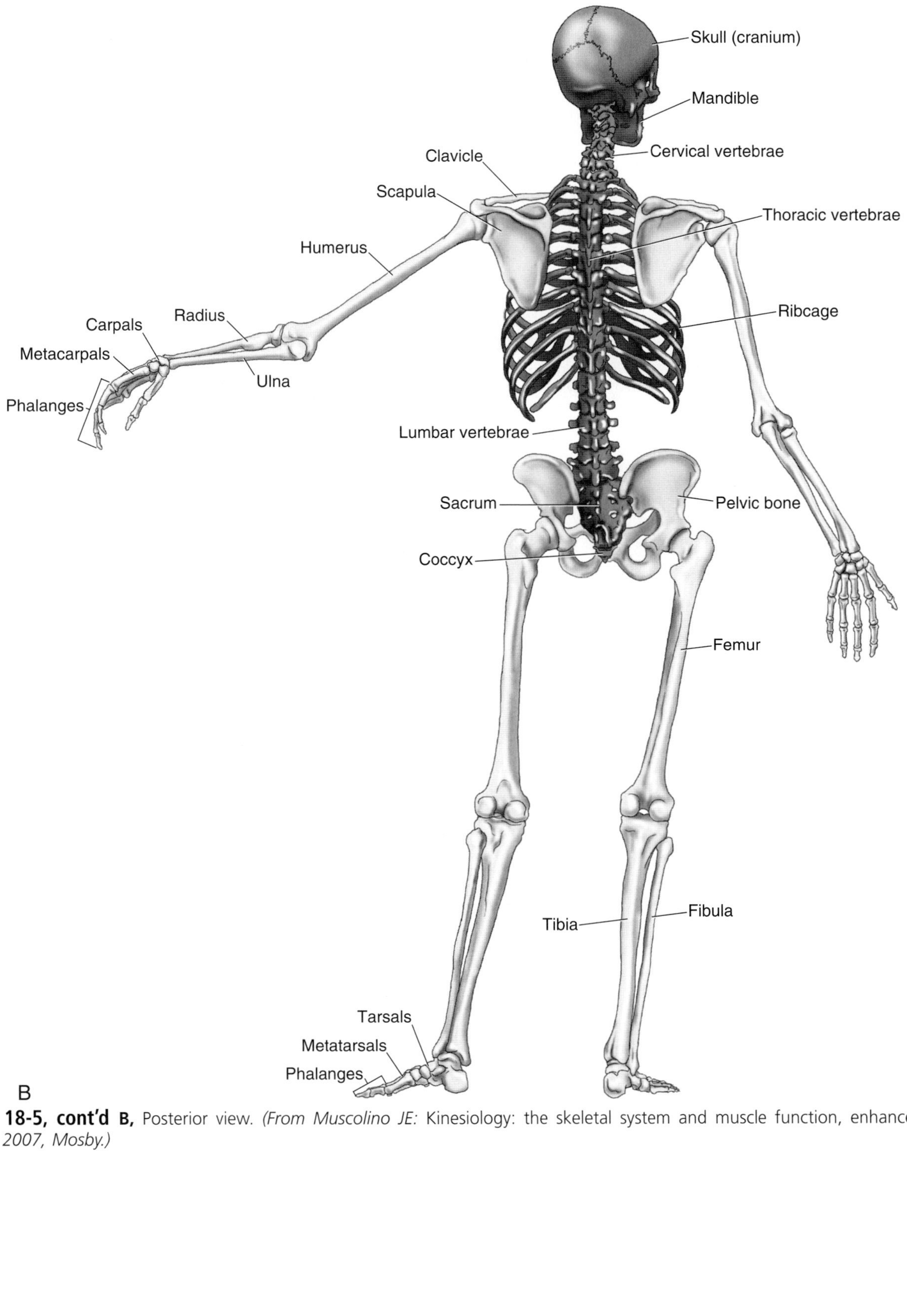

FIGURE 18-5, cont'd B, Posterior view. *(From Muscolino JE:* Kinesiology: the skeletal system and muscle function, enhanced edition, *St Louis, 2007, Mosby.)*

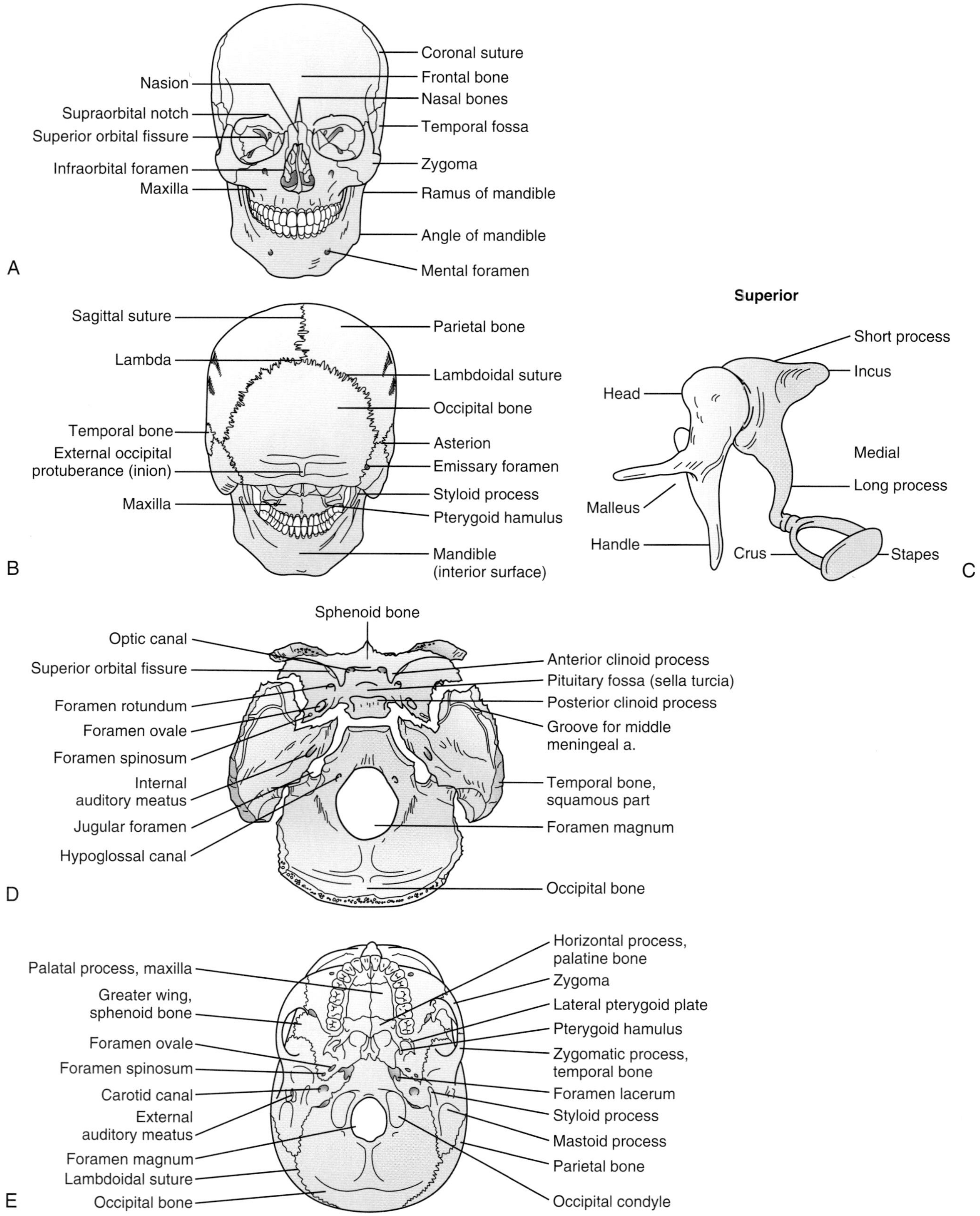

FIGURE 18-6 **A,** Anterior (frontal) view of the skull. **B,** Posterior view of the skull. **C,** The three auditory ossicles. The malleus attaches to the inner surface of the tympanic membrane (eardrum). The incus links the malleus to the stapes. The stapes is attached to the wall of the inner ear. **D,** Detailed view of the internal surface of the base of the skull. The sphenoid, occipital, and temporal bones are presented as slightly separated to show that many of the important apertures traversing the floor of the skull are found within one of these bones or along their mutual borders. **E,** Basal view of the skull, showing several of the important foramina that convey nerves and vessels in and out of the cranial cavity.

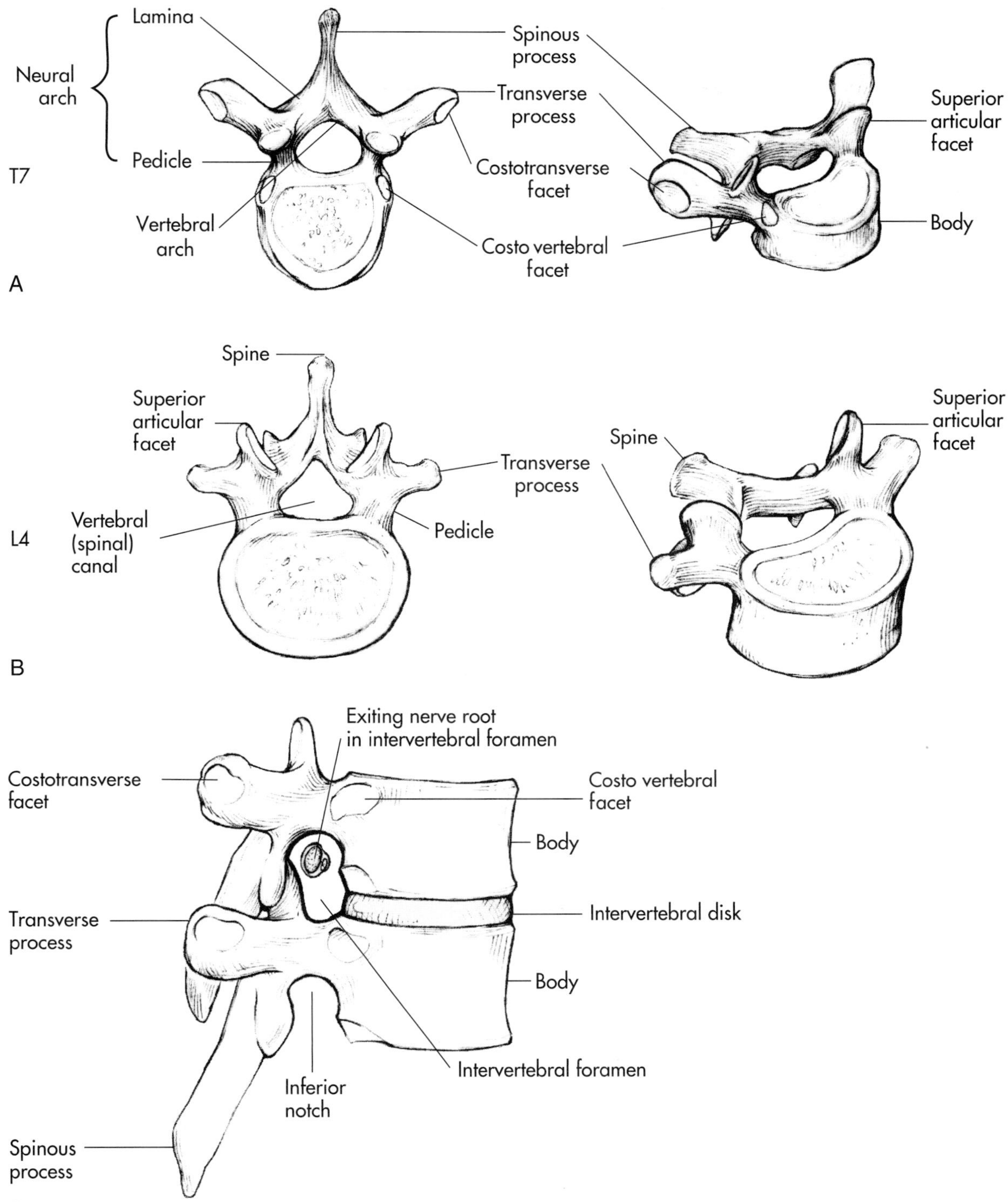

Figure 18-7 Common types of vertebrae (two views of T7 and L4 vertebrae). **A,** Superoinferior views. **B,** Right anterior oblique views. **C,** Intervertebral foramen. Vertebrae T5 and T6 have been articulated, showing the resulting intervertebral foramen with a segmental nerve in place. Blood vessels (not shown) enter and leave the interior of the vertebral canal through the intervertebral foramen. *(From Mathers LH et al: Clinical anatomy principles, St. Louis, 1996, Mosby.)*

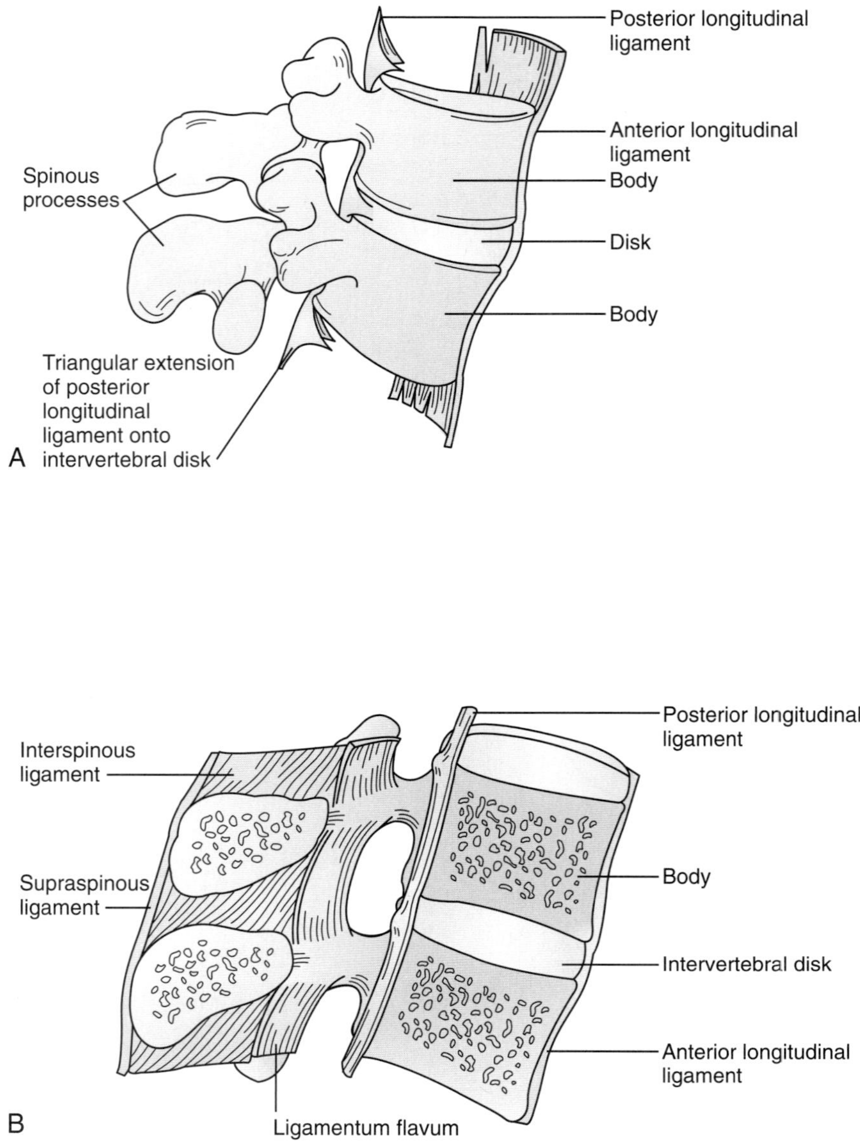

FIGURE 18-8 **A** and **B,** Vertebral ligaments.

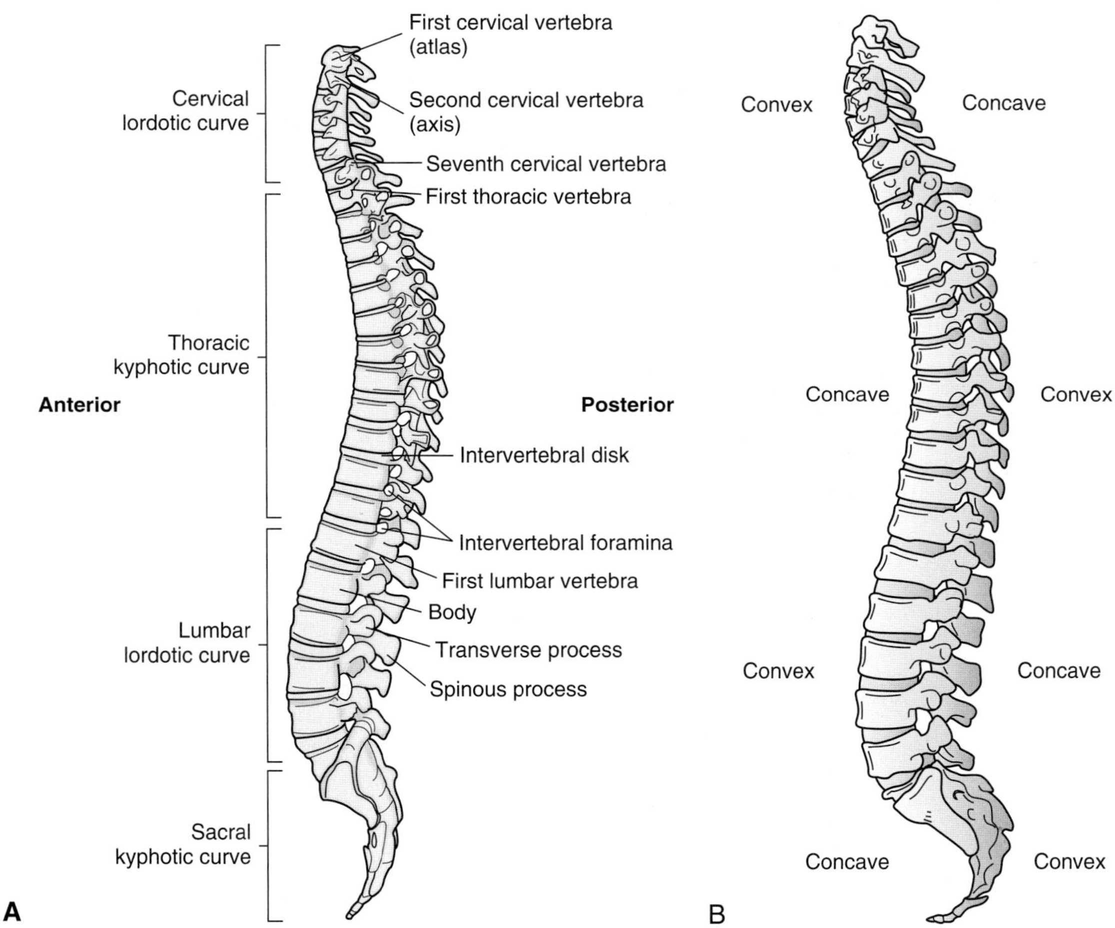

FIGURE 18-9 **A,** Vertebral column. **B,** The convex and concave curves of the vertebral column.

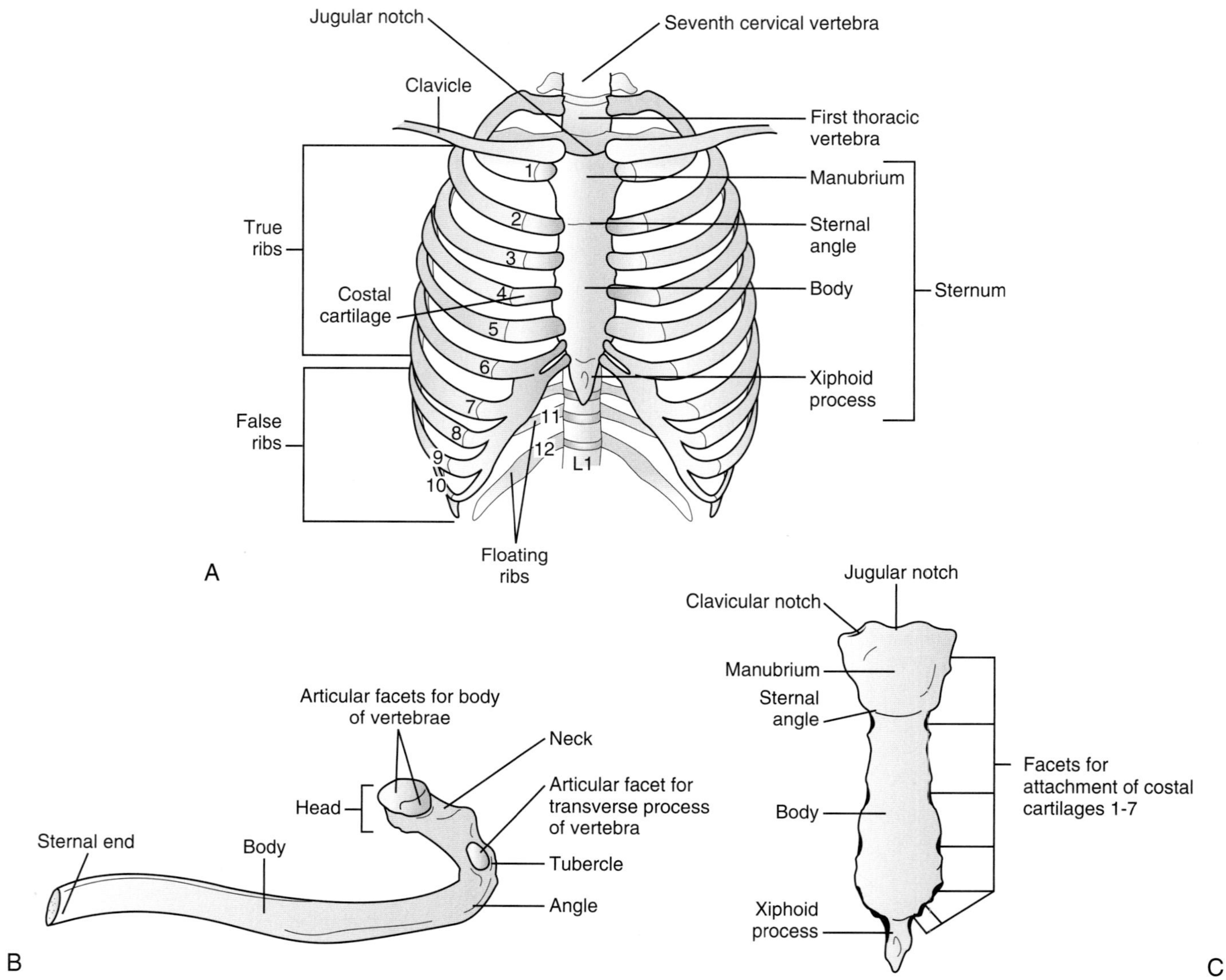

FIGURE 18-10 **A,** Rib cage. **B,** Typical rib. **C,** Sternum.

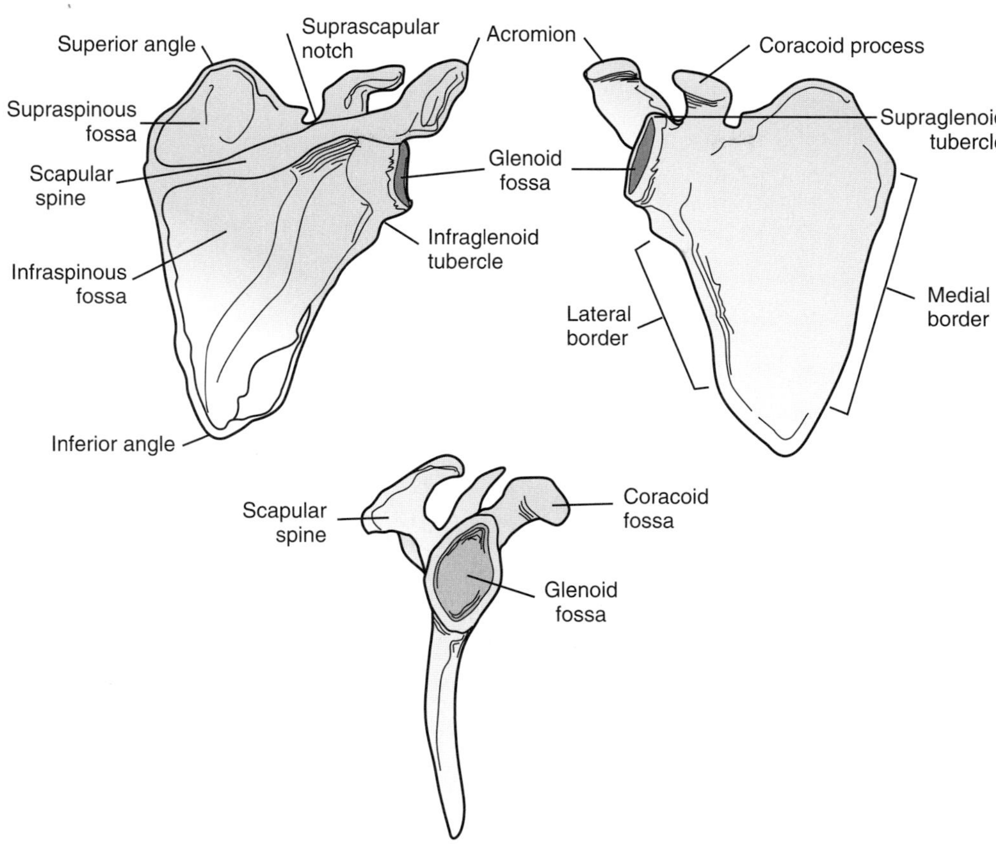

FIGURE 18-11 Scapula (three views).

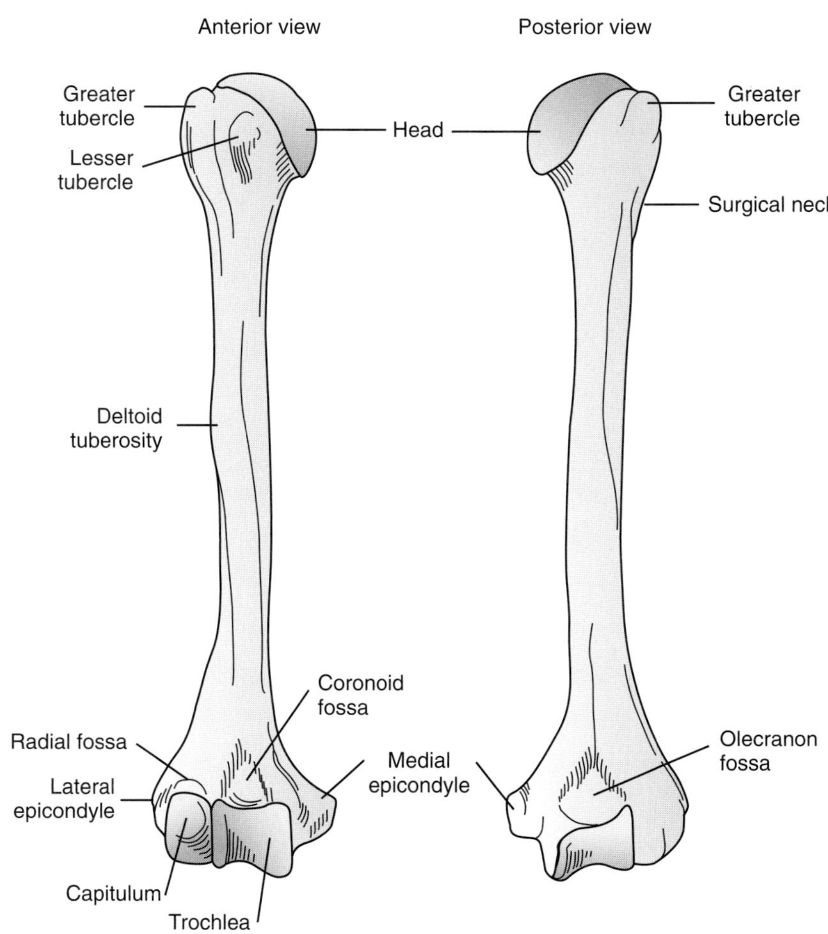

FIGURE 18-12 Anterior and posterior views of the right humerus.

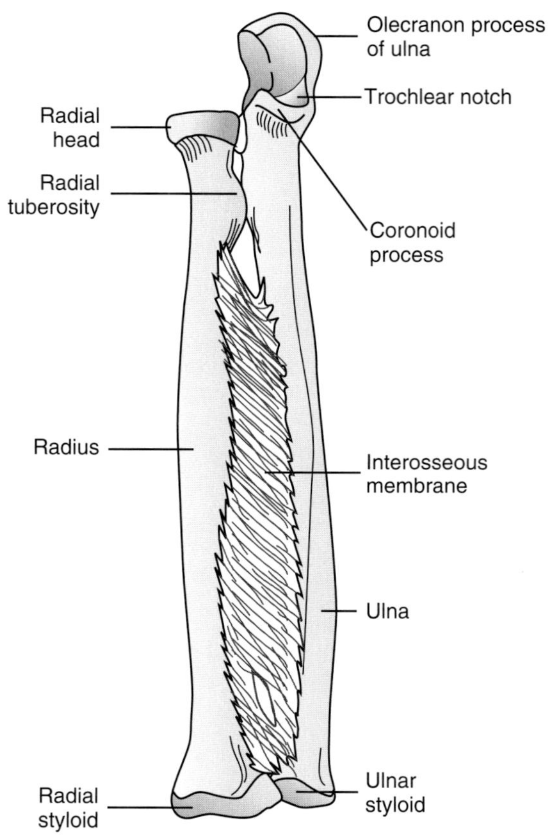

FIGURE 18-13 Anterior view of the forearm bones.

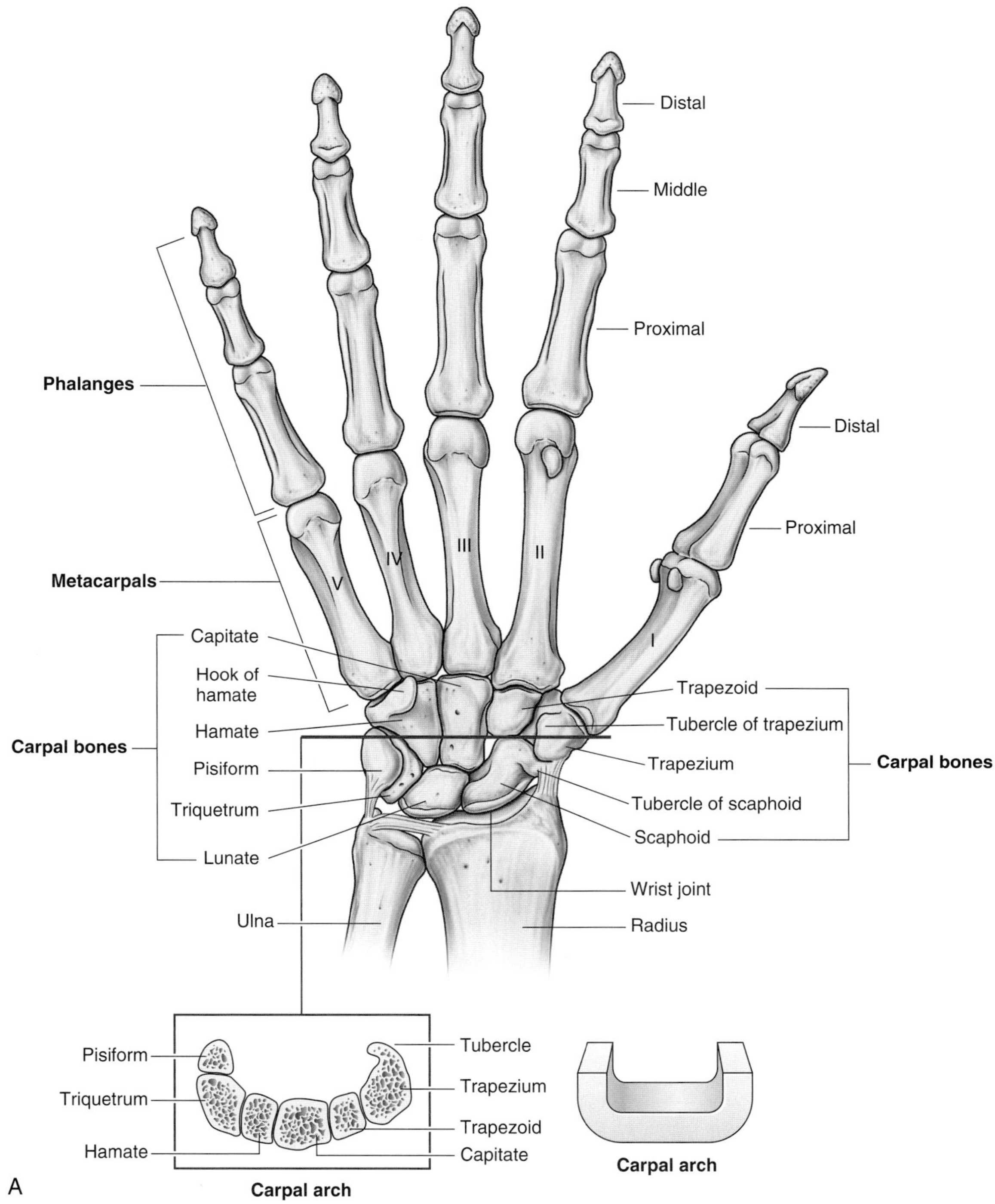

FIGURE 18-14 Anterior view of the bones of the hand.

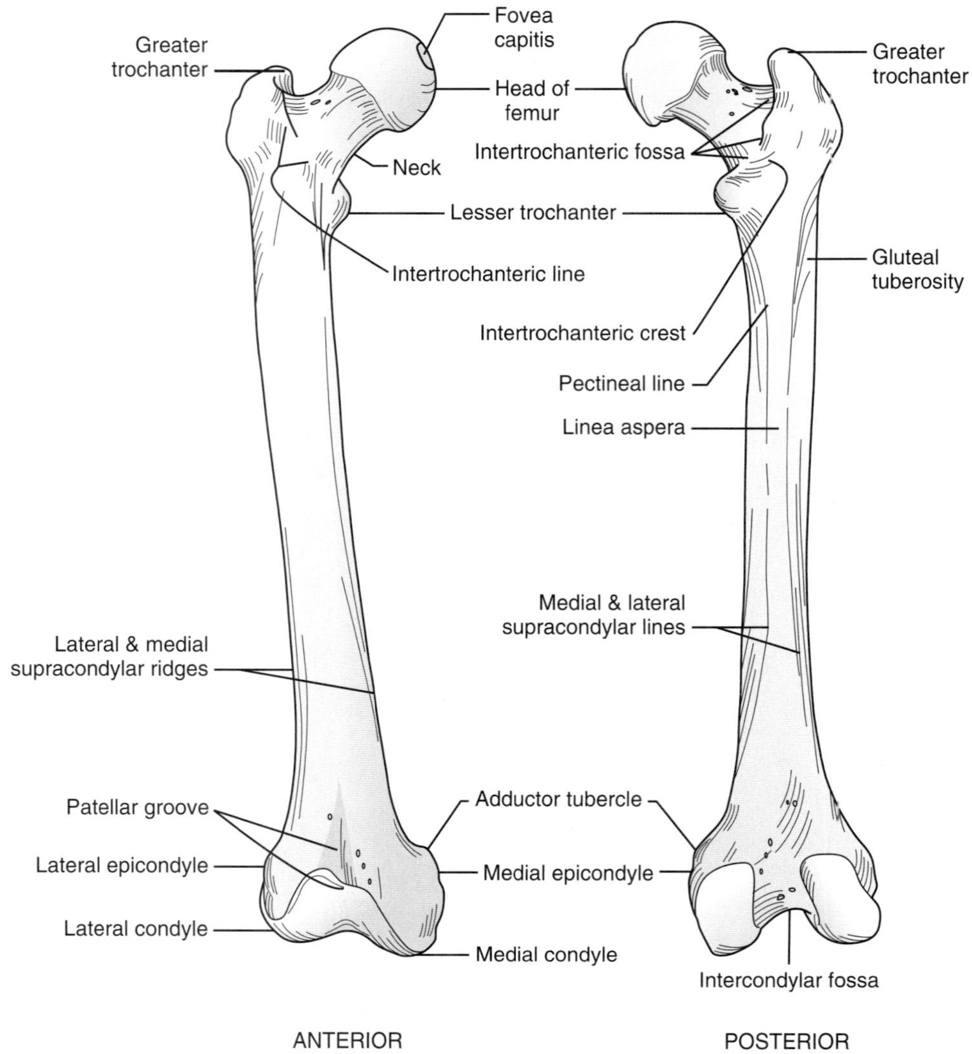

FIGURE 18-15 Anterior and posterior views of the right femur.

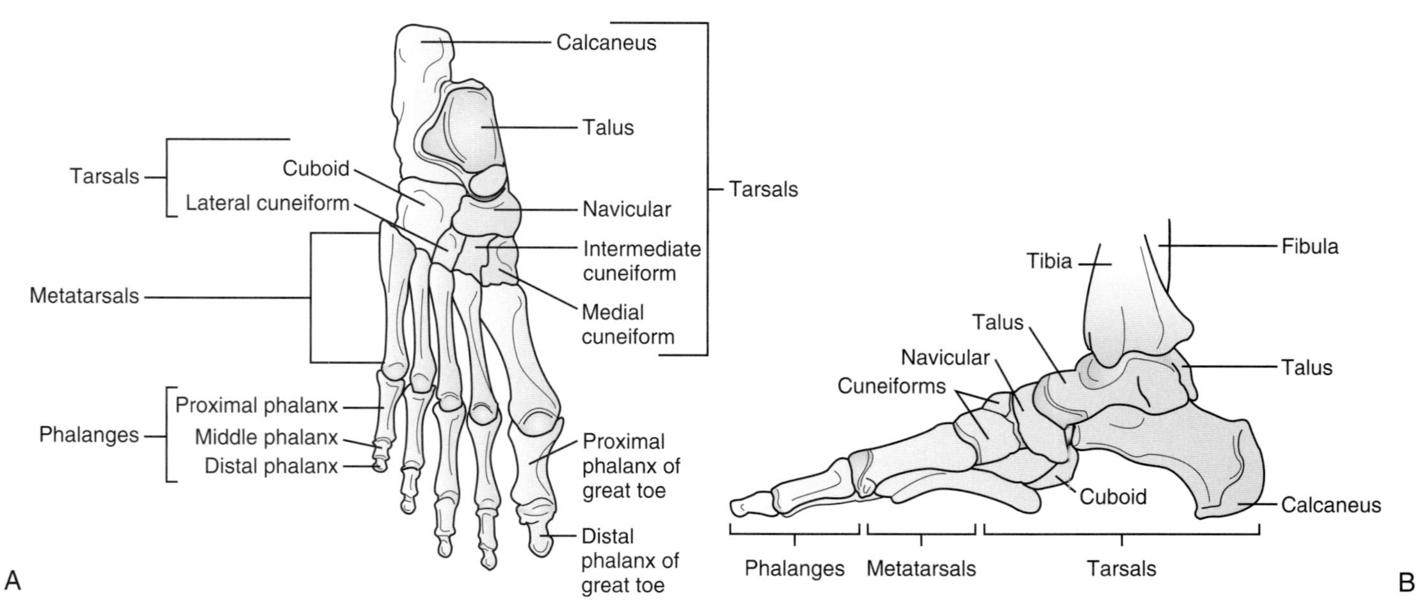

FIGURE 18-16 **A,** Dorsal view of the bones of the foot. **B,** Medial view of the bones of the foot and ankle.

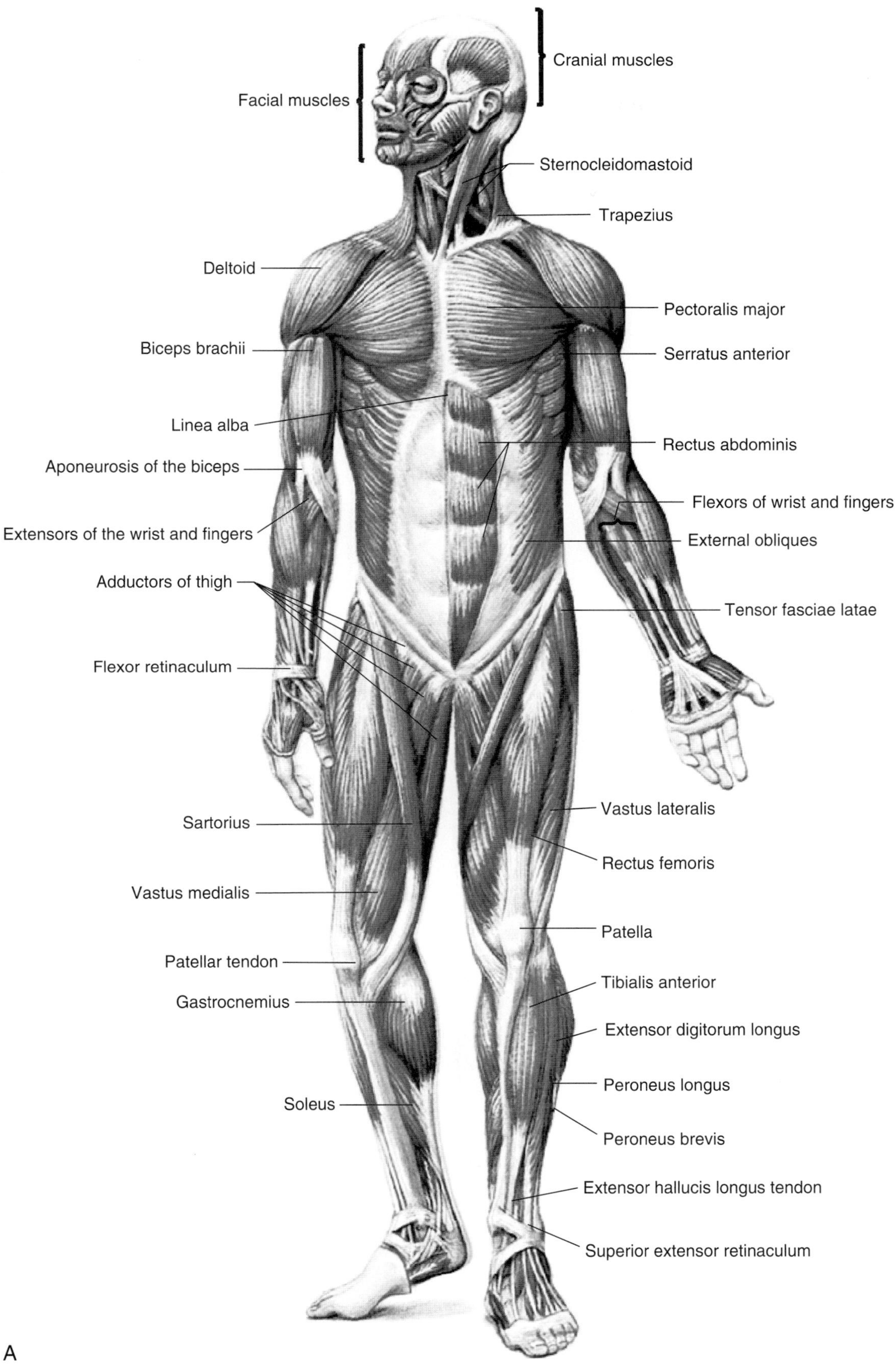

FIGURE 18-17 Surface and deep muscles. **A,** Anterior.

Continued

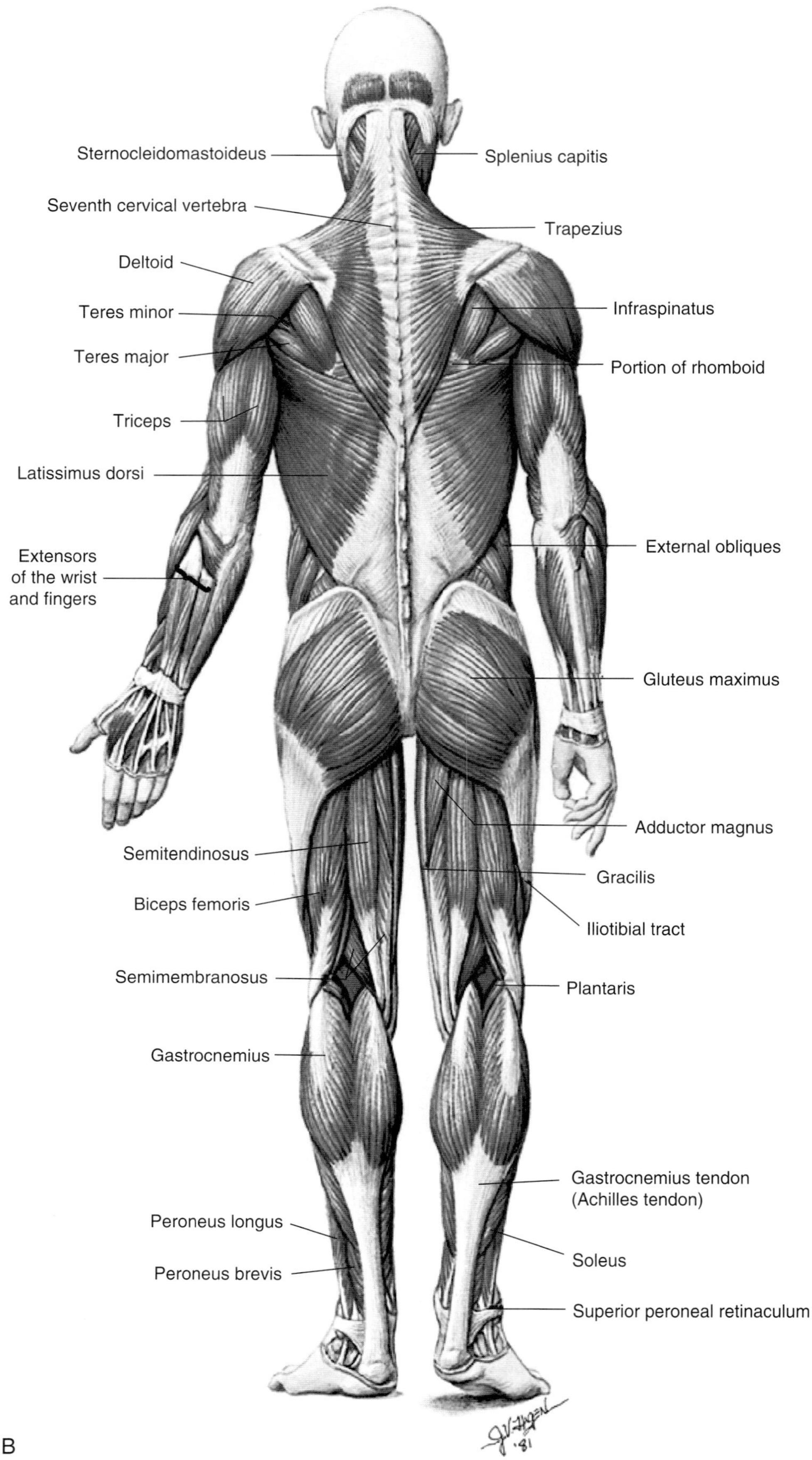

FIGURE 18-17, cont'd B, Posterior. *(From LaFleur Brooks, M:* Exploring medical language: a student-directed approach*, ed 3, St Louis, 1994, Mosby.)*

CHAPTER

19

Massage Therapy Procedures

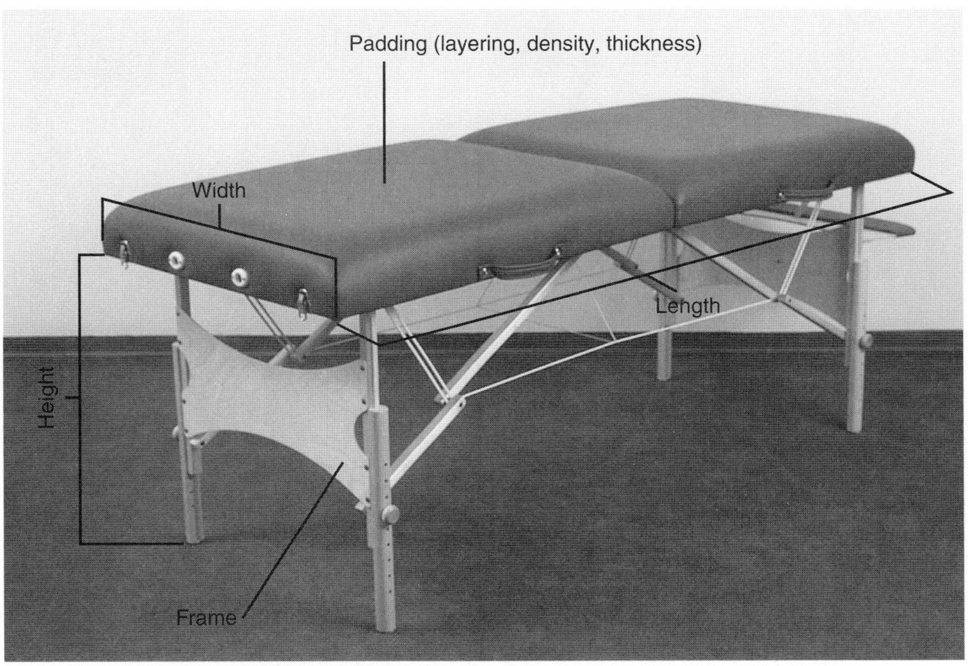

FIGURE 19-1 A typical portable massage table.

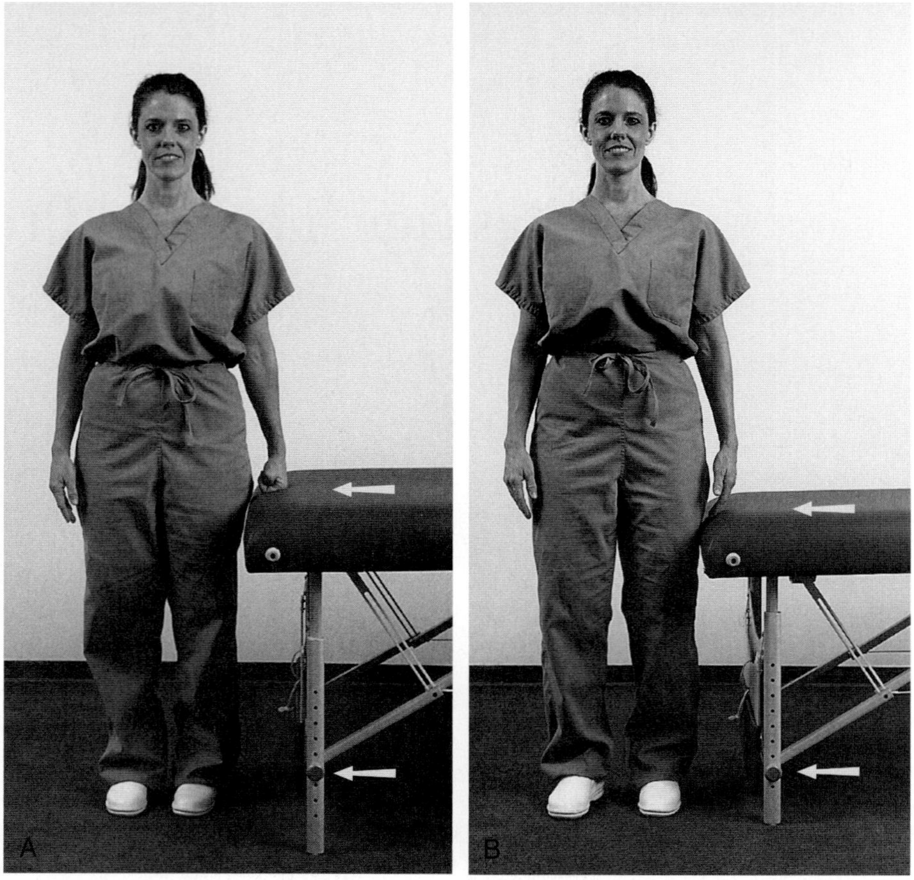

FIGURE 19-2 Two methods of determining the correct height for a massage table. **A,** Hand in a fist touching tabletop. **B,** Hand relaxed with fingertips touching tabletop.

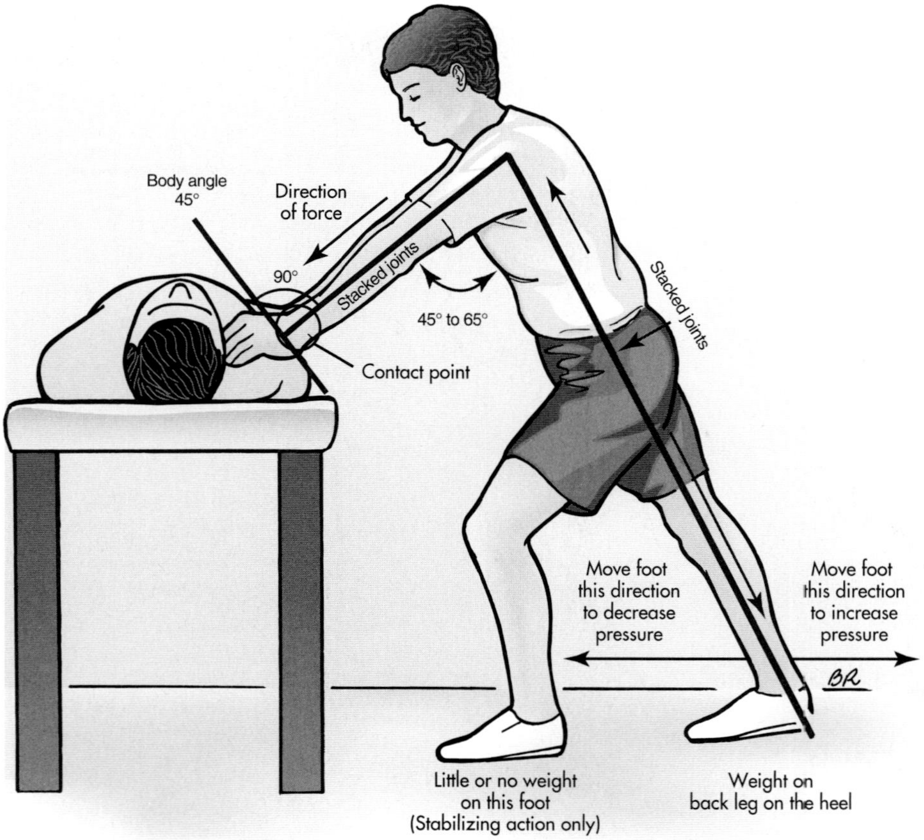

FIGURE 19-3 Correct body mechanics for compressive force required for massage.

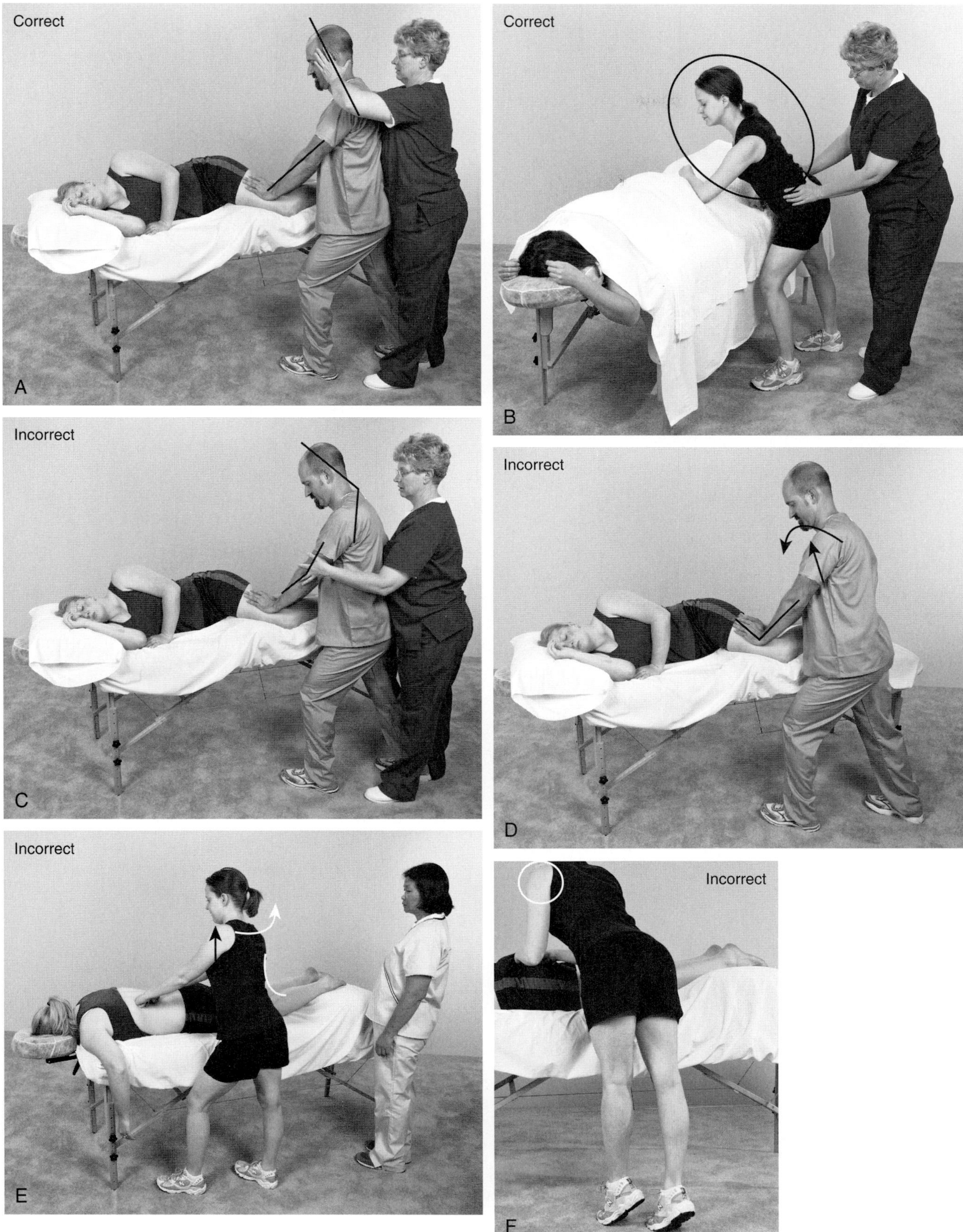

FIGURE 19-4 The neck and shoulder. **A,** Correct body mechanics: Head up, arms at 45 degrees and straight. **B,** Correct body mechanics. **C,** Incorrect body mechanics: Elbows bent, head forward. **D,** Incorrect body mechanics: Shoulders up, rotated, and forward. **E,** Incorrect body mechanics: Shoulders up and rotated with low back sway. **F,** Incorrect body mechanics.

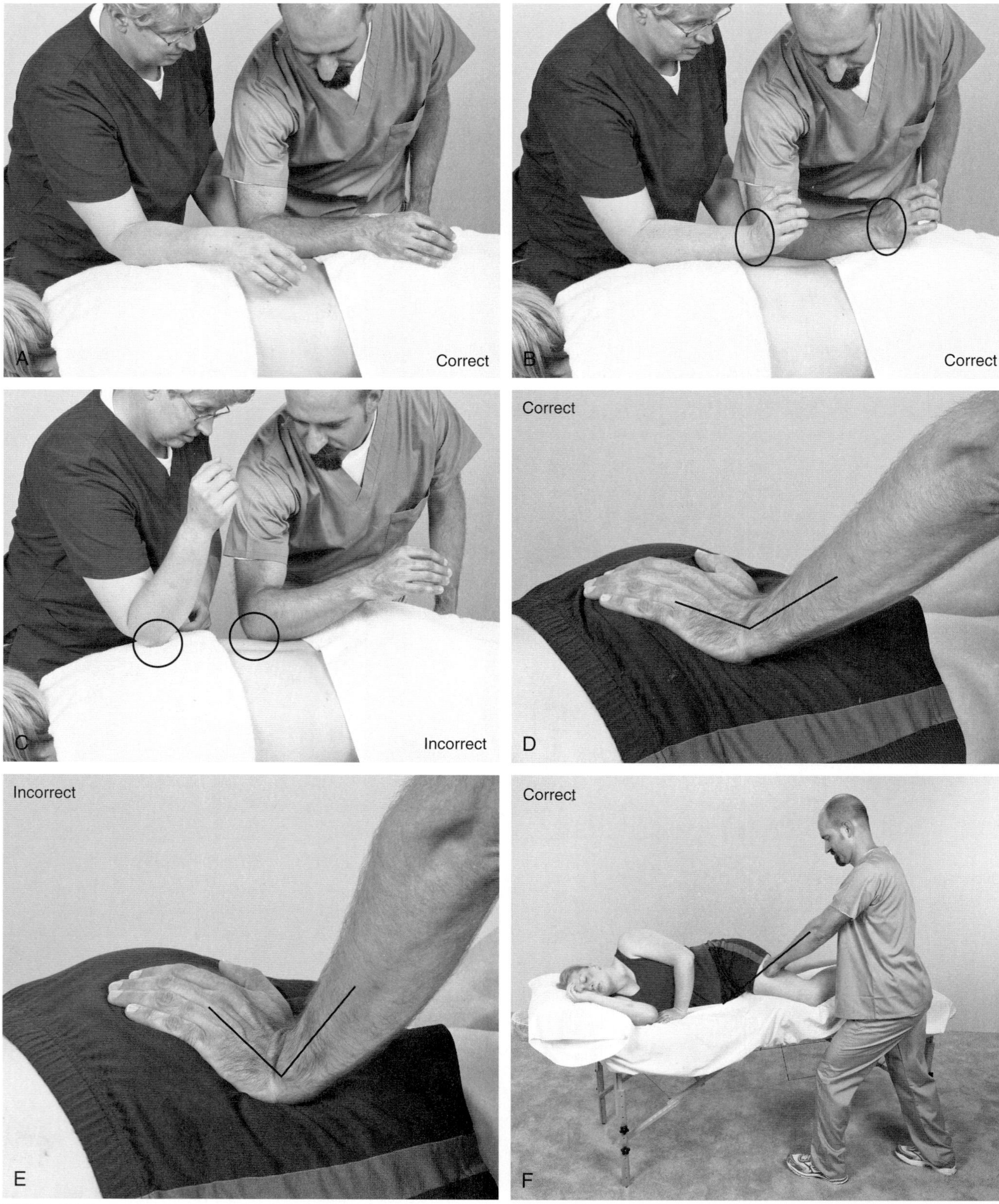

FIGURE 19-5 The forearm and wrist. **A,** Forearm. Incorrect body mechanics. Stiff wrist. **B,** Forearm. Correct body mechanics. Relaxed and flat. **C,** Forearm. Incorrect body mechanics. Using wrong point of elbow. **D,** Wrist. Correct body mechanics. **E,** Wrist. Incorrect body mechanics. **F,** Wrist. Correct body mechanics.

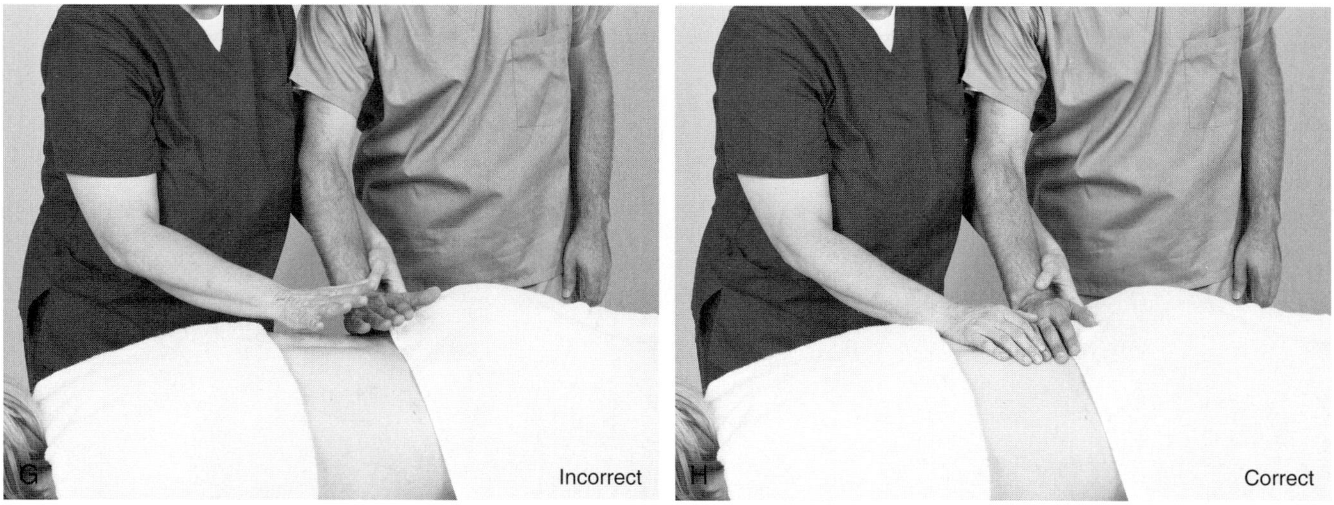

FIGURE 19-5, cont'd **G,** Wrist. Incorrect body mechanics. Hand stiff. **H,** Wrist. Correct body mechanics. Hand relaxed.

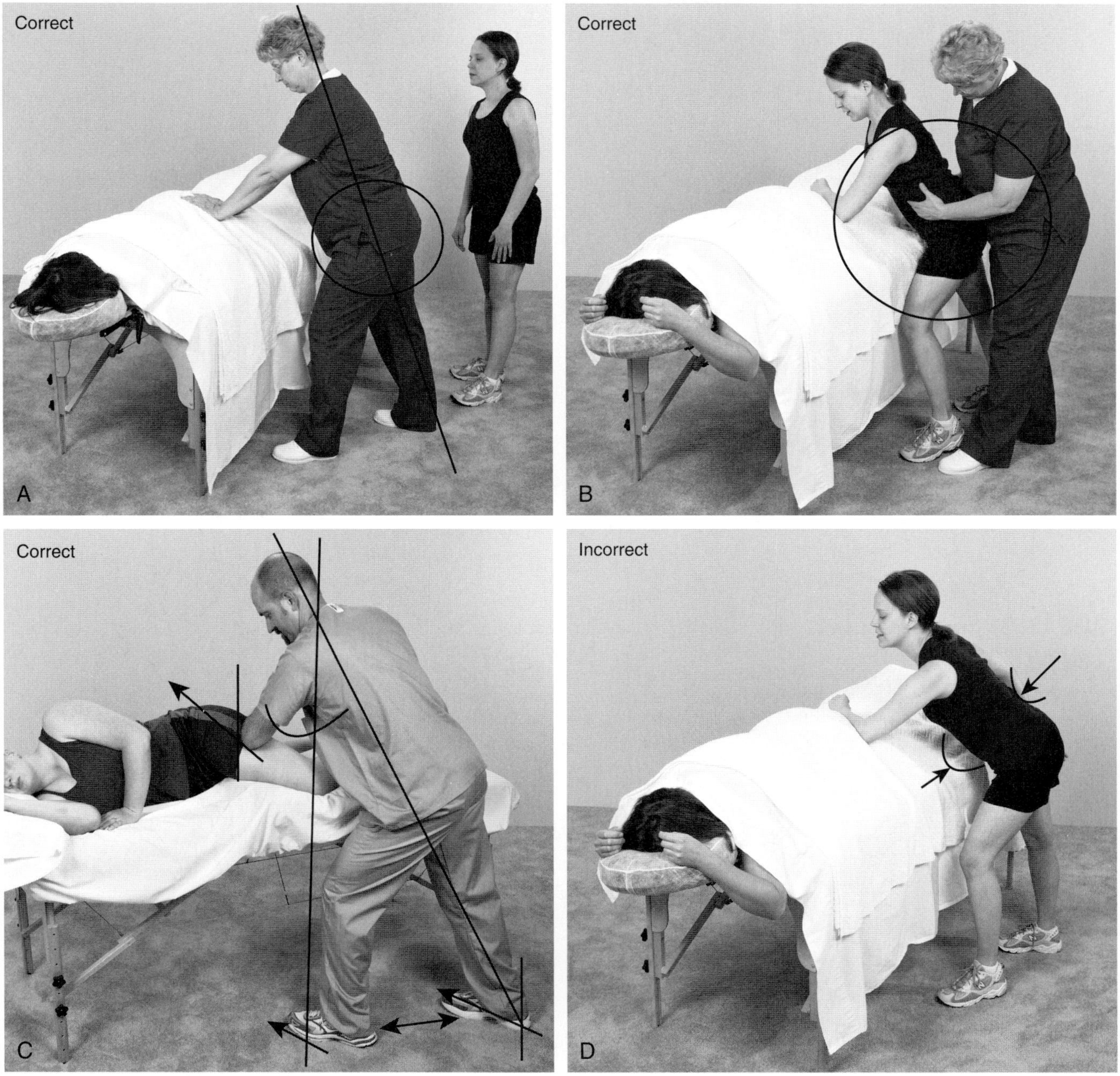

FIGURE 19-6 The low back and hips. **A,** Correct body mechanics: Back straight, core stability. **B,** Correct body mechanics: Maintaining core stability. **C,** Correct body mechanics: Back straight; feet wide enough apart and pointed in the same direction as the arm; center of gravity correct. **D,** Incorrect body mechanics: Loss of core stability.

Continued

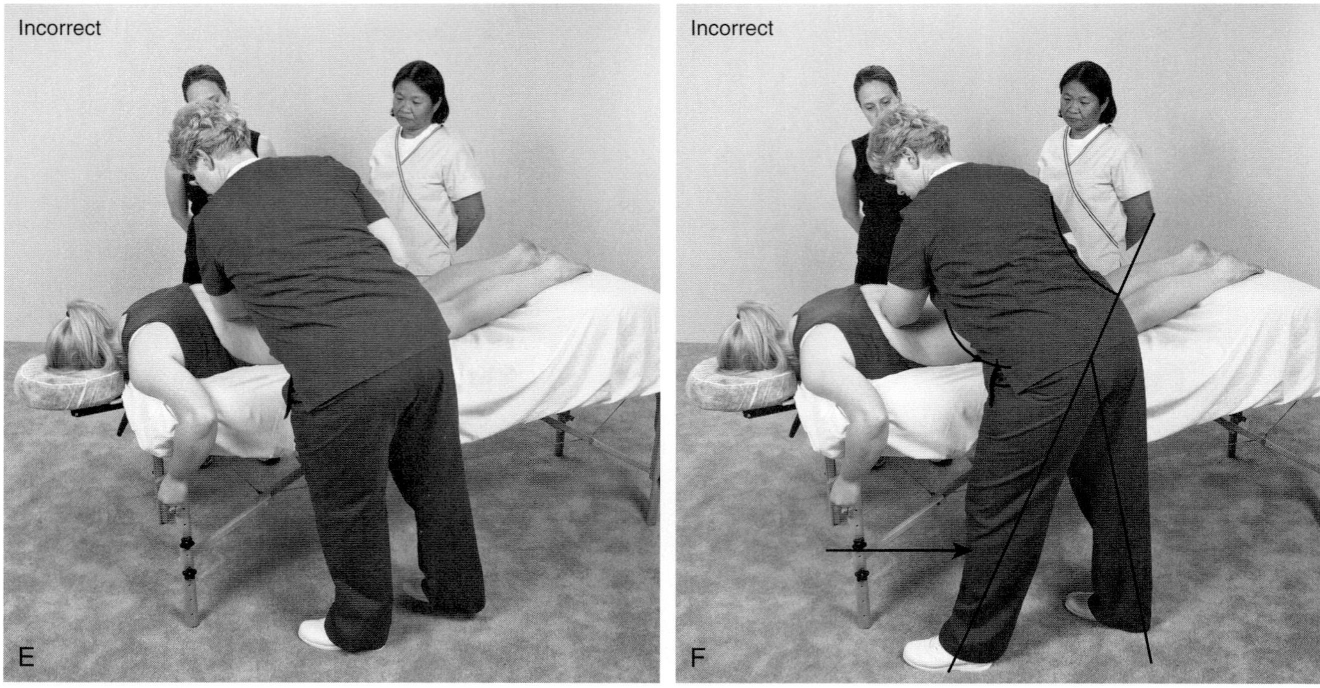

FIGURE 19-6, cont'd **E,** Incorrect body mechanics: Torsion. **F,** Incorrect body mechanics: Lower body sticks out because knee is extended; sway back; no core stability.

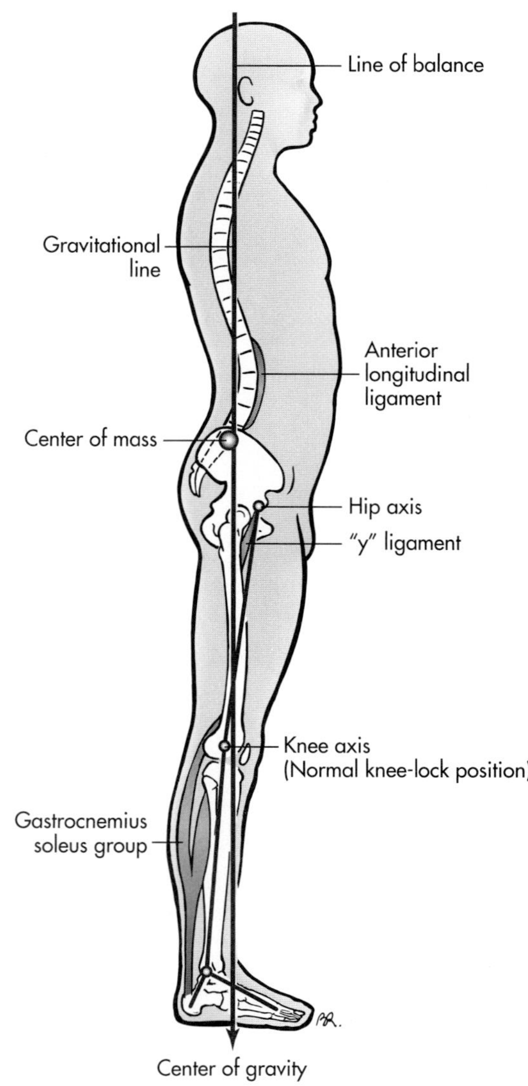

FIGURE 19-7 Relaxed standing posture that supports the gravitational line with normal knee-lock position in the last 15 degrees of extension. The gravitational force line falls behind the hip joint, in front of the knee joint, and in front of the ankle joint. The only muscle group used for balance is the gastrocnemius-soleus group. The relaxed stance involves leaning on the "y," or iliofemoral, ligament, the anterior longitudinal ligament, and the posterior knee ligaments.

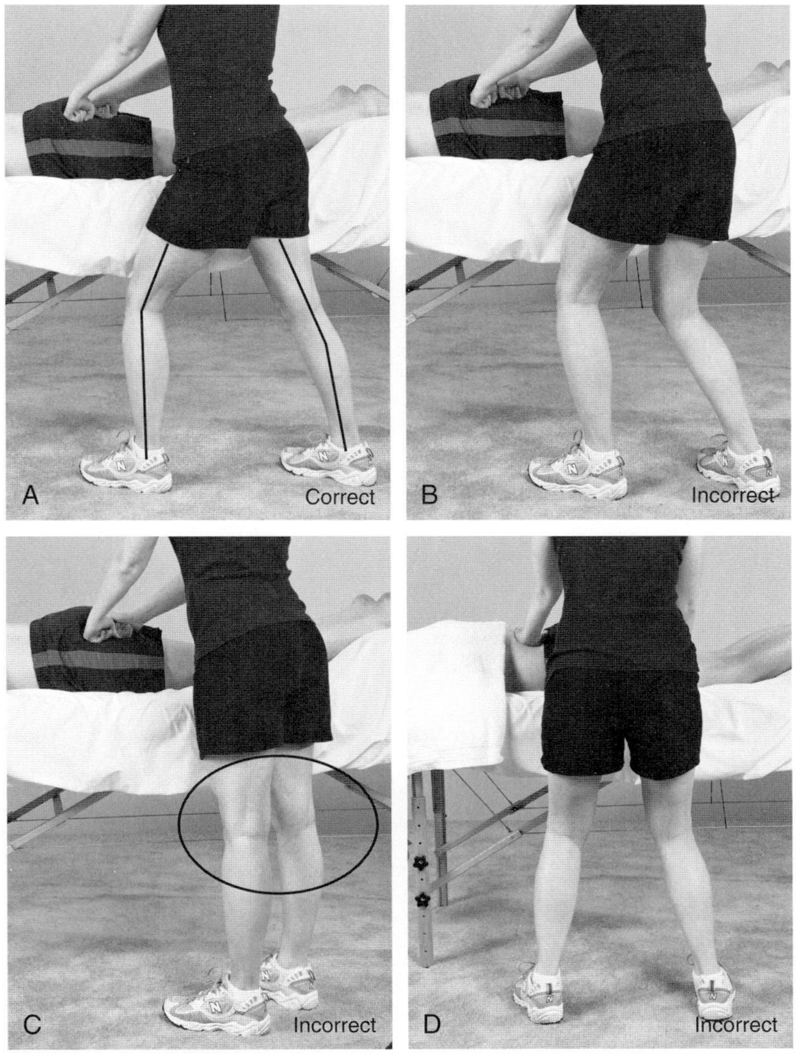

FIGURE 19-8 The knees. **A,** Correct body mechanics: Normal knee extension and flexion in asymmetric stance. **B,** Incorrect body mechanics: Bilateral flexion. **C,** Incorrect body mechanics: Bilateral hyperextension. **D,** Incorrect body mechanics: Bilateral flexion.

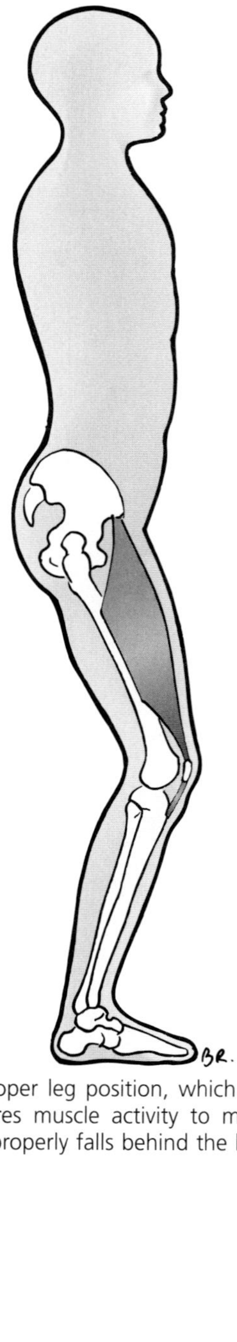

FIGURE 19-9 Improper leg position, which puts excessive strain on joints and requires muscle activity to maintain balance. The gravitational line improperly falls behind the knees.

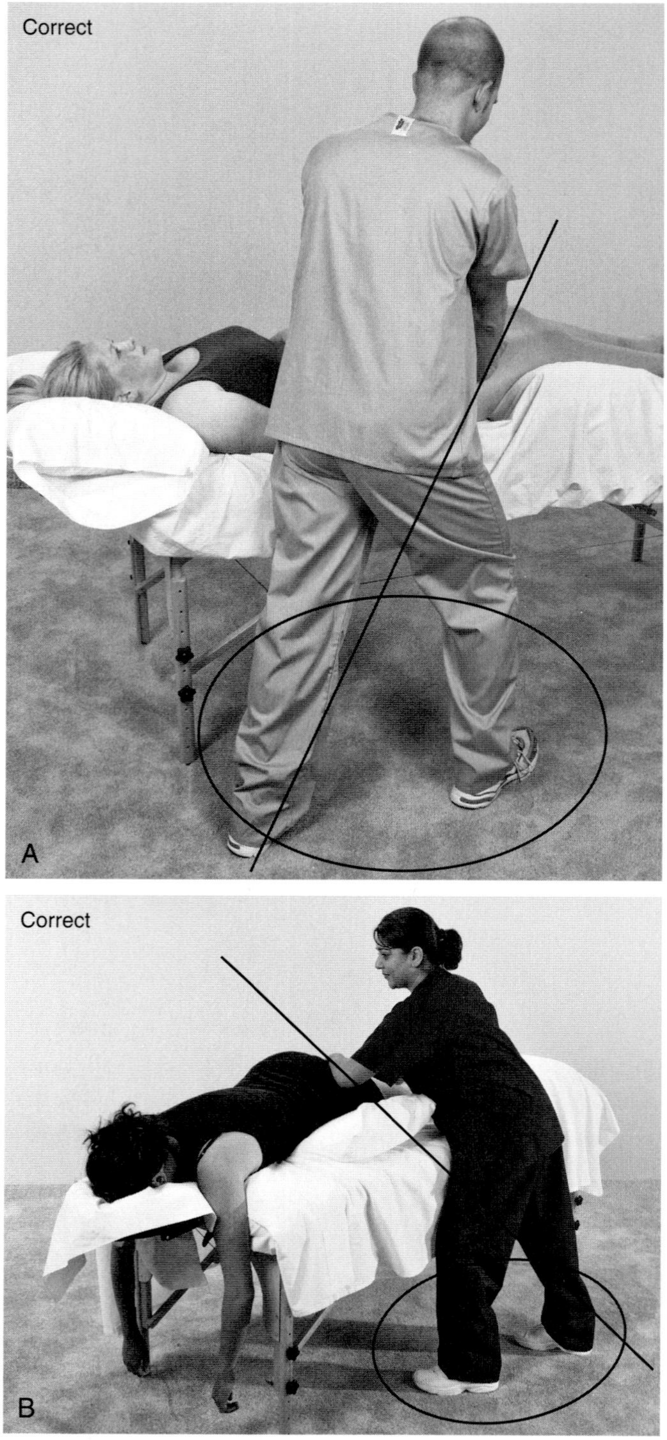

FIGURE 19-10 The ankle and foot. **A,** Correct body mechanics: Feet pointed in the direction of the stroke, asymmetric stance, feet shoulder width apart. **B,** Correct body mechanics: Feet pointed in the direction of the stroke, asymmetric stance, feet shoulder width apart.

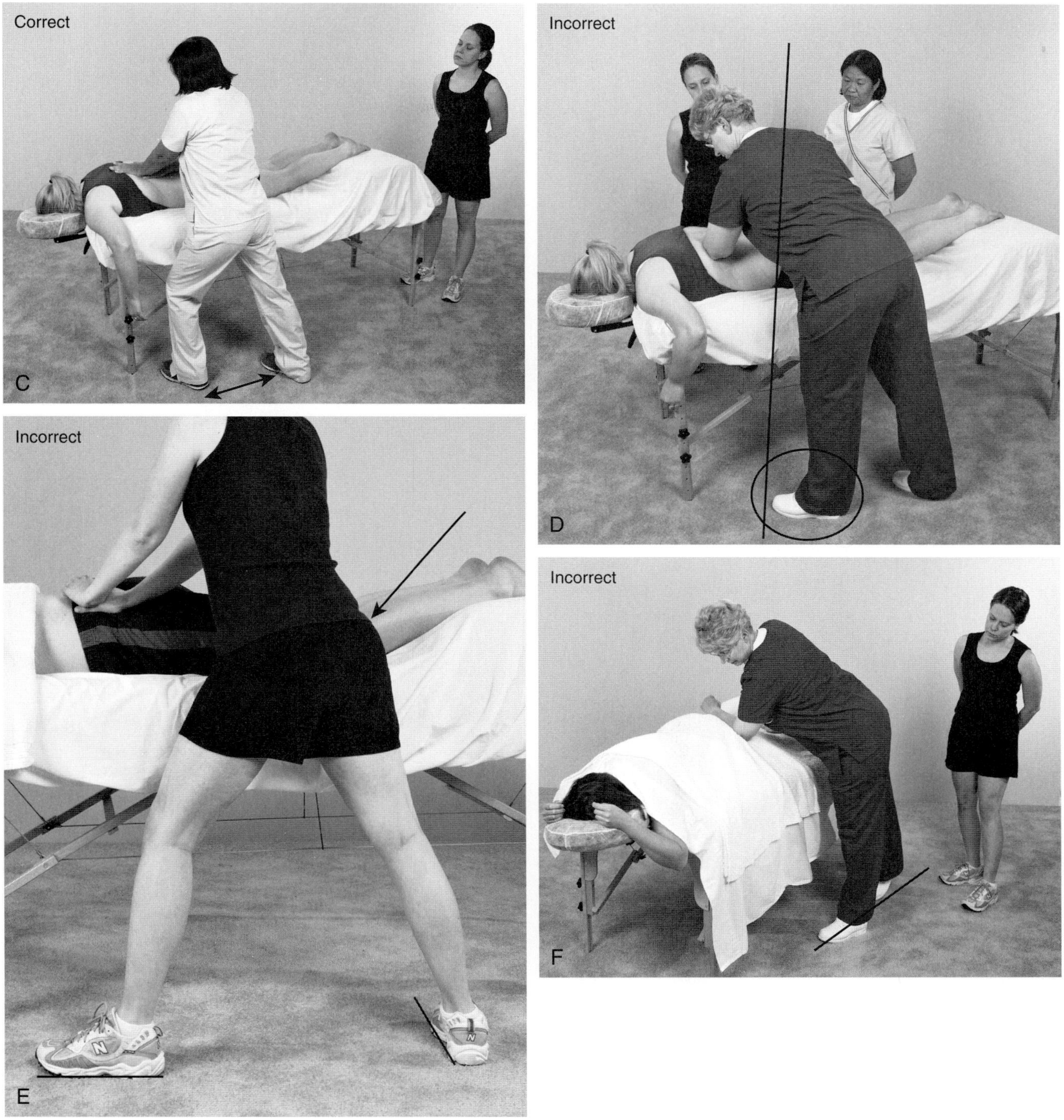

FIGURE 19-10, cont'd **C,** Correct body mechanics. **D,** Incorrect body mechanics: Weight on wrong foot. **E,** Incorrect body mechanics: Feet too far apart and not properly aligned, resulting in torsion strain. **F,** Incorrect body mechanics: Tightrope effect.

Continued

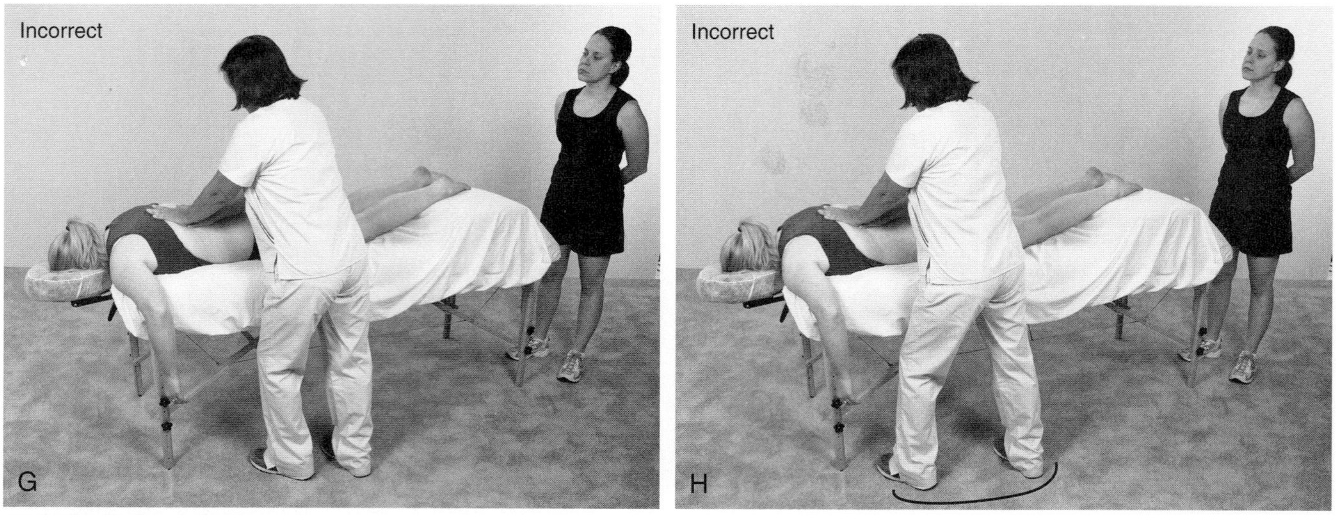

FIGURE 19-10, cont'd **G,** Incorrect body mechanics: Feet too close together. **H,** Incorrect body mechanics: Feet in symmetric stance.

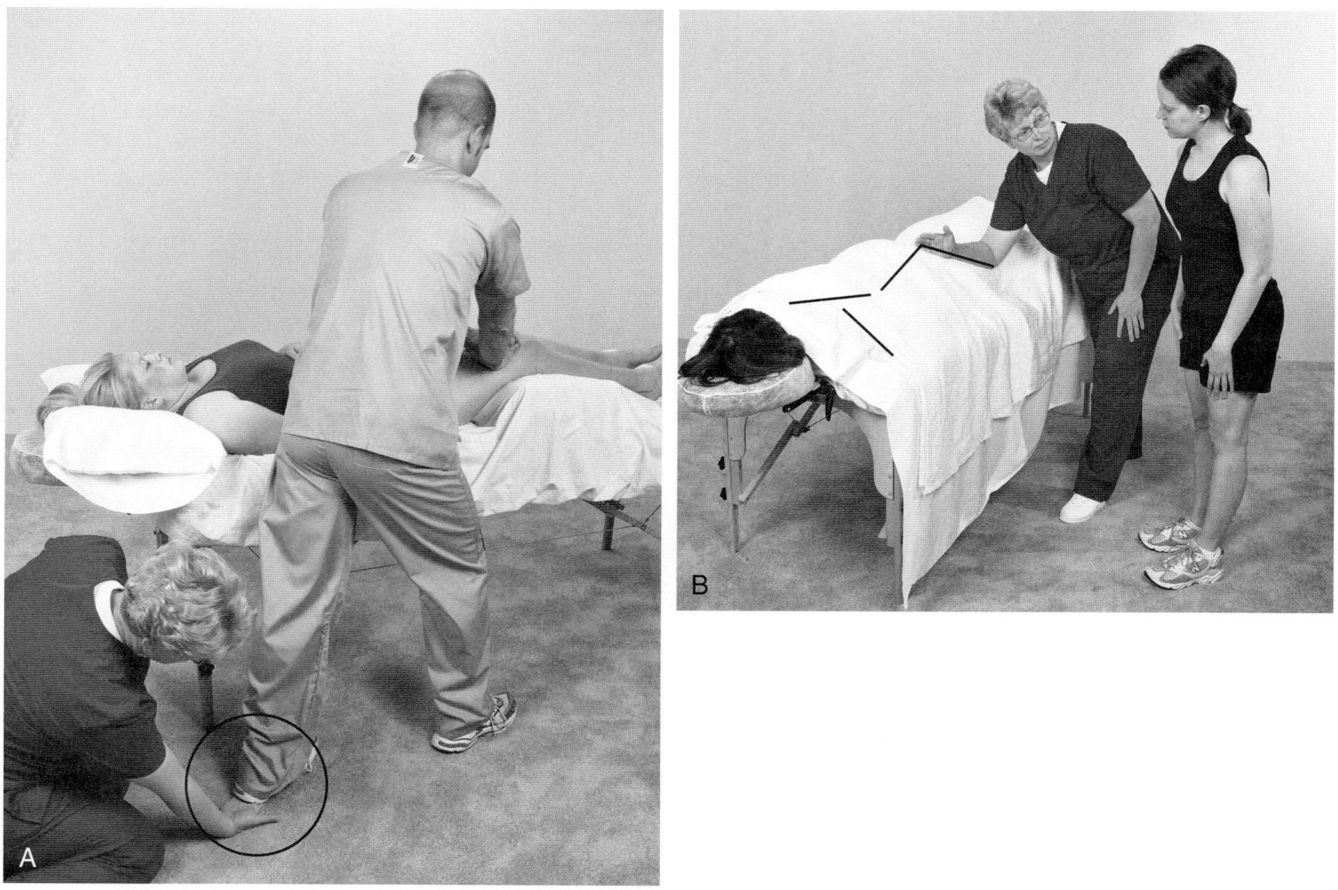

FIGURE 19-11 Basic principles of body mechanics: Correct positioning. **A,** Weight on back foot. **B,** Lean uphill.

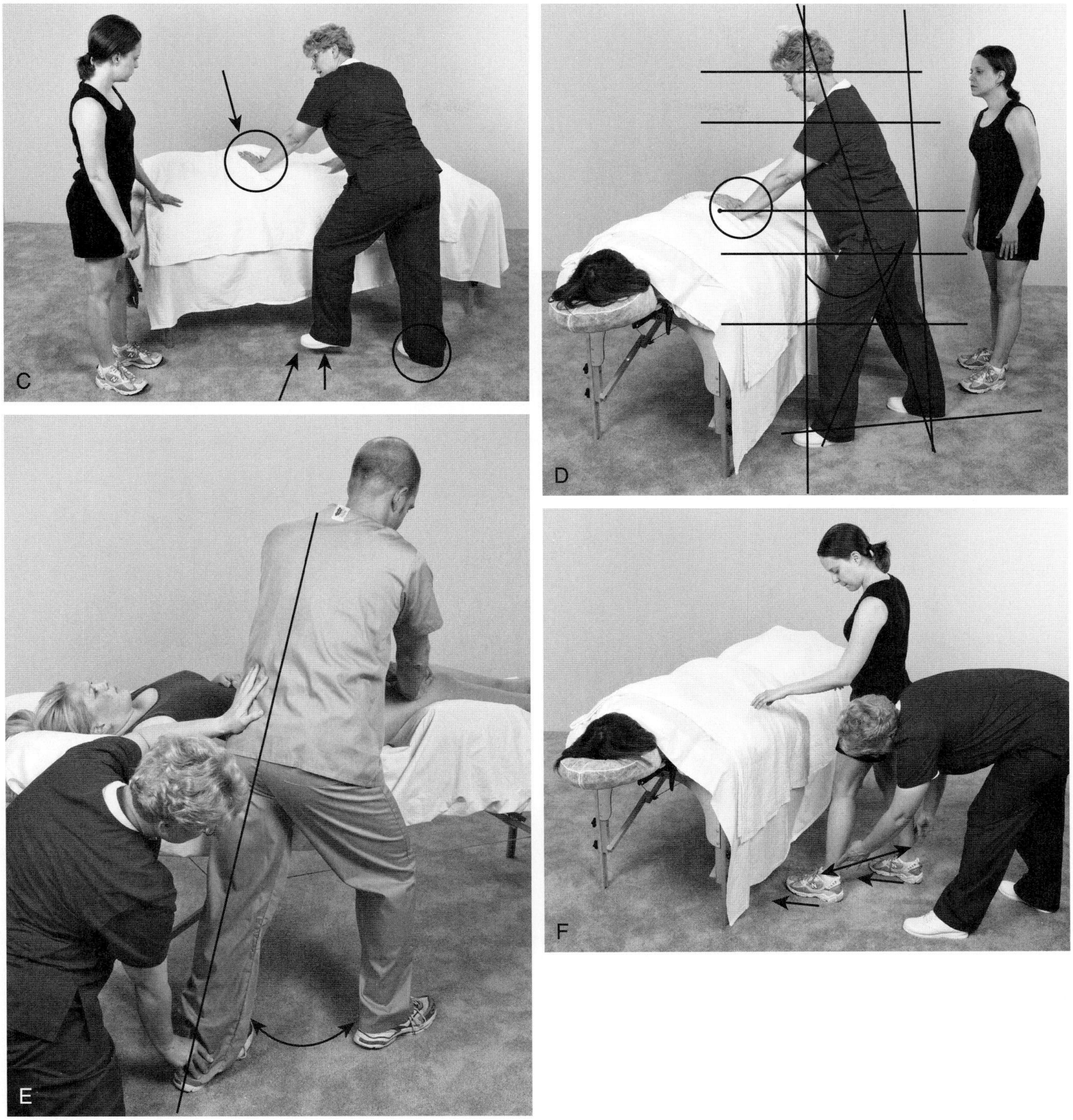

FIGURE 19-11, cont'd **C,** Weight transfer balance point. **D,** Proper alignment for body mechanics. **E,** Maintain normal knee-lock position (feet shoulder width apart) and weight on back of foot. **F,** Feet shoulder width apart, asymmetric stance.

Continued

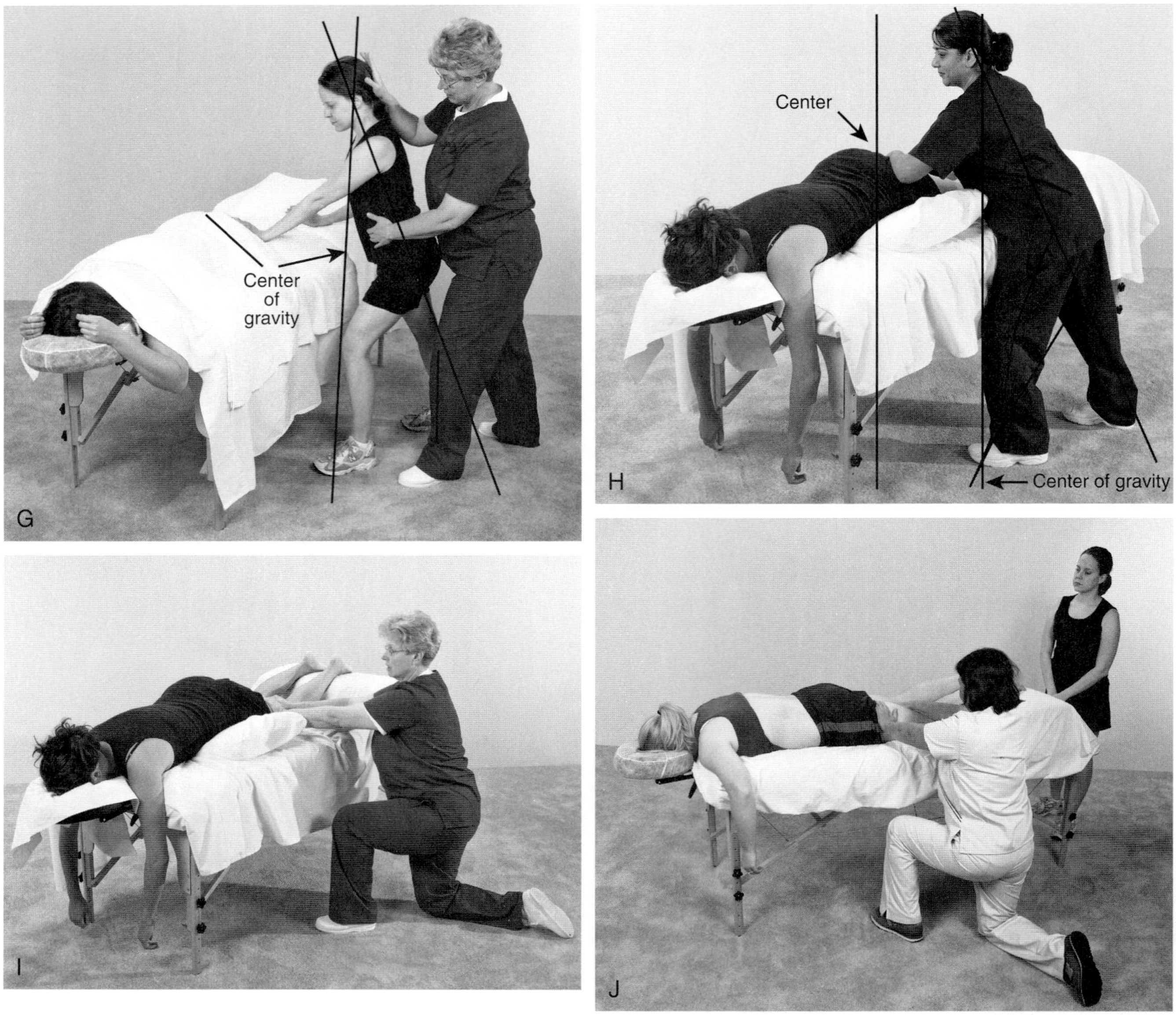

FIGURE 19-11, cont'd G, Correct center of gravity. Straight back, solid core. **H,** Center of gravity between contact on body and back, weight-bearing foot. **I,** Alternate position, kneeling. **J,** Alternate position, kneeling.

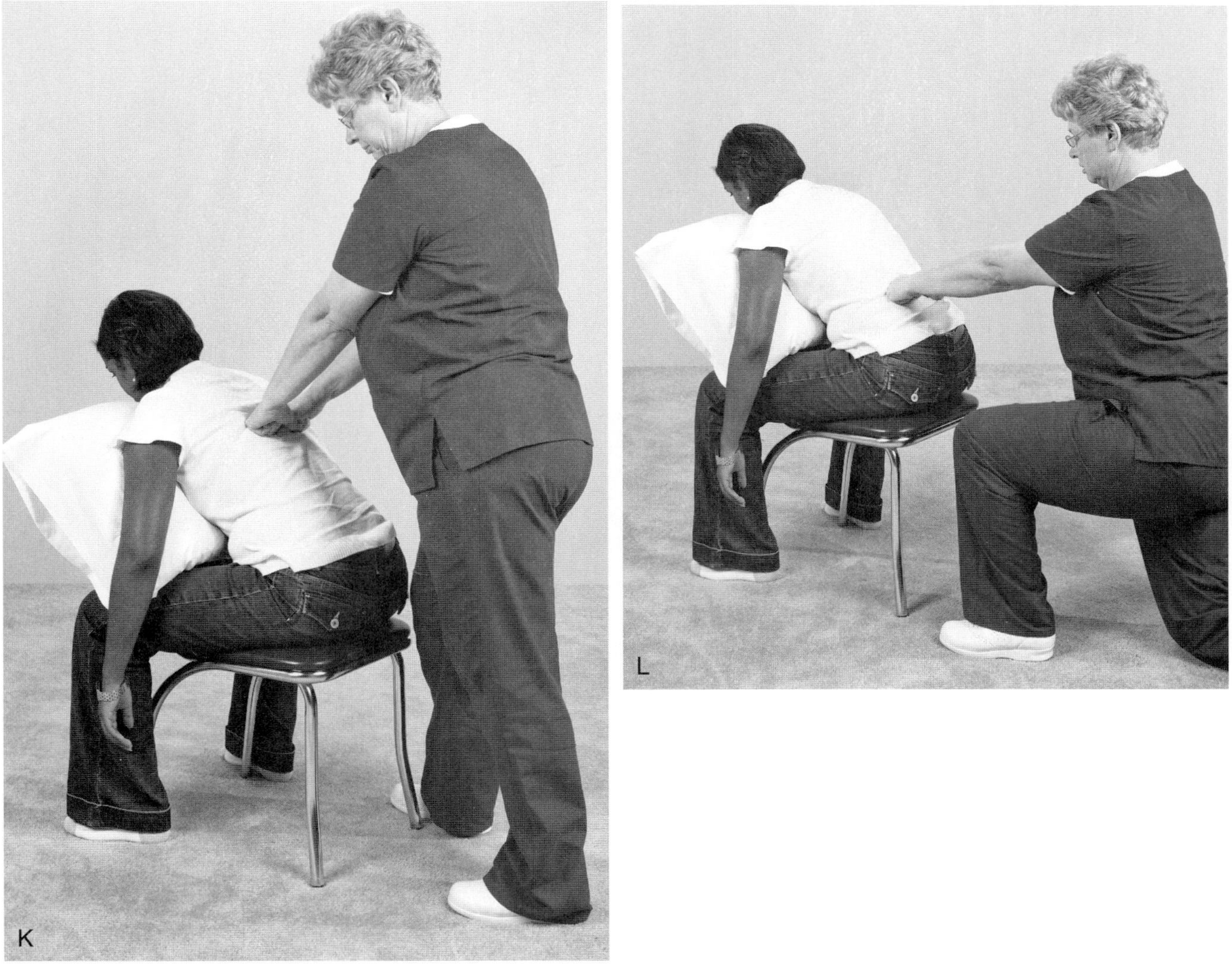

FIGURE 19-11, cont'd **K,** Body mechanics, seated position. **L,** Seated position, kneeling.

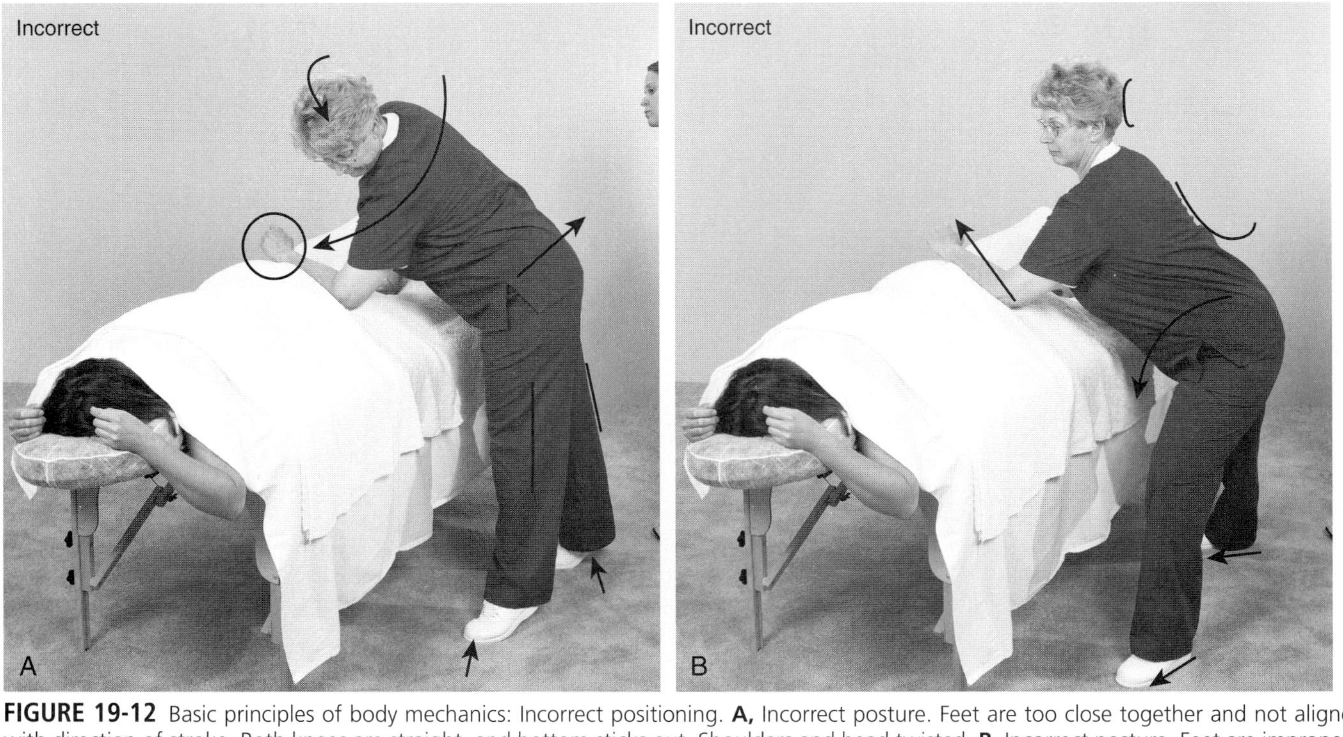

FIGURE 19-12 Basic principles of body mechanics: Incorrect positioning. **A,** Incorrect posture. Feet are too close together and not aligned with direction of stroke. Both knees are straight, and bottom sticks out. Shoulders and head twisted. **B,** Incorrect posture. Feet are improperly aligned to the direction of stroke and too far apart. Practitioner should not be bent at the hips.

Continued

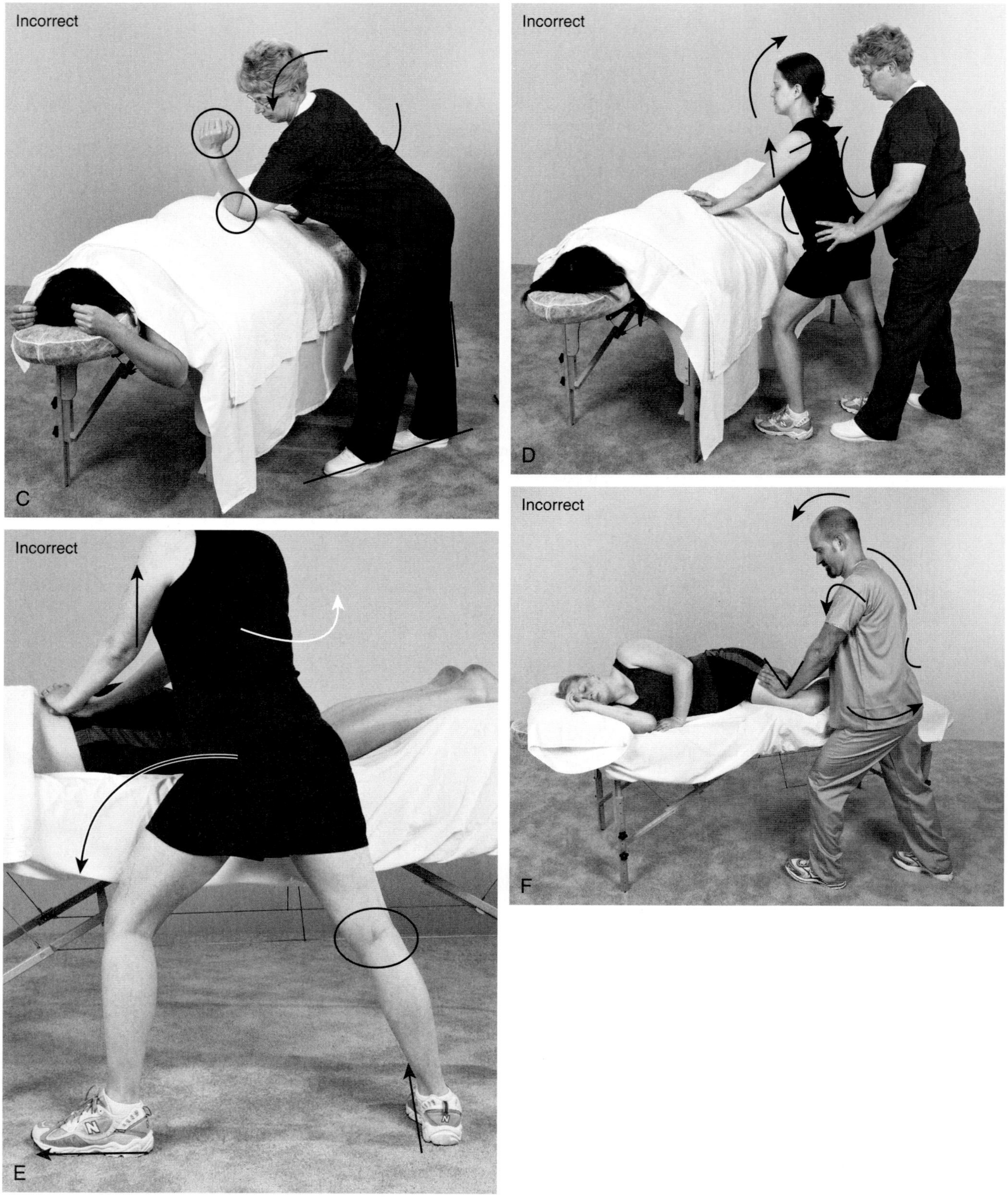

FIGURE 19-12, cont'd C, Incorrect posture. Feet should not have a "tightrope effect." Back leg knee is hyperextended and torso is twisted. **D,** Head tipped back. Sway back. Shoulder up and scapula winged. No core stability. **E,** Stance too wide. Misalignment of feet. Hyperextended knee. Torso torsion. High shoulder. **F,** Wrist angle incorrect, rounded shoulders. Sway back. Twisted torso. Head down.

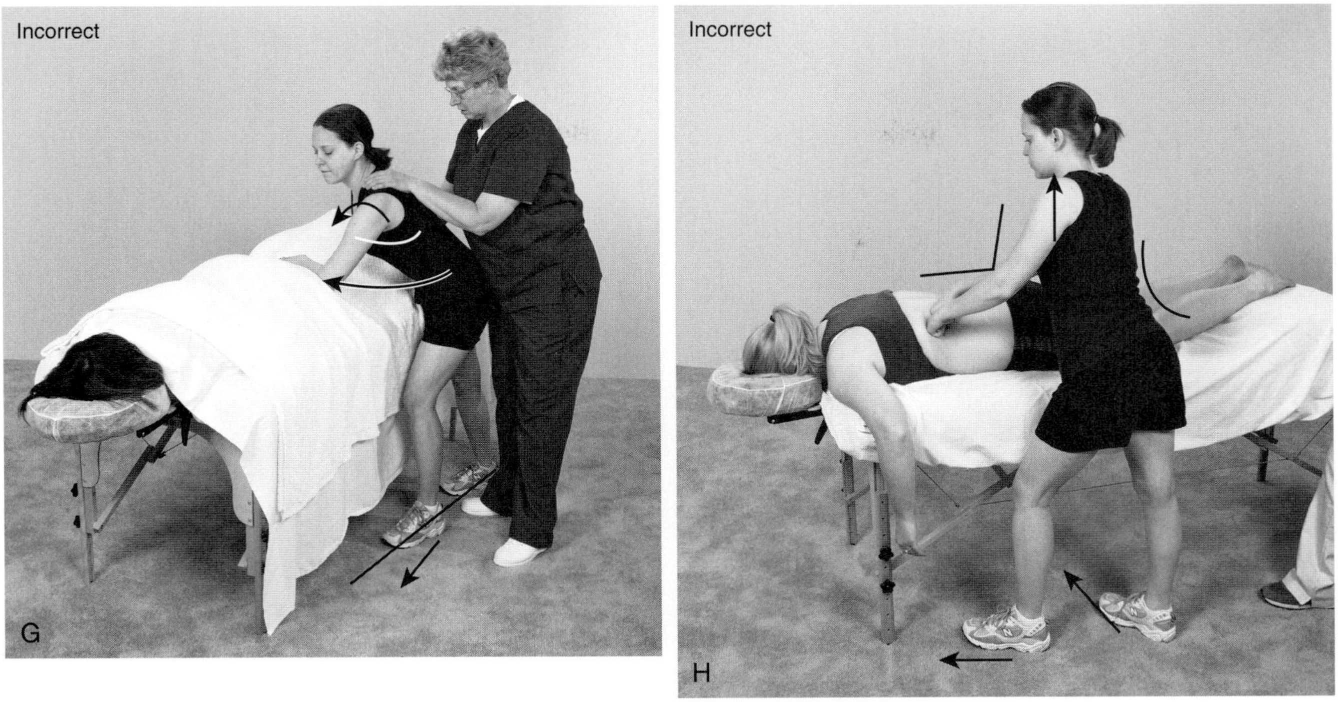

FIGURE 19-12, cont'd G, Tightrope foot placement. Twisted torso. Rounded shoulders. Arm too far in front. **H,** Bent elbow. Elevated shoulder. Sway back. Misaligned feet.

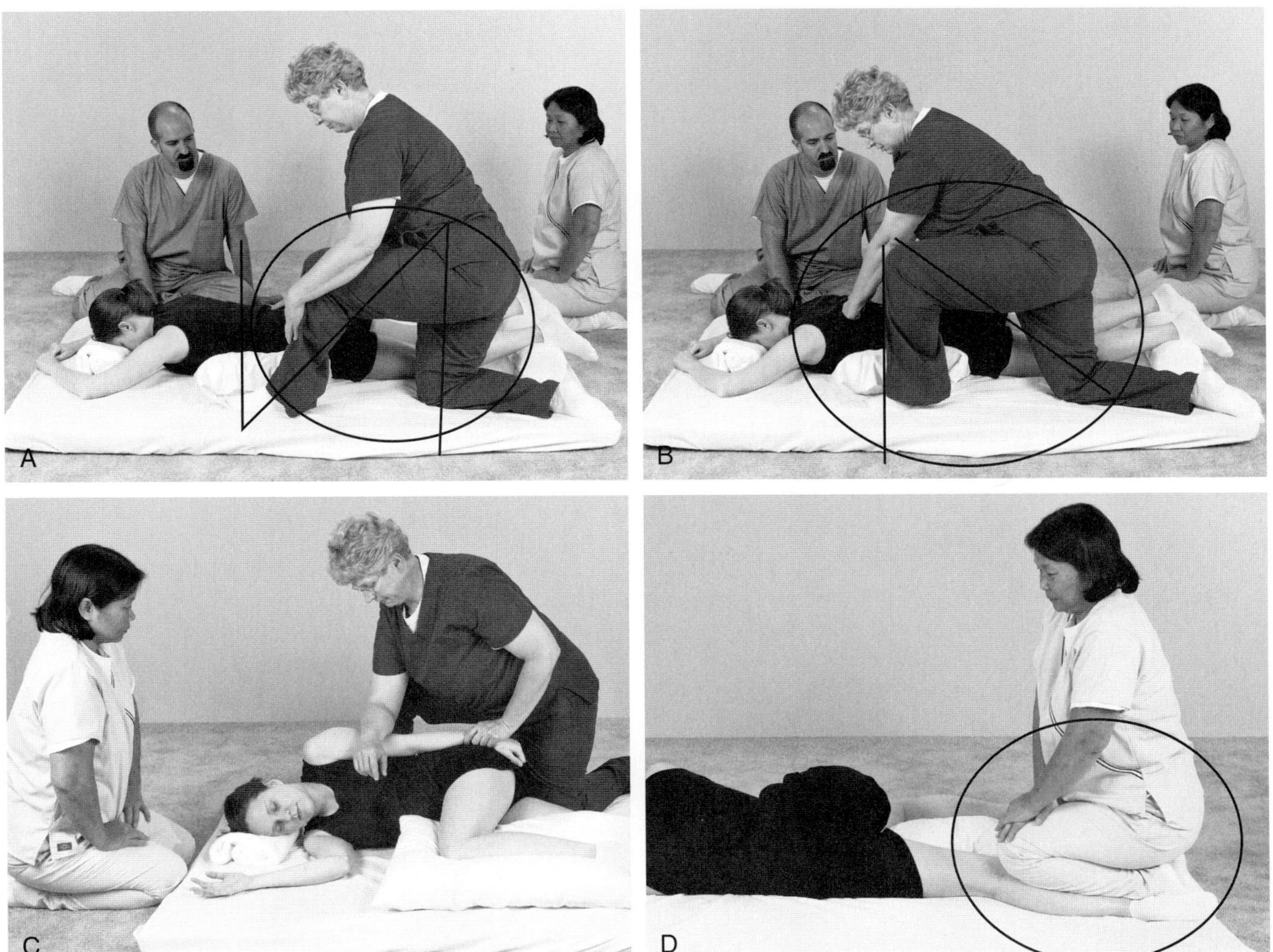

FIGURE 19-13 Body mechanics on the mat. **A,** Basic position. **B,** Correct weight transfer. **C,** Arm massage using correct body motions. **D,** Apply pressure using leg.

Continued

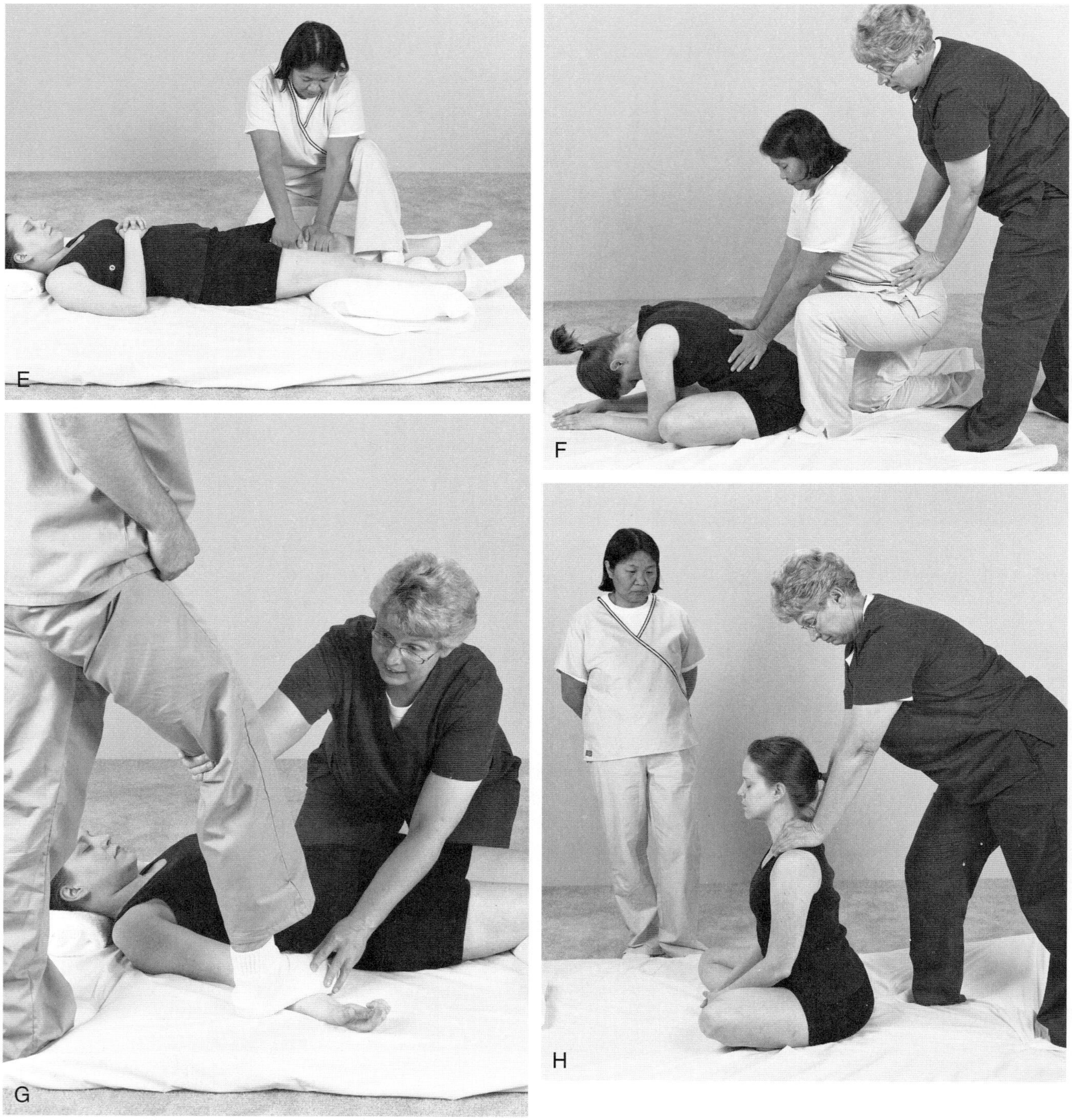

FIGURE 19-13, cont'd E, Kneading. **F,** Maintain straight back. **G,** Correct foot compression. **H,** Correct shoulder compression.

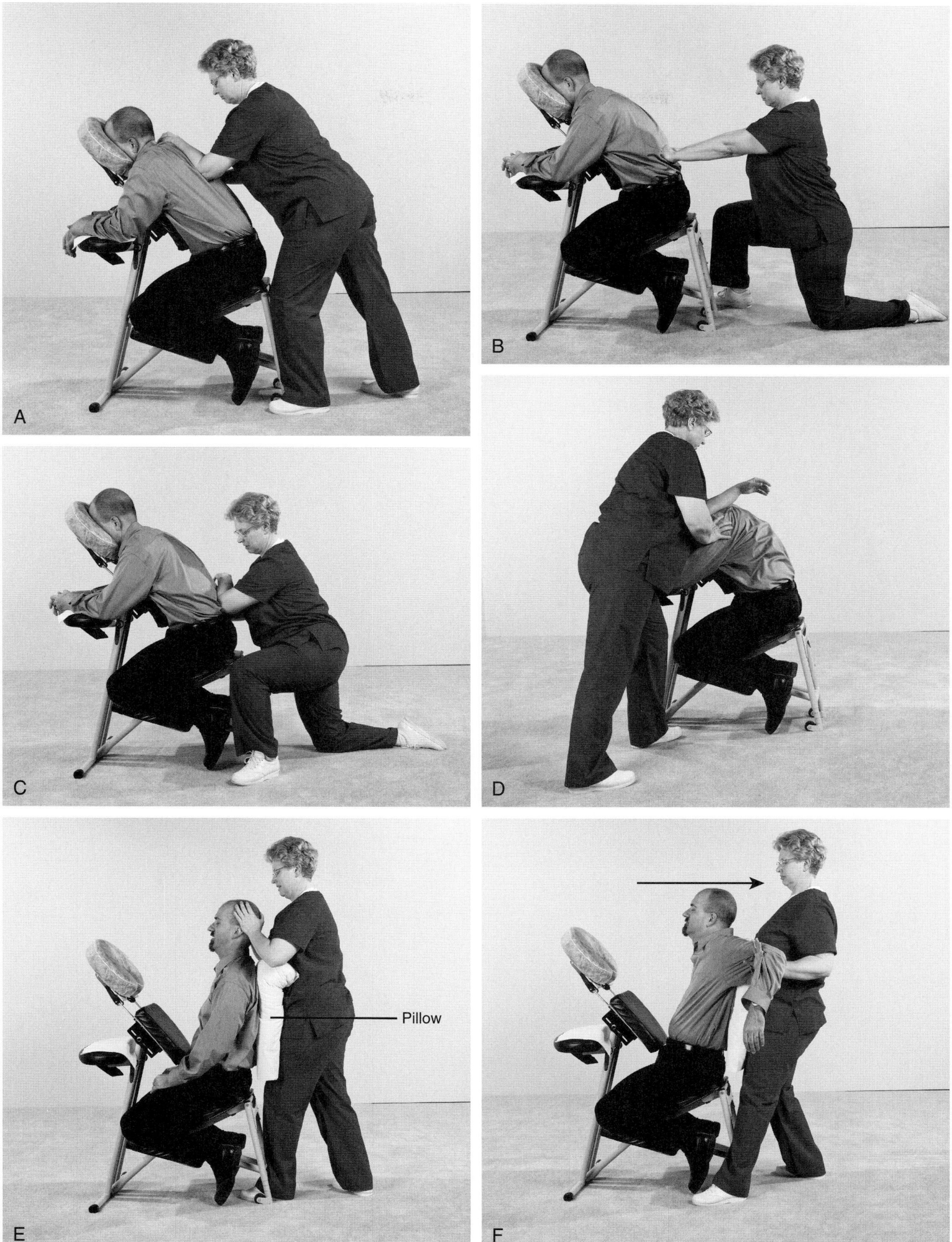

FIGURE 19-14 Body mechanics for chair massage. **A,** Forearm compression, standing. **B,** Fist compression, kneeling. **C,** Forearm position, kneeling. **D,** Forearm compression, shoulder. **E,** Position client against pillow. **F,** Stretch, lean back.

Continued

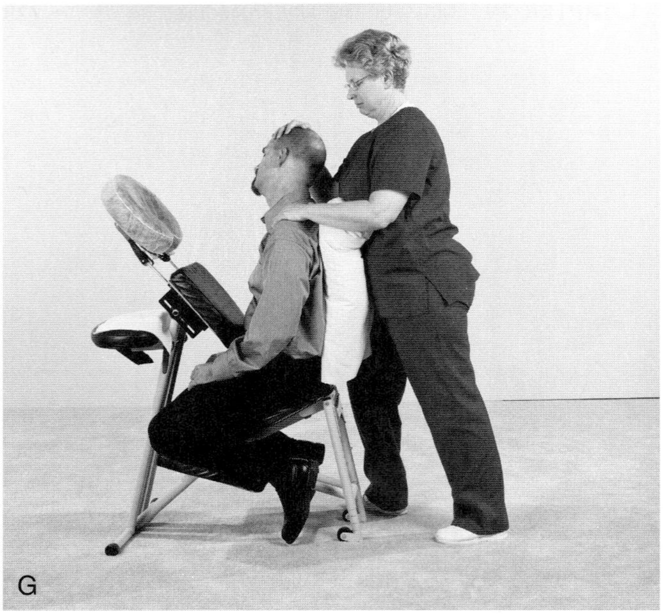

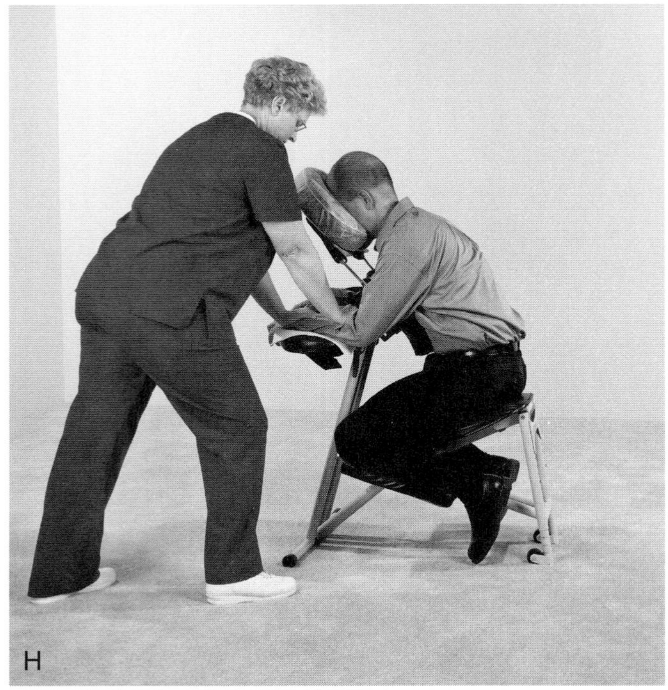

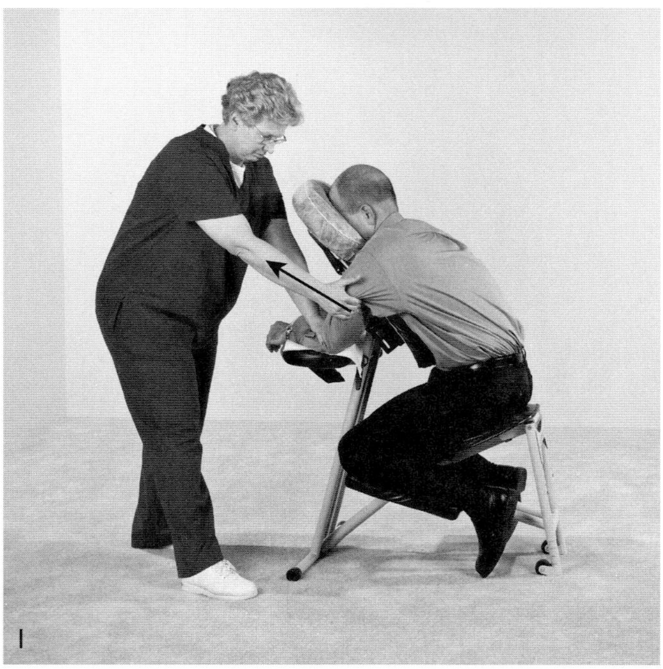

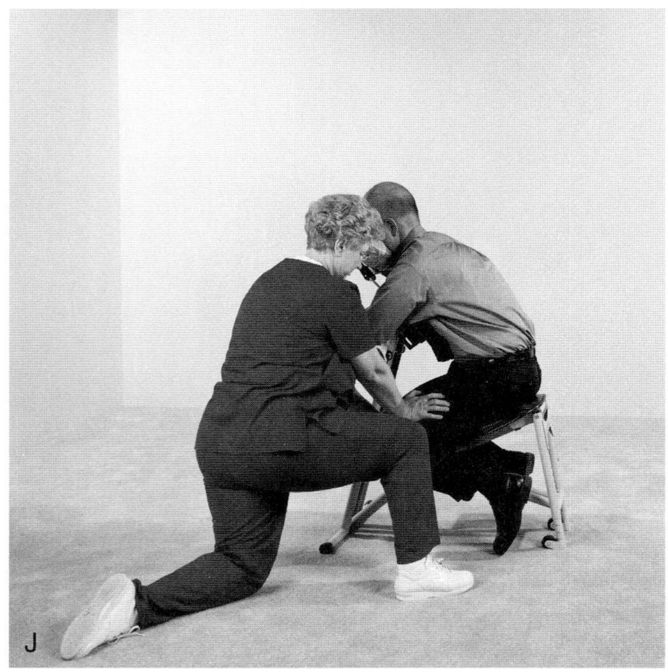

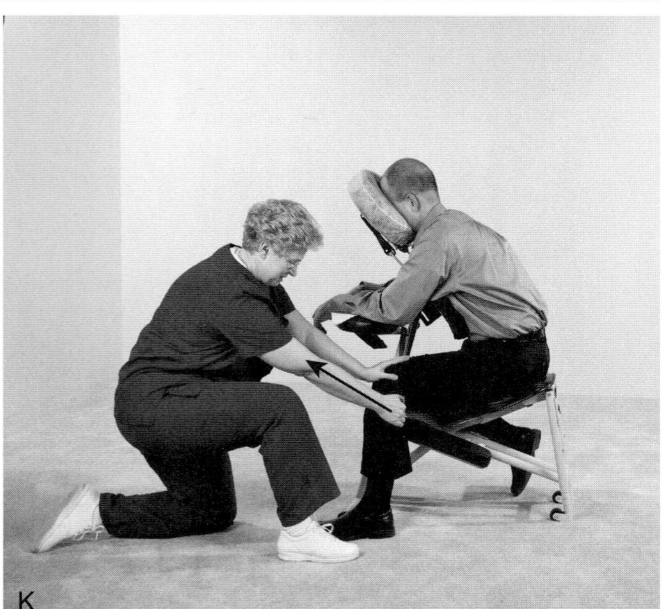

FIGURE 19-14, cont'd **G,** Movement of the neck. **H,** Palm compression, forearm. **I,** Pull back to massage upper arm. **J,** Kneel to compress thigh. **K,** Pull and lean back to massage calf.

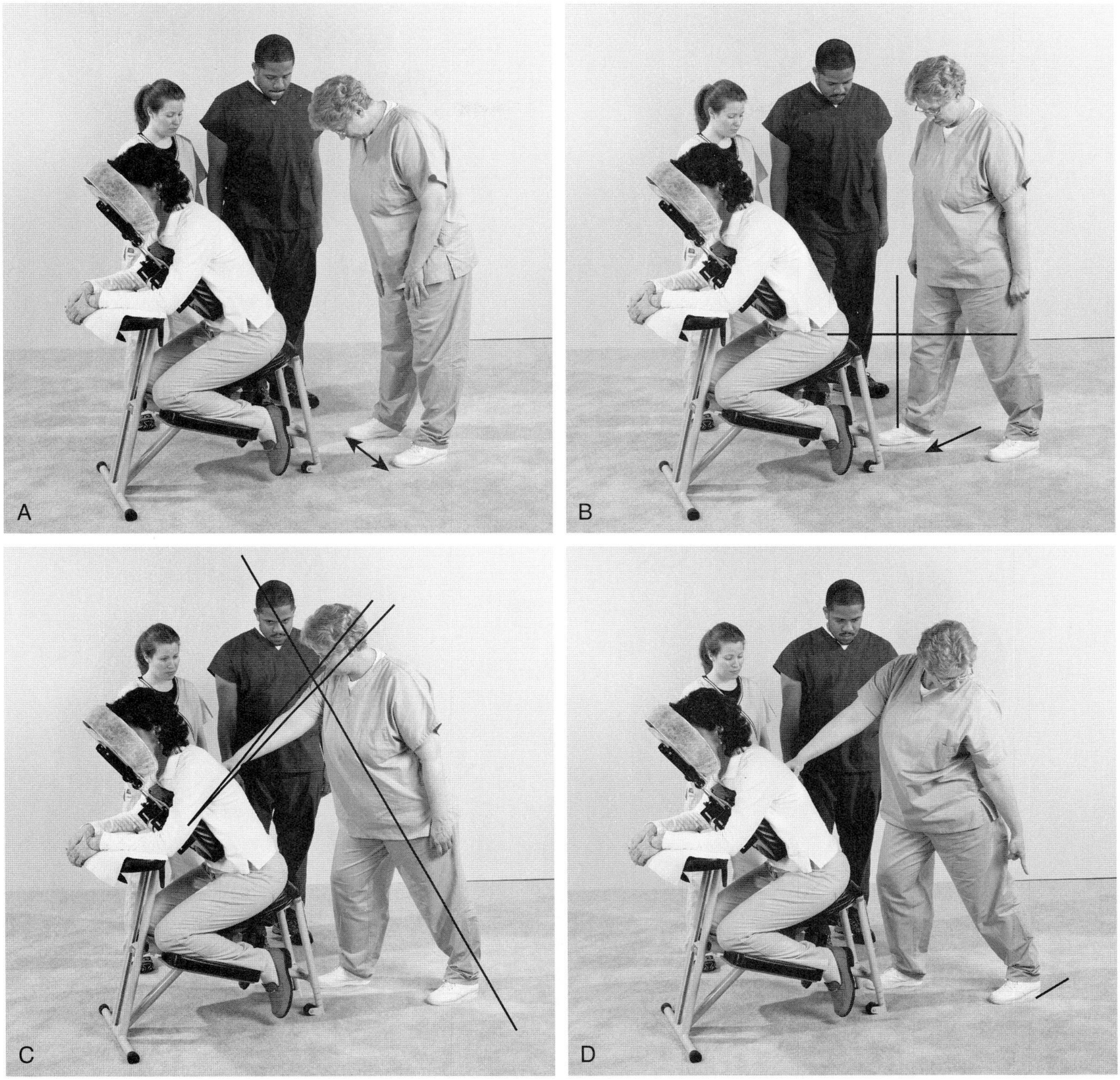

FIGURE 19-15 Body mechanics for chair/seated massage. **A,** Feet should be shoulder width apart. **B,** Bring one foot forward halfway between client and the other foot. **C,** Lean. **D,** Put weight on back foot/heel.

Continued

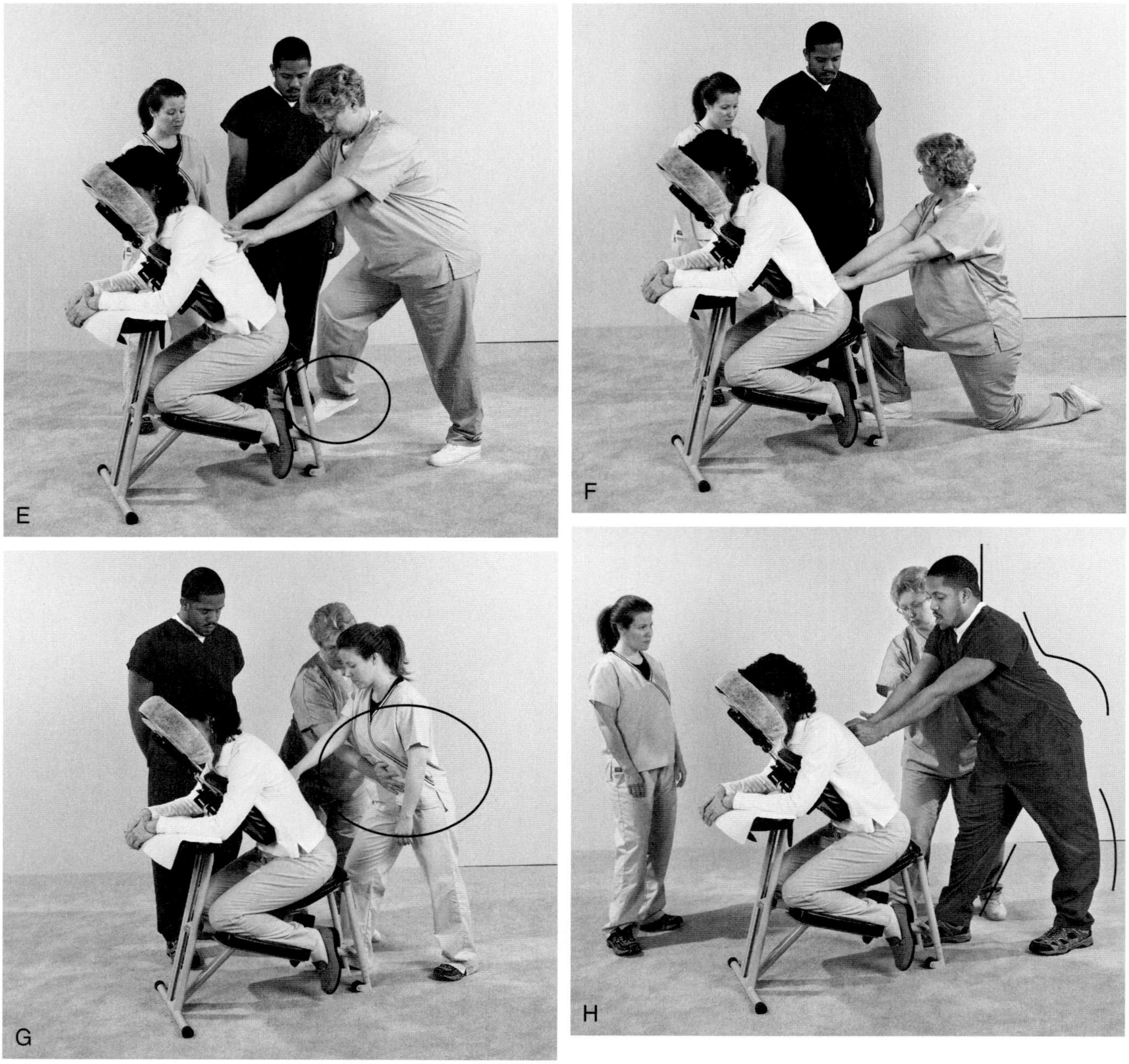

FIGURE 19-15, cont'd **E,** Front foot is non-weight bearing. **F,** Kneel; use knee pads if necessary. **G,** Maintain core stability. **H,** Incorrect stance.

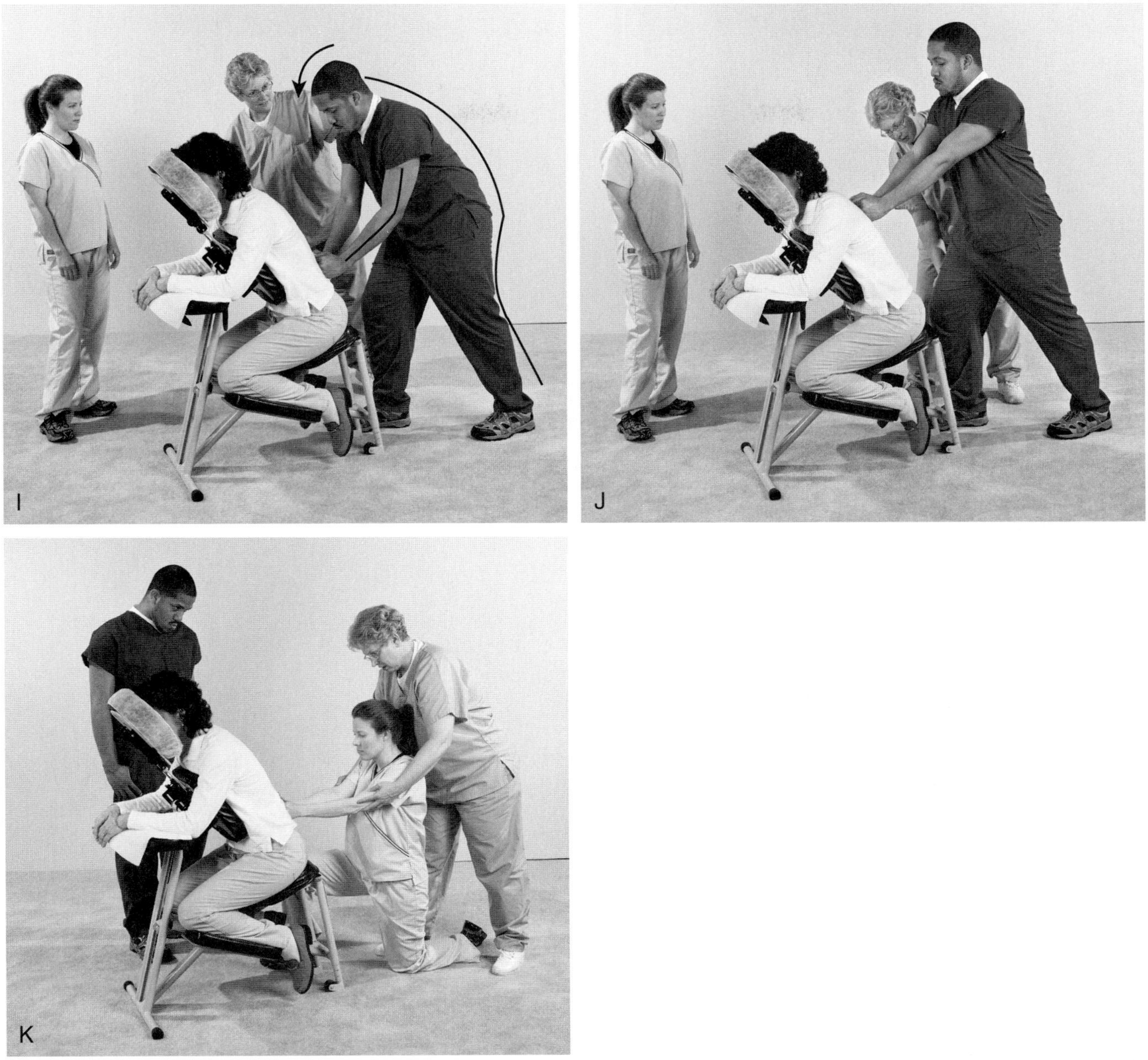

FIGURE 19-15, cont'd I, Incorrect stance. **J,** Improved body mechanics, but there is still a problem with shoulder position. **K,** Kneel to apply compression at lower back and maintain elbow stability.

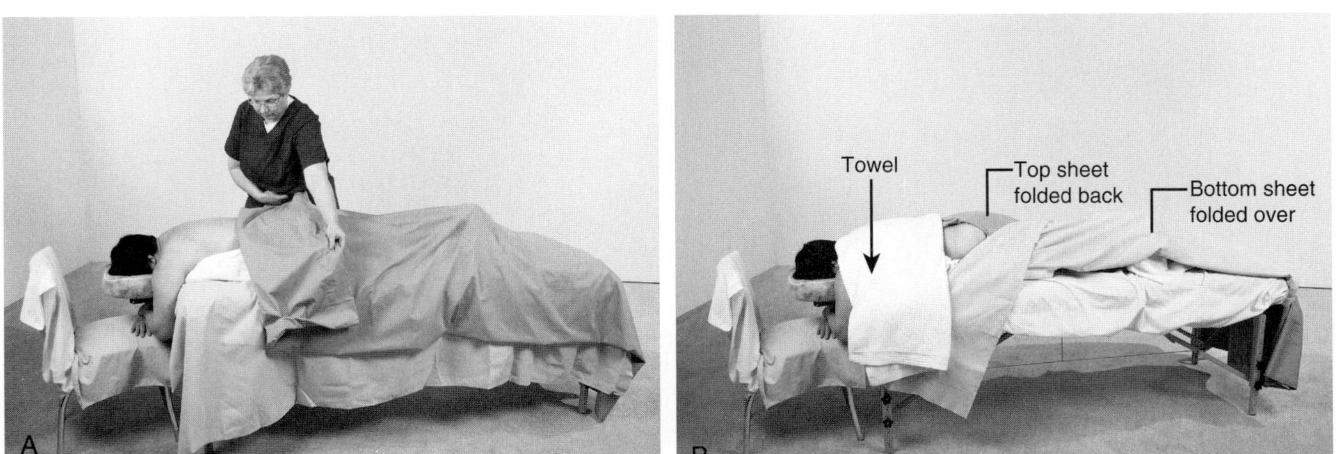

FIGURE 19-16 Draping. **A,** Prone: Undraped back. **B,** Draping for the gluteal area.

Continued

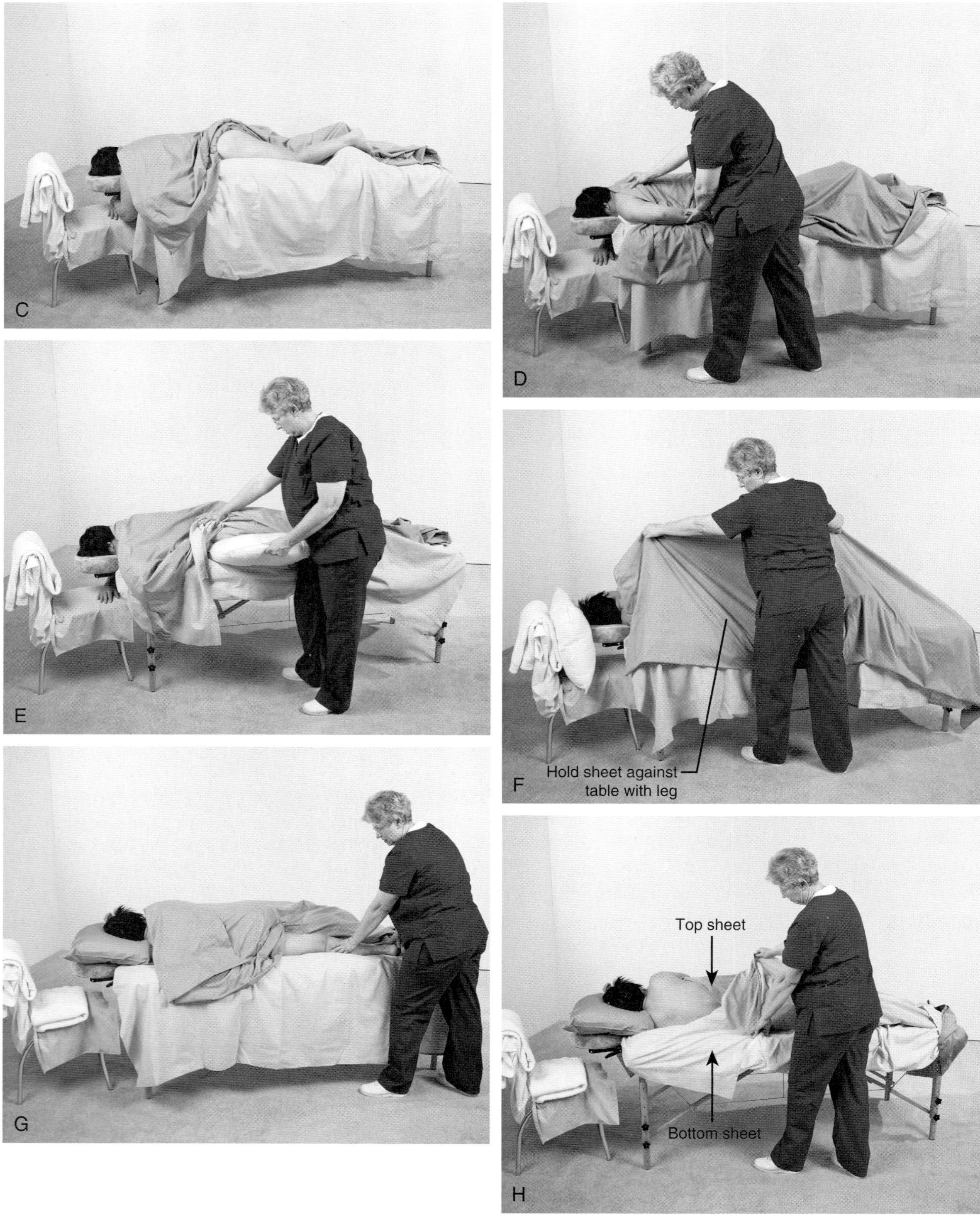

FIGURE 19-16, cont'd **C,** Prone: Draping for leg. **D,** Prone: Draping for arm. **E,** Preparation to place client in the side-lying position: remove bolster. **F,** Lift top sheet in the middle to allow client to roll. **G,** Side-lying: Draping for leg. **H,** Side-lying: Draping for back. Use bottom sheet to fold over leg and glutes.

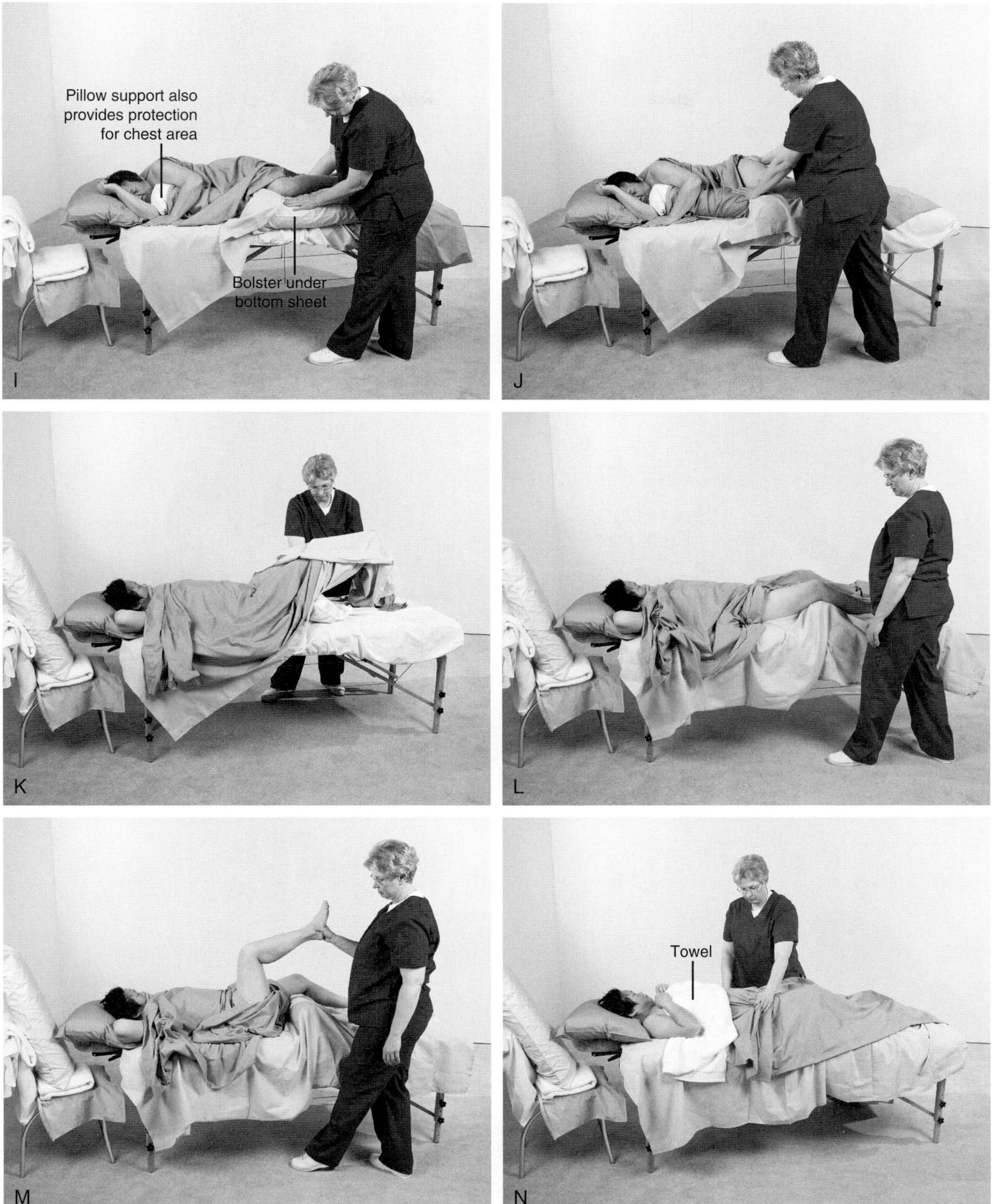

FIGURE 19-16, cont'd **I,** Side-lying: Draping for leg. **J,** Move drape to provide access to upper thigh and gluteal area. **K,** Supine: Fold bottom sheet over top sheet. Lift to position bolster. **L,** Supine: Draping for leg. **M,** Contour drape to prevent exposure of the groin area. **N,** Towel over top sheet: Client holds towel while sheet is moved.

Continued

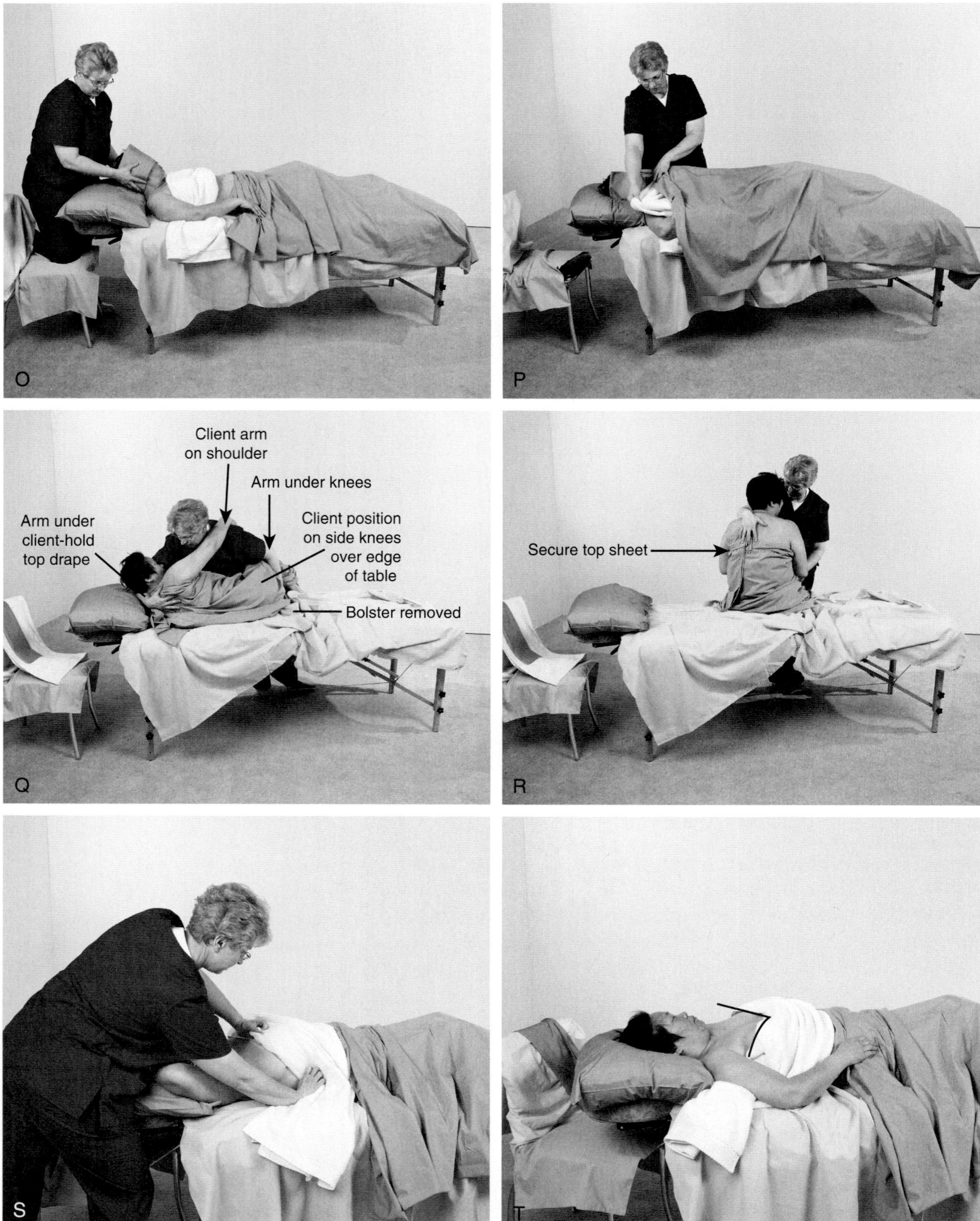

FIGURE 19-16, cont'd O, Draping for abdomen. Optional use of a pillowcase to cover the eyes. **P,** Redrape and remove towel. **Q,** Help client from the table. **R,** Lift by standing; secure drape. **S,** Working around the female breast. Use towel to move breast tissue. **T,** Contour drape around the breast.

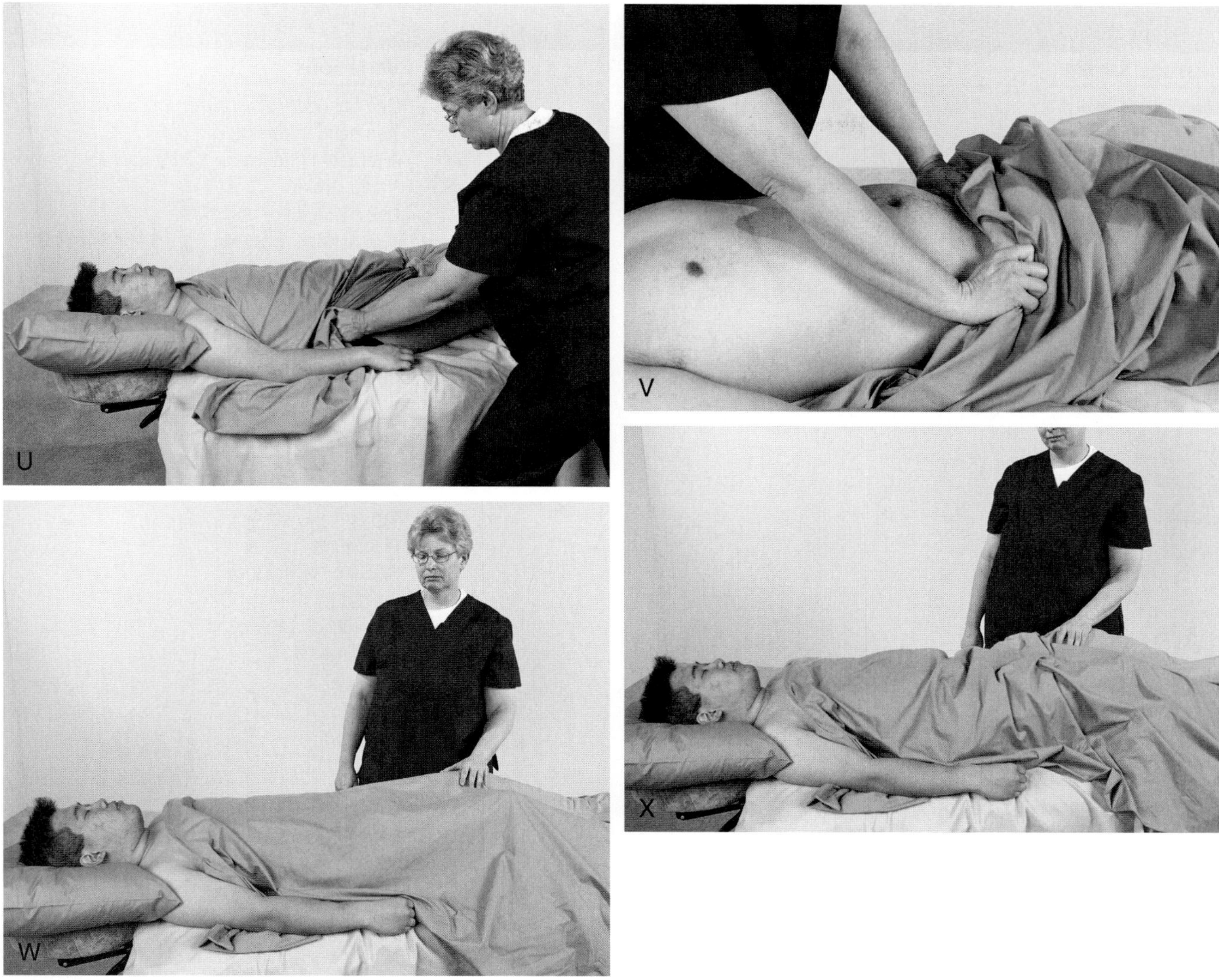

FIGURE 19-16, cont'd **U,** Working in the groin area, use a top sheet to slide drape tightly into area. For males, this will move the genitals out of the massage area. **V,** Use drape to slide to the top of the pubic bone. For males, this will move the genitals away from the massage area. **W,** Avoid flat draping on males in the supine position. **X,** Bunched sheets disguise the genital area.

TABLE 19-1 Massage Strokes and Their Variations

Massage Stroke	Variations
Effleurage *(gliding)*	One handed *(raking, ironing, circular)* Two handed *(heart, circular)* Alternate hand *(raking, circular)* Nerve stroke
Pétrissage *(kneading)*	One handed Two handed *(praying hands, ocean waves)* Alternate hand Fulling Skin rolling
Friction	Superficial warming *(sawing)* Rolling Wringing Cross-fiber Chucking Circular
Tapotement *(percussion)*	Tapping *(pulsing, raindrops)* Pincement Hacking *(quacking)* Cupping Pounding *(rapping)* Clapping Diffused
Vibration *(shaking)*	Fine Jostling Rocking

CHAPTER

20

The Client Consultation

INFORMED CONSENT PROCESS

A new client arrives for a massage.

The massage professional shows the client an informational brochure explaining massage, why it works, the procedures and process of massage, the benefits of massage, and the general contraindications. The client is asked to read the information. The massage professional then discusses the information with the client. In general terms the massage professional explains alternatives to massage, such as exercise and self-hypnosis, that provide benefits similar to massage.

The massage professional then tells the client about his or her professional background: that he or she graduated from a state-licensed massage therapy school 2 years ago, after a training program of 1,000 hours; that he or she has been nationally certified by the National Certification Board for Therapeutic Massage; that he or she has been in professional practice part time for 2 years and averages eight massages a week; and that he or she has taken additional training in myofascial approaches and massage for elderly people (approximately 100 hours for each). The client also is given information on methods of reporting misconduct of the massage therapist to state agencies, national professional organizations, and the police.

The client is given the policy and procedures booklet or statement and is asked to read it. After the client has done so, the massage professional goes over the booklet with the client, point by point, so that he or she understands the rules and requirements of the massage therapist. The massage professional makes sure that the requirements to report abuse and threat of deadly harm, as well as the release of files by court order, are discussed.

The massage professional hands the client a form that states the following:

I, (client's name) ______________________________, have received a copy of the rules and regulations for Massage Works operated by Sue and John Grey. I have read the rules and regulations, and I understand them. The massage procedures, information about massage in general, general benefits of massage, contraindications to massage, and possible alternatives have been explained to me. The qualifications of the massage professional and reporting measures for misconduct have been disclosed to me.

I understand that the massage I receive is for the purpose of stress reduction and relief from muscular tension, spasm, or pain and to increase circulation. If I experience any pain or discomfort, I will immediately inform the massage practitioner so that the pressure or methods can be adjusted to my comfort level. I understand that massage professionals do not diagnose illness or disease or perform any spinal manipulations, nor do they prescribe any medical treatments, and nothing said or done during the session should be construed as such. I acknowledge that massage is not a substitute for medical examination or diagnosis and that I should see a health care provider for those services. Because massage should not be performed under certain circumstances, I agree to keep the massage practitioner updated as to any changes in my health profile, and I release the massage professional from any liability if I fail to do so.

Client's signature ______________________________ Date ____________

Therapist's signature ______________________________ Date ____________

Consent to Treat a Minor

By my signature I authorize (therapist's name) to provide therapeutic massage to my child or dependent.

Signature of Parent or Guardian ______________________________ Date ____________

For clients who will have several sessions, the next step is completion of the needs assessment and initial treatment plan (presented in detail in Chapter 3).

Modified Informed Consent Form for Single Session

For clients who will be seen only once (as might occur if the professional is working on a cruise ship, doing sports massage at an event, or doing promotional chair massage at a health fair), the following modification in informed consent can be made.

I, (client's name) ______________________________, have received a copy of the rules and regulations for (name of business) ______________________________, operated by (owner) ______________________________. I have read the rules and regulations, and I understand them. The general benefits of massage and contraindications to massage have been explained to me. I have disclosed to the therapist any condition I have that would contraindicate massage. Other than to determine contraindications, I understand that no specific needs assessment has been performed. The qualifications of the massage professional and reporting measures for misconduct have been disclosed to me.

I understand that the massage I receive is for the purpose of stress reduction and relief from muscular tension, spasm, or pain and to increase circulation. If I experience any pain or discomfort, I will immediately inform the massage practitioner so that the pressure or methods can be adjusted to my comfort level. I understand that massage professionals do not diagnose illness or disease or perform any spinal manipulations, nor do they prescribe any medical treatments. I acknowledge that massage is not a substitute for medical examination or diagnosis and that I should see a health care provider for those services.

I understand that a single massage session or massage used on a random basis is limited to providing a general, nonspecific massage approach using standard massage methods and does not include any methods to address soft tissue structure or function specifically.

Client's signature ______________________________ Date ____________

Therapist's signature ______________________________ Date ____________

Consent to Treat a Minor

By my signature I authorize (therapist's name) to provide massage work to my child or dependent.

Signature of Parent or Guardian ______________________________ Date ____________

MASSAGE ASSESSMENT/PHYSICAL OBSERVATION/PALPATION AND GAIT

PRE
POST

Client Name: ______________________ **Date:** ______________________

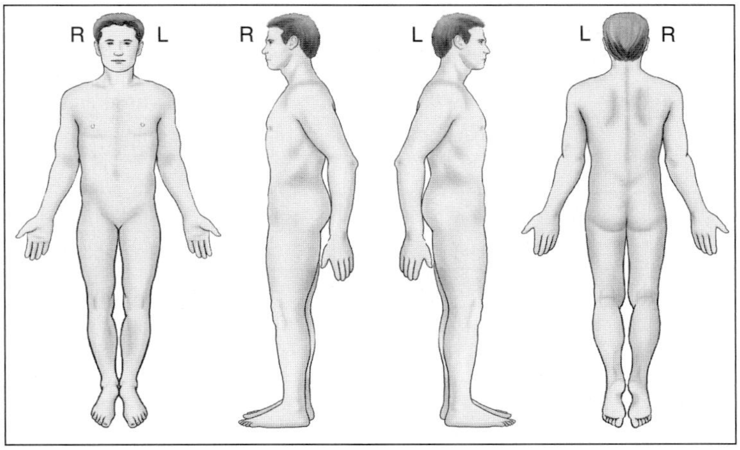

OBSERVATION & PALPATION		
ALIGNMENT	**RIBS**	**SCAPULA**
Chin in line with nose, sternal notch, navel	Even	Even
Other:	Springy	Move freely
HEAD	Other:	Other:
Tilted (L)	**ABDOMEN**	**CLAVICLES**
Tilted (R)	Firm and pliable	Level
Rotated (L)	Hard areas	Other:
Rotated (R)	Other:	**ARMS**
EYES	**WAIST**	Hang evenly (internal) (external)
Level	Level	(L) rotated ☐ medial ☐ lateral
Equally set in socket	Other:	(R) rotated ☐ medial ☐ lateral
Other:	**SPINE CURVES**	**ELBOWS**
EARS	Normal	Even ☐
Level	Other:	Other:
Other:	**GLUTEAL MUSCLE MASS**	**WRISTS**
SHOULDERS	Even	Even
Level	Other:	Other:
(R) high / (L) low	**ILIAC CREST**	**FINGERTIPS**
(L) high / (R) low	Level	Even
(L) rounded forward	Other:	Other:
(R) rounded forward	**KNEES**	**PATELLA**
Muscle development even	Even/symmetrical	(L) ☐ movable ☐ rigid
Other:	Other:	(R) ☐ movable ☐ rigid

FIGURE 20-1 A sample physical assessment form. This information is obtained by observing (looking and feeling) and measuring. The key to completing the form is: identify what is the same on the two sides of the body and what is different.

Continued

	ANKLES		**TRUNK**		**LEGS**
	Even		Remains vertical		Swing freely at hip
	Other:		Other:		Other:
	FEET		**SHOULDERS**		**KNEES**
	Mobile		Remain level		Flex and extend freely through stance and swing phase
	Other:		Rotate during walking		Other:
	ARCHES		Other:		**FEET**
	Even		**ARMS**		Heel strikes first at start of stance
	Other:		Motion is opposite leg swing		Plantar flexed at push-off
	TOES		Motion is even (L) and (R)		Foot clears floor during swing phase
	Straight		Other:		Other:
	Other:		(L) swings freely		**STEP**
	SKIN		(R) swings freely		Length is even
	Moves freely and resilient		Other:		Timing is even
	Pulls/restricted		**HIPS**		Other:
	Puffy/baggy		Remain level		**OVERALL**
	Other:		Other:		Rhythmic
	HEAD		Rotate during walking		Other:
	Remains steady/eyes forward		Other:		
	Other:				

FIGURE 20-1, cont'd

TREATMENT PLAN

Client Name: ______________________________

Choose One: ☐ Original plan ☐ Reassessment date ______________

Short-term client goals:
Quantitative: ______________________________
Qualitative: ______________________________

Long-term client goals:
____
____

Therapist objectives:
____
____

1) Frequency, 2) length, and 3) duration of visits:
1) __________ 2) __________ 3) __________

Progress measurements to be used: (Ex.— pain scale, range of motion, increased ability to perform function)
____
____

Dates of reassessment:
____

Categories of massage methods to be used: (Ex.— general constitutional, stress reduction, circulatory, lymphatic, neuromuscular, connective tissue, neurochemical, etc.)
____
____

Additional notes:
____
____
____

Client Signature: ______________________ Date: __________

Therapist Signature: ______________________ Date: __________

FIGURE 20-2 A sample form for a care/treatment plan.

SESSION NOTES
SOAP CHARTING FORM

Client Name: ______________________________ Date: ______________
Practitioner Name: ______________________________

Subjective

<u>CLIENT STATUS</u>

- **Information from client, referral source, or reference books:**

1) Current conditions/changes from last session: ______________________________

Objective

2) Information from <u>assessment</u> (physical, gait, palpation, muscle testing): ______________________________

<u>CONTENT OF SESSION</u>

- **Generate goal (possibilities) from analysis of information in <u>client status</u>.**

1) Goals worked on this session. (Base information on client status this session and goals previously established in Treatment Plan): ______________________________

What was <u>done</u> this session: ______________________________

Analysis

<u>RESULTS</u>

- **Analyze results of session in relationship to what was done and how this relates to the session goals. (This is based on <u>cause</u> and <u>effect</u> of methods used and the effects on the persons involved).**

1) What worked/what didn't: (Based on measurable and objective Post Assessment) ______________________________

Plan

<u>PLAN:</u> Plans for next session, what client will work on, what next massage will reassess and continue to assess: ______________________________

CLIENT COMMENTS: ______________________________

Time In: ______________ Time Out: ______________

Therapist signature: ______________________________

FIGURE 20-3 A SOAP charting form modified for student learning. The key to completing the form is: answer the questions based on what happened during the massage.

APPENDIX A

HIPAA Compliance and Privacy*

COMPLIANCE DEFINED

Compliance in the health care industry is the process of meeting regulations, recommendations, and expectations of federal and state agencies that pay for health care services and regulate the industry. Health care compliance encompasses the claims reimbursement processes, managed care procedures, Occupational Safety and Health Administration (OSHA), Clinical Laboratory Improvement Amendments (CLIA), licensure, and due diligence in obeying the law.

Any business that is involved with the health care industry must conform its practices to follow the principles and practices as identified by state and federal agencies. The professional elements of the principles and practices include:

- Regulations and recommendations to protect individuals
- Streamline processes
- Supporting system-wide stability

A compliance strategy provides a standardized process for handling business functions, much like a "user's manual." This will enable consistent and effective management and staff performance. Failure to comply with mandates leads to sanctions and fines from state and federal agencies. Failure to follow guidelines potentially results in more fraud and abuse in the claims reimbursement cycle.

HEALTH INFORMATION USING ELECTRONIC TECHNOLOGIES

Over the past decade, the United States health care system has undergone rapid change with regard to the separate issues of privacy, security, and claims processing. A number of organizations have participated to help standardize and improve the delivery and quality of health care.

Some code systems and additional terminology have been created by the adoption of the many federal statutes. In this chapter you will learn some important key terms related to health information as it pertains to compliance and its role in electronic technology. You will also get acquainted with important initiatives that control the use of health information.

e-Health Information Management

e-Health information management, more commonly seen as eHIM, is a term coined by the American Health Information Management Association's eHealth Task Force to describe any and all transactions in which health care information is accessed, processed, stored, and transferred using electronic technologies.

National Health Information Infrastructure

The National Health Information Infrastructure (NHII) is an initiative set forth to improve patient safety and the quality of health care, as well as to better inform individuals regarding their own health information and to help them understand health care costs. It has also encouraged the use of computers and standardized electronic financial transactions.

NHII is overseen by the Department of Health and Human Services with the National Committee on Vital and Health Statistics (NCVHS) serving as a public advisory committee .

HEALTH INSURANCE PORTABILITY AND ACCOUNTABILITY ACT

The Health Insurance Portability and Accountability Act of 1996 (HIPAA), Public Law 104-191, has significant impact on both individuals and health care providers.

*This paper is intended to promote awareness. It is not all-encompassing in regard to HIPAA and OIG compliance. It is not intended to replace policy and procedures manuals and similar policy documents. Definitions from the *Federal Register* are excerpts, used for ease of understanding.

Among five titles, two provisions of HIPAA relate most to health care, *Title I: Insurance Reform* and *Title II: Administrative Simplification*. HIPAA projects long-term benefits that include lowered administrative costs, increased accuracy of data, increased patient and customer satisfaction, and reduced revenue cycle time, ultimately improving financial management.

Title I: Health Insurance Reform

The primary purpose of HIPAA *Title I: Insurance Reform* is to provide continuous insurance coverage for workers and their insured dependents when they change or lose jobs. This aspect of HIPAA affects individuals as consumers, not particularly as patients. Previously, when an employee left or lost a job and changed insurance coverage, a "preexisting" clause prevented or limited coverage for certain medical conditions. HIPAA now limits the use of preexisting condition exclusions, prohibits discrimination for past or present poor health, and guarantees certain employers and individuals the right to purchase new health insurance coverage after losing a job. Additionally, HIPAA allows renewal of health insurance coverage regardless of an individual's health condition that is covered under the particular policy.

Title II: Administrative Simplification

The goals of HIPAA *Title II: Administrative Simplification* focus on the health care practice setting and aim to reduce administrative costs and burdens. Standardizing electronic transmissions of administrative and financial information will reduce the number of forms and methods used in the claims processing cycle and reduce the nonproductive effort that goes into processing paper or nonstandard electronic claims. Additional provisions are meant to ensure the privacy and security of an individual's health data.

Two parts of the Administrative Simplification provisions are as follows:

1. Development and implementation of standardized electronic transactions using common sets of descriptors (i.e., standard code sets). These must be used to represent health care concepts and procedures when performing health-related financial and administrative activities electronically (i.e., standard transactions). HIPAA has been part of a great shift in processing electronic data. Transaction standards apply to the following, which are called covered entities under HIPAA: health care third-party payers, health care providers, and health care clearinghouses. A **clearinghouse** is an independent organization that receives insurance claims from the physician's office, performs software edits, and redistributes the claims electronically to various third-party payers.
2. Implementation of privacy and security procedures to prevent the misuse of health information by ensuring:
   - Privacy and confidentiality
   - Security of health information

Administrative simplification has created uniform sets of standards that protect and place limits on how confidential health information can be used. For years, health care providers have locked medical records in file cabinets and refused to share patient health information. Patients now have specific rights regarding how their health information is used and disclosed because federal and state laws regulate the protection of an individual's privacy. Knowledge and attention to the rights of patients are important to the compliance endeavor in a health care practice. Providers are entrusted with health information and are expected to recognize when certain health information can be used or disclosed.

Patients have the legal right to request (1) access and amendments to their health records, (2) an accounting of those who have received their health information, and (3) restrictions on who can access their health records. Understanding the parameters concerning these rights is crucial to complying with HIPAA.

Health care providers and their employees can be held accountable for using or disclosing patient health information inappropriately. HIPAA regulations will be enforced, as clearly stated by the U.S. government. The revolution of HIPAA will take time to understand and implement correctly, but as the standards are put into action, both within the practice setting and across the many different fields comprising the health industry, greater benefits will be appreciated by the health care provider, staff, and patients.

Defining Roles and Relationships: Key Terms

HIPAA legislation required the *U.S. Department of Health and Human Services* (DHHS or HHS*) to establish national standards and identifiers for electronic transactions, as well as implement privacy and security standards. In regard to HIPAA, *Secretary* refers to the HHS Secretary or any officer or employee of HHS to whom the authority involved has been delegated.

The *Centers for Medicare and Medicaid Services* (CMS), previously known as the Health Care Financing Administration (HCFA), will enforce the insurance portability and transaction and code set requirements of HIPAA for Medicare and Medicaid programs.

*Both DHHS and HHS are used throughout the textbook as abbreviations for Department of Health and Human Services.

The *Office for Civil Rights* (OCR) will enforce privacy standards.

Electronic media refers to the mode of electronic transmission, including the following:

- Internet (online mode—wide open)
- Extranet or private network using Internet technology to link business parties
- Leased telephone or dial-up telephone lines, including fax modems (speaking over telephone is not considered an electronic transmission)
- Transmissions that are physically moved from one location to another using magnetic tape, disk, or compact disk media

A **transaction** refers to the transmission of information between two parties to carry out financial or administrative activities related to health care.

Refer to Box A-1 for titles of additional entities that oversee the HIPAA-related functions.

BOX A-1 Overseers of HIPAA Functions

A covered entity transmits health information in electronic form in connection with a *transaction* covered by HIPAA. The covered entity may be (1) a health care coverage carrier such as Blue Cross/Blue Shield, (2) a health care clearinghouse through which claims are submitted, or (3) a health care provider such as the primary care physician.

A **business associate** is a person who, on behalf of the covered entity, performs or assists in the performance of a function or activity involving the use or disclosure of individually identifiable health information, including claims processing or administration, data analysis, processing or administration, utilization review, quality assurance, billing, benefit management, practice management, and repricing. For example, if a provider's practice contracts with an outside billing company to manage its claims and accounts receivable, the billing company would be a business associate of the provider (the covered entity).

A **health care provider** is a person trained and licensed to provide care to a patient, and also a place that is licensed to give health care, such as a hospital, skilled nursing facility, inpatient/outpatient rehabilitation facility, home health agency, hospice program, physician, diagnostic department, outpatient physical or occupational therapy, rural clinic, or home dialysis supplier.

Privacy and security officers oversee the HIPAA-related functions. These individuals may or may not be employees of a particular health care practice. A **privacy officer** or **privacy official (PO)** is designated to help the provider remain in compliance by setting policies and procedures (P&P) and by training and managing the staff regarding HIPAA and patient rights, and the PO is usually the contact person for questions and complaints.

A **security officer** protects the computer and networking systems within the practice and implements protocols such as password assignment, backup procedures, firewalls, virus protection, and contingency planning for emergencies.

HIPAA in the Practice Setting

The individuals mentioned in Box A-1 create relationships that guide the health care provider and the practice. A health care provider can be a physician's assistant, nurse practitioner, social worker, chiropractor, radiologist, or dentist; HIPAA does not affect only medical physicians. The health care provider is designated as a HIPAA-mandated covered entity under certain conditions. It is important to remember that health care providers who transmit any health information in electronic form in connection with a HIPAA transaction are covered entities. Electronic form or media can include floppy disk, compact disk (CD), or file transfer protocol (FTP) over the Internet. Voice-over-modem faxes, meaning a telephone line, are not considered electronic media, although a fax from a computer (e.g., WinFax program) is considered an electronic medium.

HIPAA requires the designation of a privacy officer or privacy official (PO) to develop and implement the organization's policies and procedures (P&P). The PO for an organization may hold another position within the practice or may not be an employee of the practice at all. Often, the PO is a contracted professional and available to the practice through established means of contact.

The business associate is often considered an extension of the provider practice. If an office function is outsourced with use or disclosure of individually identifiable health information, the organization that is acting on behalf of the health care provider is considered a business associate. For example, if the office's medical transcription is performed by an outside service, the transcription service is a business associate of the covered entity (the health care provider/practice).

HIPAA privacy regulations as a federal mandate will apply unless the state laws are contrary or more stringent with regard to privacy. A state law is contrary if it is impossible to comply with the state law while complying with federal requirements or if the state law stands as an obstacle to the purposes of the federal law. **State preemption**, a complex technical issue not within the scope of the health care provider's role, refers to instances when state law takes precedence over federal law. The PO determines when the need for preemption arises.

THE PRIVACY RULE: CONFIDENTIALITY AND PROTECTED HEALTH INFORMATION

What I may see or hear in the course of the treatment or even outside of the treatment in regard to the life of men, which on no account one must spread abroad, I will keep to myself holding such things shameful to be spoken about.

Hippocrates, 400 BC

The Hippocratic Oath, federal and state regulations, professional standards, and ethics all address patient privacy. Because current technology allows easy access to health care information, HIPAA imposes new requirements for health care providers. Since computers have become indispensable for the health care office, confidential health data have been sent across networks, e-mailed over the Internet, and even exposed by hackers, with few safeguards taken to protect data and prevent information from being intercepted or lost. With the implementation of standardizing electronic transactions of health care information, the use of technologies will pose new risks for privacy and security. These concerns were addressed under HIPAA, and regulations now closely govern how the industry handles its electronic activities.

Privacy is the condition of being secluded from the presence or view of others. **Confidentiality** is using discretion in keeping secret information. Integrity plays an important part in the health care setting. Staff members of a health care organization need a good understanding of HIPAA's basic requirements and must be committed to protecting the privacy and rights of the practice's patients.

Disclosure means the release, transfer, provision of access to, or divulging in any other manner of information outside the entity holding the information. An example of a disclosure is giving information to the hospital's outpatient surgery center about a patient you are scheduling for a procedure.

Consent is the verbal or written agreement that gives approval to some action, situation, or statement. A **consent form** is not required before physicians use or disclose protected health information (PHI) for treatment, payment, or routine health care operations (TPO).

Treatment includes coordination or management of health care between providers or referral of a patient to another provider. PHI can be disclosed to obtain reimbursement. Other health care operations include performance reviews, audits, training programs, and certain types of fundraising (Figures A-1 through A-4).

Keep in mind that a HIPAA privacy consent is not the same as a consent to treat. Exceptions may be based on specific state law requirements, on an emergency situation, on a language barrier that makes it impossible to obtain, or when treating prison inmates.

Under the HIPAA Privacy Rule, **authorization** is an individual's formal, written permission to use or disclose his or her personally identifiable health information for purposes other than treatment, payment, or health care operations. For some "extra" activities, including marketing, research, and psychotherapy notes, an **authorization form** is necessary for use and disclosure of PHI that is not included in any existing consent form agreements. Documentation pertaining to psychiatric counseling is kept with the patient's medical records, but psychotherapy notes should be kept separate.

Individually identifiable health information (IIHI) is any part of an individual's health information, including demographic information (e.g., address, date of birth), collected from the individual that is created or received by a covered entity. This information relates to the individual's past, present, or future physical or mental health or condition; the provision of health care to the individual; or the past, present, or future payment for the provision of health care. IIHI data identify the individual or establish a reasonable basis to believe the information can be used to identify the individual. For example, if you as a health care provider are talking to an insurance representative, you will likely give information such as the patient's date of birth and last name. These pieces of information would make it reasonably easy to identify the patient. If you are talking to a pharmaceutical representative about a drug assistance program that covers a new pill for heartburn and you say that your practice has a patient living in your town who is indigent and has stomach problems, you are not divulging information that would identify the patient.

Protected health information (PHI) is any information that identifies an individual and describes his or her health status, age, sex, ethnicity, or other demographic characteristics, whether or not that information is stored or transmitted electronically. It refers to IIHI that is transmitted by electronic media, maintained in electronic form or transmitted, or maintained in any other form or medium. PHI does not include IIHI in education records covered by the Family Educational Right and Privacy Act.

Traditionally, the focus was on protecting paper medical records and documentation that held patient's health information, such as laboratory results and radiology reports. HIPAA Privacy Regulation expands these protections to apply to PHI. The individual's health information is protected regardless of the type of medium in which it is maintained. This includes paper, the health care provider's computerized practice management and billing system, spoken words, and x-ray films.

Use means the sharing, application, utilization, examination, or analysis of IIHI within an organization that holds such information. When a patient's billing record is accessed to review the claim submission history, the individual's health information is in "use."

HIPAA imposes requirements to protect not only disclosure of PHI outside of the organization, but also for internal uses of health information. PHI may not be used or disclosed without permission of the patient or someone authorized to act on behalf of the patient, unless the use or disclosure is specifically required or permitted by the regulation (e.g., TPO). The two types of disclosure required by HIPAA Privacy Rule are to the individual who is the subject of the PHI and to the Secretary or DHHS to investigate compliance with the rule.

REQUIRED ELEMENTS OF HIPAA AUTHORIZATION

Identification of person (or class) authorized to request

Identification of person (or class) to whom covered entity is to use/disclose

Description of information to be released with specificity to allow entity to know which information the authorization references

Description of each purpose of the requested use or disclosure

Expiration date, time period, or event

Statement that is revocable by written request

Individual's (patient's) signature and date

Statement of representative's authority

Authorization for Release of Information

PATIENT NAME: Levy (LAST) Chloe (FIRST) E. (MI) ______ (MAIDEN OR OTHER NAME)

DATE OF BIRTH: 02 - 12 - 1950 (MO DAY YR) SS# 320 - 21 - 3408 MEDICAL RECORD #: 3075

ADDRESS: 3298 East Main Street CITY: Woodland Hills STATE: XY ZIP: 12345-0001

DAY PHONE: 013-340-9800 EVENING PHONE: 013-549-8708

I hereby authorize Gerald Practon, MD **(Print Name of Provider) to release information from my medical record as indicated below to:**

NAME: Margaret L. Lee, MD

ADDRESS: 328 Seward Street CITY: Anytown STATE: XY ZIP: 45601-0731

PHONE: 013-219-7698 FAX: 013-290-9877

INFORMATION TO BE RELEASED:

	DATES:
☒ History and physical exam	6-8-20XX
☐ Progress notes	
☐ Lab reports	
☐ X-ray reports	
☐ Other: ______	

I specifically authorize the release of information relating to:
- ☐ Substance abuse (including alcohol/drug abuse)
- ☐ Mental health (including psychotherapy notes)
- ☐ HIV related information (AIDS related testing)

X ______
SIGNATURE OF PATIENT OR LEGAL GUARDIAN DATE

PURPOSE OF DISCLOSURE: ☐ Changing physicians ☒ Consultation/second opinion ☐ Continuing care ☐ Legal ☐ School ☐ Insurance ☐ Workers Compensation ☐ Other (please specify): ______

1. I understand that this authorization will expire on 09/01/20XX (Print the Date this Form Expires) days after I have signed the form.
2. I understand that I may revoke this authorization at any time by notifying the providing organization in writing, and it will be effective on the date notified except to the extent action has already been taken in reliance upon it.
3. I understand that information used or disclosed pursuant to this authorization may be subject to redisclosure by the recipient and no longer be protected by Federal privacy regulations.
4. I understand that if I am being requested to release this information by Gerald Practon, MD (Print Name of Provider) for the purpose of:
   ______
   a. By authorizing this release of information, my health care and payment for my health care will not be affected if I do not sign this form.
   b. I understand I may see and copy the information described on this form if I ask for it, and that I will get a copy of this form after I sign it.
   c. I have been informed that Gerald Practon, MD (Print Name of Provider) will/will not receive financial or in-kind compensation in exchange for using or disclosing the health information described above.
5. I understand that in compliance with XY (Print the State Whose Laws Govern the Provider) statute, I will pay a fee of $ 5.00 (Print the Fee Charged). There is no charge for medical records if copies are sent to facilities for ongoing care or follow up treament.

Chloe E. Levy 6/1/XX OR ______
SIGNATURE OF PATIENT DATE PARENT/LEGAL GUARDIAN/AUTHORIZED PERSON DATE

RECORDS RECEIVED BY ______ DATE ______ RELATIONSHIP TO PATIENT ☐ ______

FOR OFFICE USE ONLY
DATE REQUEST FILLED ______ BY: ______
IDENTIFICATION PRESENTED ______ FEE COLLECTED $______

FIGURE A-1 Completed authorization for release of information form for a patient relocating to another city. The figure indicates the required elements for HIPAA authorization. Note: This form is used on a one-time basis for reasons other than treatment, payment, or health care operations. When the patient arrives at the new physician's office, a consent for treatment, payment, or health care operations form will need to be signed. *(From Federal Register, Vol. 64, No. 212, Appendix to Subpart E of Part 164: Model Authorization Form, November 3, 1999.)*

NAME OF FACILITY
Consent for Release of Information

Date May 16, 20XX

1. I hereby authorize College Hospital (Name of Institution) to release the following information from the health record(s) of Martha T. Jacobson (Patient name)

   52 East Rugby Street, Woodland Hills, XY 12345 (Address)

   covering the period(s) of hospitalization from:

   Date of Admission January 3, 20XX
   Date of Discharge January 5, 20XX
   Hospital # 278-1200 Birthdate June 27, 1960
2. Information to be released:
   - ☐ Copy of (complete) health record(s)
   - ☐ History and physical
   - ☐ Other ______
   - ☑ Discharge summary
   - ☐ Operative report
3. Information is to be released to: Michael Hotta, MD
   260 West Main Street, Woodland Hills, XY 12345
4. Purpose of disclosure June 14, 20XX consultation
5. I understand this consent can be revoked at any time except to the extent that disclosure made in good faith has already occurred in reliance to this consent.
6. Specification of the date, event, or condition upon which this consent expires:
   December 31, 20XX
7. The facility, its employees and officers, and attending physician are released from legal responsibility or liability for the release of the above information to the extent indicated and authorized herein.

Signed *Martha T. Jacobson*
(Patient or Representative)

______
(Relationship to Patient)

May 16, 20XX
(Date of Signature)

FIGURE A-2 Consent for Release of Information form to a hospital. *(Reprinted with permission from the American Health Information Management Association. Copyright © 2010 by the American Health Information Management Association. All rights reserved.)*

Confidential Information

The insurance billing specialist must be responsible for maintaining confidentiality of patients' health information when working with patients and their medical records. Example A-1 lists some of the PHI that is typical in a medical office that falls under HIPAA compliance regulations.

EXAMPLE A-1

Protected Health Information in a Medical Office

- Intake forms
- Laboratory work requests
- Physician-patient conversations
- Conversations that refer to patients by name
- Physician dictation tapes
- Telephone conversations with patients
- Encounter sheets
- Physician's notes
- Prescriptions
- Insurance claim forms
- X-rays
- E-mail messages

The patient record and any photographs obtained are confidential documents and require an authorization form that must be signed by the patient to release information (see Figures A-1 through A-4). If the form is a photocopy, it is necessary to state that the photocopy is approved by the patient, or write to the patient and obtain an original signed document.

Exceptions to HIPAA

Unauthorized release of information is called **breach of confidential communication** and is considered a HIPAA violation, which may lead to fines.

Confidentiality between the physician and patient is automatically waived in the following situations:

1. When the patient is a member of a managed care organization (MCO) and the physician has signed a contract with the MCO that has a clause that says "for quality care purposes, the MCO has a right to access the medical records of their patients, and for

COLLEGE CLINIC
4567 Broad Avenue
Woodland Hills, XY 12345-0001
Phone: 555/486-9002
Fax: 555/487-8976

CONSENT TO THE USE AND DISCLOSURE OF HEALTH INFORMATION

I understand that this organization originates and maintains health records which describe my health history, symptoms, examination, test results, diagnoses, treatment, and any plans for future care or treatment. I understand that this information is used to:

- plan my care and treatment
- communicate among health professionals who contribute to my care
- apply my diagnosis and services, procedures, and surgical information to my bill
- verify services billed by third-party payers
- assess quality of care and review the competence of healthcare professionals in routine healthcare operations

I further understand that:

- a complete description of information uses and disclosures is included in a *Notice of Information Practices* which has been provided to me
- I have a right to review the notice prior to signing this consent
- the organization reserves the right to change their notice and practices
- any revised notice will be mailed to the address I have provided prior to implementation
- I have the right to object to the use of my health information for directory purposes
- I have the right to request restrictions as to how my health information may be used or disclosed to carry out treatment, payment, or health care operations
- the organization is not required to agree to the restrictions requested
- I may revoke this consent in writing, except to the extent that the organization has already taken action in reliance thereon.

☐ I request the following restrictions to the use or disclosure of my health information.

____

Date	Notice Effective Date
Signature of Patient or Legal Representative	Witness
Signature	Title
Date ____________	__ Accepted __ Rejected

FIGURE A-3 An example of a consent form used to disclose and use health information for treatment, payment, or health care operations. This is not required under HIPAA, but you may find that some medical practices use it. *(From Fordney MT, French L: Medical insurance billing and coding: a worktext, Philadelphia, 2003, Elsevier.)*

utilization management purposes," the MCO has a right to audit those patients' financial records. Other managed care providers need to know about the patients if involved in the care and treatment of members of the MCO.

2. When patients have certain communicable diseases that are highly contagious or infectious and state health agencies require providers to report, even if the patient does not want the information reported.
3. When a medical device breaks or malfunctions, the Food and Drug Administration requires providers to report certain information.
4. When a patient is suspect in a criminal investigation or to assist in locating a missing person, material witness, or suspect, police have the right to request certain information.
5. When the patient's records are subpoenaed or there is a search warrant. The courts have the right to order providers to release patient information.

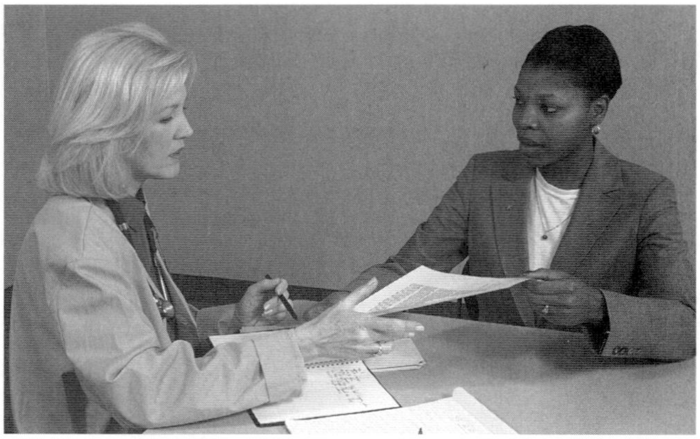

FIGURE A-4 Patient signing a consent form.

6. When the patient is suing someone, such as an employer, and wishes to protect herself or himself.
7. When there is a suspicious death or suspected crime victim, providers must report cases.
8. When the physician examines a patient at the request of a third party who is paying the bill, as in workers' compensation cases.
9. When state law requires the release of information to police that is for the good of society, such as reporting cases of child abuse, elder abuse, domestic violence, or gunshot wounds.

The purpose of the Privacy Rule is to ensure that patients who receive medical treatment may have control in the manner in which specific information is used and to whom it is disclosed. **Confidential communication** is a privileged communication that may be disclosed only with the patient's permission. Everything you see, hear, or read about patients remains confidential and does not leave the office. Never talk about patients or data contained in medical records where others may overhear. Some employers require employees to sign a confidentiality agreement. Such agreements should be updated periodically to address issues raised by the use of new technologies.

Privileged Information. **Privileged information** is related to the treatment and progress of the patient. The patient must sign an authorization to release this information or selected facts from the medical record. Some states have passed laws allowing certain test results (e.g., disclosure of the presence of the human immunodeficiency virus [HIV] or alcohol or substance abuse) and other information to be placed separate from the patient's medical record. A special authorization form is used to release this information.

Nonprivileged Information. **Nonprivileged information** consists of ordinary facts unrelated to treatment of the patient, including the patient's name, city of residence, and dates of admission or discharge. This information must be sensitized against unauthorized disclosure under the privacy section of HIPAA. The patient's authorization is not necessary for the purposes of treatment, payment, or health care operations, unless the record is in a specialty hospital (e.g., alcohol treatment) or a special service unit of a general hospital (e.g., psychiatric unit). Professional judgment is required. The information is disclosed on a legitimate need-to-know basis, meaning that the medical data should be revealed to the attending physician because the information may have some effect on the treatment of the patient.

Patients' Rights

Right to Privacy. All patients have a right to privacy. It is important never to discuss patient information other than with the physician, an insurance company, or an individual who has been authorized by the patient. If a telephone inquiry is made and you need to verify that callers are who they say they are:

- Ask for one or more of the following items: patient's full name, home address, date of birth, Social Security number, mother's maiden name, or dates of service.
- Ask for a call-back number and compare it with the number on file.
- Ask the patient to fax a sheet with his or her signature on it so that you can compare it with one on file.
- Some hospitals may assign a code word or number that may be a middle name or date that is easy for patients to remember. If a patient does not know the code word, then ask for personal identifying information as mentioned.

If a telephone inquiry is made about a patient, ask the caller to put the request in writing and include the patient's signed authorization. If the caller refuses, have the physician return the call. If a relative telephones asking about a patient, have the physician return the call. When you telephone a patient about an insurance matter and reach voice mail, use care in the choice of words when leaving the message in the event the call was inadvertently received at the wrong number. Leave your name, the office name, and the return telephone number. Never attempt to interpret a report or provide information about the outcome of laboratory or other diagnostic tests to the patient. Let the physician do it.

Do's and Don'ts of Confidentiality

Don't. Discuss a patient with acquaintances, yours or the patient's.

Don't. Leave patients' records or appointment books exposed on your desk. If confidential documents are on your desk and patients can easily see them as they walk by, either turn the documents over or lock them in a secure drawer when you leave your desk, even if you are gone for only a few moments.

Don't. Leave a computer screen with patient information visible, even for a moment, if another patient may see the data. If patient information is on your computer, either turn the screen off or save it on disk, lock the disk in a secure place, and clear the information from the screen.

DO. Properly dispose of notes, papers, and memos by using a shredding device.

DO. Be careful when using the copying machine because it is easy to forget to remove the original insurance claim or medical record from the document glass.

DO. Use common sense and follow the guidelines mentioned in this chapter to help you keep your professional credibility and integrity.

Privacy Rules: Patient Rights Under HIPAA

Patients are granted the following six federal rights that allow them to be informed about PHI and to control how their PHI is used and disclosed:

1. *Right to* ***Notice of Privacy Practices*** *(NPP)*, a document in plain language that is usually given to the patient at the first visit or at enrollment. The staff must make a reasonable "best effort" to obtain a signature from the patient acknowledging receipt and this must be done once only. If the patient cannot or will not sign, this should be documented in the patient's health record. The NPP must be posted at every service delivery site and available in paper form for those who request it. A provider's website must have the NPP placed on the site and must deliver a copy electronically on request.
2. *Right to request restrictions on certain uses and disclosures of PHI.* Patients have the right to ask for restrictions on how a medical office uses and discloses PHI for TPO (e.g., a patient had a successfully treated sexually transmitted disease many years before and requests that, whenever possible, this material not be disclosed). A provider is not required to agree to these requests but must have a process to review the requests, accept and review any appeal, and give a sound reason for not agreeing to the request. Restrictions must be documented and followed. See Box A-2, which details the regulations for disclosing the minimum necessary PHI, de-identification of PHI, marketing related to the patient, and fundraising activities related to patients.
3. *Right to request confidential communications* by alternative means or at an alternative location (e.g., call at work rather than at the residence or test results sent in writing instead of by telephone). The patient does not need to explain the reason for the request. The health care office must have a process in place to both evaluate requests and appeals and respond to the patient. Patients may be required by the office to make their request in writing. Such a document protects the practice's compliance endeavors.
4. *Right to access (inspect and obtain a copy of) PHI.* Privacy regulations allow the provider to require the patient make the request for access in writing. Generally, a request must be acted on within 30 days. A reasonable, cost-based fee for copies of PHI may only include the costs for supplies and labor for copying, postage when mailed, and preparing a summary of the PHI if the patient has agreed to this instead of complete access. If a digital office copier is used, be sure precautions are taken to digitally shred information after every copy, print scan, or fax job so that information is kept secure.

Under HIPAA Privacy Regulation, patients do not have the right to access the following:

- Psychotherapy notes
- Information compiled in reasonable anticipation of, or for use in, legal proceedings
- Information exempted from disclosure under the Clinical Laboratory Improvements Amendment (CLIA)

The office may deny patient access for the previously mentioned reasons without giving the patient the right to review the denial.

If the health care provider has determined that the patient would be endangered (or cause danger to another person) from accessing the confidential health information, access may be denied. In this case, the patient has the right to have the denial reviewed by another licensed professional who did not participate in the initial denial decision.

Regarding psychotherapy notes, HIPAA gives special protection to PHI. Disclosure of a patient's mental health records requires specific patient permission. This means that when an insurance payer requests the health records to review the claim, a patient authorization is required.

Certain clinical data are excluded from the definition of psychotherapy notes. In other words, when an individual is using the services of a mental health professional, not all information gathered and recorded in the health record of the mental health provider is considered psychotherapy notes. The law lists specific items that are excluded from such notes:

- Medication prescription and monitoring
- Counseling session start and stop times
- Modalities and frequencies of treatment furnished
- Results of clinical tests
- Any summary of the following items: diagnosis, functional status, treatment plan, symptoms, prognosis, and progress to date

BOX A-2 HIPAA Help

You will find key terms addressed in the Notice of Privacy Practices (NPP) that apply to the patient's right to request restrictions on certain uses and disclosures of PHI.

- **Minimum Necessary**. Privacy regulations require that use or disclosure of only the minimum amount of information necessary to fulfill the intended purpose be permitted. There are some exceptions to this rule. You do not need to limit PHI for disclosures in regard to health care providers for treatment, the patient, DHHS for investigations of compliance with HIPAA, or as required by law.

Minimum Necessary determinations for *uses of PHI* must be determined within each organization, and reasonable efforts must be made to limit access to only the minimum amount of information needed by identified staff members. In smaller offices, employees may have multiple job functions. If a medical assistant helps with the patient examination, documents vital signs, and then collects the patient's copayment at the reception area, the assistant will likely access clinical and billing records. Simple procedure and policy (P&P) about appropriate access to PHI may be sufficient to satisfy the Minimum Necessary requirement. Larger organizations may have specific restrictions on who should have access to different types of PHI because staff members tend to have a more targeted job role. Remain knowledgeable about your office's policy regarding Minimum Necessary. If you are strictly scheduling appointments, you may not need access to the clinical record. An x-ray technician will likely not need to access the patient billing records.

Minimum Necessary determinations for *disclosures of PHI* are distinguished by two categories within the Privacy Rule:

1. For disclosures made on a routine and recurring basis, you may implement policies and procedures, or standard protocols, for what will be disclosed. These disclosures would be common in your practice. Examples may include disclosures for workers' compensation claims or school physical forms.
2. For other disclosures that would be considered nonroutine, criteria should be established for determining the Minimum Necessary amount of PHI and to review each request for disclosure on an individual basis. A staff member (e.g., PO, medical records supervisor) will likely be assigned to determine this situation when the need arises.

As a general rule, remember that you must limit your requests to access PHI to the Minimum Necessary to accomplish the task for which you will need the information.

- **De-identification of Confidential Information**. Other requirements relating to uses and disclosures of PHI include health information that does not identify an individual or leaves no reasonable basis to believe that the information can be used to identify an individual. This "de-identified" information is no longer individually identifiable health information (IIHI). Most providers will never have the need to de-identify patient information, and the requirements for de-identifying PHI are lengthy. The regulations give specific directions on how to ensure all pieces of necessary information are removed to fit the definition. De-identified information is not subject to the privacy regulations because it does not specifically identify an individual.
- **Marketing**. When communicating about a product or service, the goal is to encourage patients to purchase or use the product or service. For instance, a dermatologist may advertise for a discount on facial cream when you schedule a dermabrasion treatment. You will likely not be involved in marketing, but keep in mind the general rule that PHI (including names and addresses) cannot be used for marketing purposes without specific authorization of the patient. Sending appointment reminders and general news updates about your organization and the services you provide would not be considered marketing and would not require patient authorization.
- **Fundraising**. Again, you will likely not be involved in fundraising activities, but HIPAA allows demographic information and dates of care to be used for fundraising purposes without patient authorization. The disclosure of any additional information requires patient authorization. Your organization's NPP will state that patients may receive fundraising materials and are given the opportunity to opt out of receiving future solicitations.

In general, the major difference between what are and what are not considered psychotherapy notes is the information that is the *recorded (in any manner) documentation and/or analysis of conversation*. This information should also be kept separate from the medical section of the patient health record to be distinguished as psychotherapy notes. For example, Jane Doe tells her psychologist the details of her childhood trauma. The documented conversation specific to her trauma (e.g., what occurred, how she felt) is considered the psychotherapy notes and cannot be released without specific permission from Jane Doe.

It is also important to understand that patients do not have the right to obtain a copy of psychotherapy notes under HIPAA. However, the treating mental health provider may decide when a patient may obtain access to this health information.

State law must always be considered. Some states allow patients access to their psychotherapy notes; therefore state law would take precedence over HIPAA as a result of the state preemption allowance.

5. *Right to request an amendment of PHI*. Patients have the right to request that their PHI be amended. As with the other requests, the provider may require the request to be in writing. The provider must have a process to accept and review both the request and any appeal in a timely fashion. The health care provider may deny this request in the following circumstances:
   - The provider who is being requested to change the PHI is not the creator of the information (e.g., office has records sent by referring physician).
   - The PHI is believed to be accurate and complete as it stands in the provider's records.
   - The information is not required to be accessible to the patient (see Right to Access, Inspect, and Obtain PHI).

Generally, the office must respond to a patient's request for amendment within 60 days. If a request is denied, the patient must be informed in writing of the reason for the denial. The patient must also be given the opportunity to file a statement of disagreement.

6. *Right to receive an accounting of disclosures of PHI.* Providers should maintain a log of disclosures of PHI, either on paper or within the organization's computer system, of all disclosures other than those made for TPO, facility directories, and some national security and law enforcement agencies. The process for providing an accounting should be outlined in the practice's policy manual. Patients may request an accounting (or tracking) of disclosures of their confidential information and are granted the right to receive this accounting once a year without charge. Additional accountings may be assessed a cost-based fee.

These accountings were required to start on April 14, 2003, when privacy regulations became enforceable. Items to be documented must include the following:

- Date of disclosure
- Name of the entity or person who received the PHI including their address, if known
- Brief description of the PHI disclosed
- Brief statement of the purpose of the disclosure

The patient is entitled to one accounting per year free of charge. Additional accountings may be assessed a cost-based fee.

Verification of Identity and Authority

Before any disclosure, you must verify the identity of persons requesting PHI if they are unknown to you. You may request identifying information such as date of birth, Social Security number, or even a code word stored in your practice management system that is unique to each patient. Public officials may show you badges, credentials, official letterheads, and other legal documents of authority for identification purposes.

Additionally, you must verify that the requestor has the right and the need to have the PHI.

Exercising professional judgment will fulfill your verification requirements for most disclosures because you are acting on "good faith" in believing the identity of the individual requesting PHI. It is good practice, when making any disclosure to note, to note the "authority" of the person receiving the PHI and how this was determined. This evidence of due diligence on your part would enforce a needed structure on your staff and dampen any complaints that might arise.

Validating Patient Permission

Before making any uses or disclosures of confidential health information other than for the purposes of TPO, your office must have appropriate patient permission. Always check for conflicts between various permissions your office may have on file for a given patient. This information should be maintained either in your practice management system or in the medical chart, where it can be easily identified and retrieved.

For example, if a covered entity has agreed to a patient's request to limit how much of the PHI is sent to a consulting physician for treatment, but then received the patient's authorization to disclose the entire medical record to that physician, this would be a conflict. In general, the more restrictive permission would be the deciding factor. Privacy regulations allow resolving conflicting permissions by either obtaining new permission from the patient or communicating orally or in writing with the patient to determine the patient's preference. Be sure to document any form of communication in writing.

Guidelines for HIPAA Privacy Compliance

As an insurance billing specialist, you will likely answer the telephone and speak during the course of your business, and there will be questions about what you can and cannot say. Reasonable and appropriate safeguards must be taken to ensure that all confidential health information in your office is protected from unauthorized and inappropriate access, including both verbal and written forms.

Some of the following situations may be referred to as incidental disclosures, and this topic is discussed in further detail with additional examples later in this chapter.

1. Consider that conversations occurring throughout the office could be overheard. The reception area and waiting room are often linked, and it is easy to hear the scheduling of appointments and exchange of confidential information. It is necessary to observe areas and maximize efforts to avoid unauthorized disclosures. Simple and affordable precautions include using privacy glass at the front desk and having conversations away from settings where other patients or visitors are present. Health care providers can move their dictation stations away from patient areas or wait until no patients are present before dictating. Telephone conversations by providers in front of patients, even in emergency situations, should be avoided. Providers and staff must use their best professional judgment.
2. Be sure to check in the patient medical record and in your computer system to determine whether there

are any special instructions for contacting the patient regarding scheduling or reporting test results. Follow these requests as agreed by the office.

3. Patient sign-in sheets are permissible, but limit the information you request when a patient signs in and change it periodically during the day. A sign-in sheet must not contain information such as reason for visit or the patient's medical condition because some providers specialize in treating patients with sensitive issues. Thus showing that a particular individual has an appointment with your practice may pose a breach of patient confidentiality.
4. Make sure you have patients sign a form acknowledging receipt of the NPP. The NPP allows you to release the patient's confidential information for billing and other purposes. If your practice has other confidentiality statements and policies besides HIPAA mandates, these must be reviewed to ensure they meet HIPAA requirements.
5. Formal policies for transferring and accepting outside PHI must address how your office keeps this information confidential. When using courier services, billing services, transcription services, or e-mail, you must ensure that transferring PHI is done in a secure and compliant manner.
6. Computers are used for a variety of administrative functions including scheduling, billing, and managing medical records. Computers are typically present at the reception area. Keep the computer screen turned so that viewing is restricted to authorized staff. Screen savers should be used to prevent unauthorized viewing or access. The computer should automatically log off the user after a period of being idle, requiring the staff member to reenter his or her password.
7. Keep your user name and password confidential and change them often. Do not share this information. An authorized staff member such as the PO will have administrative access to reset your password if you lose it or if someone discovers it. Also, practice management software can track users and follow their activity. Do not set yourself up by giving out your password. Safeguards include password protection for electronic data and storing paper records securely.
8. Safeguard your work area; do not place notes with confidential information in areas that are easy to view by nonstaff. Cleaning services will access your building, usually after business hours; ensure that you safeguard PHI.
9. Place medical record charts face down at reception areas so that the patient's name is not exposed to other patients or visitors to your office. Also, when placing medical records on the door of an examination room, turn the chart so that identifying information faces the door. If you keep medical charts in the office on countertops or in receptacles, it is your duty to ensure that nonstaff persons will not access the records. Handling and storing medical records will certainly change because of HIPAA guidelines.
10. Do not post the health care provider's schedule in areas viewable by nonstaff individuals. The schedules are often posted for convenience of the professional staff, but this may be a breach in patient confidentiality.
11. Fax machines should not be placed in patient examination rooms or in any reception area where nonstaff persons may view incoming or sent documents. Only staff members should have access to the faxes.
12. If you open your office mail or take telephone calls pertaining to medical record requests, direct these issues to the appropriate staff member.
13. If you are involved in coding and billing, be sure to recognize, learn, and use HIPAA TCS.
14. Send all privacy-related questions or concerns to the appropriate staff member.
15. Immediately report any suspected or known improper behavior to your supervisor or the PO so that the issue may be documented and investigated.
16. If you have questions, contact your supervisor or the PO.

Health care organizations face challenges in implementing the HIPAA requirements; do not let these overwhelm you. Your office is required to take reasonable steps to build protections specific to your health care organization. Compliance is an ongoing endeavor involving teamwork. Understand your office's established P&P. Monitor your own activities to ensure you are following the required procedures. Do not take shortcuts when your actions involve patient privacy and security.

Be alert to other activities in your office. Help your co-workers change work habits that do not comply with HIPAA. Do not ignore unauthorized uses and disclosures of PHI, and do not allow unauthorized persons to access data. You have an obligation to your employer and the patients you serve.

CONSEQUENCES OF NONCOMPLIANCE WITH HIPAA

The prosecution of HIPAA crimes is handled by different governing bodies. HHS handles issues regarding TCS and security. Complaints can be filed against a covered entity for not complying with these rules. The OCR oversees privacy issues and complaints, referring criminal issues to the Office of Inspector General (OIG). The OIG provides the workup for referral cases, which may involve the Federal Bureau of Investigation (FBI) and other agencies.

Civil Monetary Penalties Law (42 US Code §320a-27a)

The U.S. Congress enacted the Civil Monetary Penalty (CMP) statute to provide administrative remediation to combat health care fraud and abuse. HIPAA's Final Rule includes civil monetary penalties when there is a pattern of upcoded claims or billing for medically unnecessary services. CMP imposes civil monetary penalties and assessments against a person or organization for making false or improper claims against any federal health care program.

Serious civil and criminal penalties apply for HIPAA noncompliance. A civil penalty is a fine assessed for violation of a law or regulation, whereas a criminal penalty is fine and imprisonment for criminal violation of a federal or state law. General noncompliance with the privacy, security, and transaction regulations results in a $100 fine per violation and up to $25,000 per person for identical violations in a given calendar year. Specific to the Privacy Rule is a $50,000 fine and imprisonment for 1 year if one knowingly obtains or discloses IIHI. The person who obtains or discloses such health information under false pretenses is subject to a $100,000 fine. If one obtains or discloses PHI with the intent to sell, transfer, or use it for commercial advantage, personal gain, or malicious harm, a maximum fine of $250,000 and up to 10 years' imprisonment may be applied.

OFFICE OF INSPECTOR GENERAL

The mission of the OIG is to safeguard the health and welfare of the beneficiaries of HHS programs and to protect the integrity of HHS programs (Medicare and Medicaid). The OIG was established to identify and eliminate fraud, abuse, and waste and "to promote efficiency and economy in departmental operations." HIPAA legislation has radically changed the focus and mission within OIG. HIPAA pushed OIG into a new era, guaranteeing funds for the OIG programs and mandating initiatives to protect the integrity of all health care programs. The OIG undertakes nationwide audits, as well as investigations and inspections to review the claim submission processes of providers and reimbursement patterns of the programs. Recommendations are made to the HHS Secretary and the U.S. Congress on correcting problematic areas addressed in the federal programs according to the OIG.

Efforts to combat fraud were consolidated and strengthened under Public Law 104-191, the Health Insurance Portability and Accountability Act of 1996 (HIPAA). The act established a comprehensive program to combat fraud committed against all health plans, both public and private. The legislation required the establishment of a national Health Care Fraud and Abuse Control Program (HCFAP), under the joint direction of the Attorney General and the Secretary of the Department of Health and Human Services (HHS) acting through the Department's Inspector General (HHS/OIG). The HCFAP program is designed to coordinate federal, state, and local law enforcement activities with respect to health care fraud and abuse. The act requires HHS and the Department of Justice (DOJ) to detail in an annual report the amounts deposited and appropriated to the Medicare Trust Fund, as well as the source of such deposits.

Health care providers must be aware of the potential liabilities when submitting claims for payment that are deemed to be "fraudulent" or inappropriate by the government. The government may impose significant financial and administrative penalties when health care claims are not appropriately submitted, including criminal prosecution against the offending party. Fraud, according to the OIG, can result from deliberate unethical behavior or simply from mistakes and miscues that cause excessive reimbursement. The OIG is the professional health care provider's (and his or her agents') "partner" in fighting fraud and abuse.

Compliance Program Guidance recommendations from the OIG must be the guiding principle of a health care practice in regard to the potential for unethical behavior or the mistakes that may occur within the organization. The *OIG Compliance Program for Individual and Small Group Physician Practices* and the *OIG Compliance Program Guidance for Third-Party Medical Billing Companies* are two publications in a series for the health care industry that provide guidance and acceptable principles for business operations. See Internet Resources at the end of this chapter.

If you are involved in the claims processing procedures in your organization, note the importance and urgency in following the legal and ethical path when performing your duties. Your "honest mistake" could lead to a situation that puts the health care provider at risk for investigation of fraud, waste, or abuse if it continues and is not corrected.

Fraud and Abuse Laws

Fraud can occur when deception is used in a claim submission to obtain payment from the payer. Individuals who knowingly, willfully, and intentionally submit false information to benefit themselves or others commit fraud. Fraud can also be interpreted from mistakes that result in excessive reimbursement. No proof of "specific intent to defraud" is required for fraud to be considered. Fraud usually involves careful planning. Examples of fraud can be found in Box A-3.

Abuse means incidents or practices by physicians, not usually considered fraudulent, that are inconsistent with accepted sound medical business or fiscal practices.

BOX A-3 Examples of Fraud

- Bill for services or supplies not provided (phantom billing or invoice ghosting) or for an office visit if a patient fails to keep an appointment and is not notified ahead of time that this is office policy.
- Alter fees on a claim form to obtain higher payment.
- Forgive the deductible or copayment.
- Alter medical records to generate fraudulent payments.
- Leave relevant information off a claim (e.g., failing to reveal whether a spouse has health insurance coverage through an employer).
- Upcode (e.g., submitting a code for a complex fracture when the patient had a simple fracture).
- Shorten (e.g., dispensing less medication than billed for).
- Split billing schemes (e.g., billing procedures over a period of days when all treatment occurred during one visit).
- Use another person's insurance card in obtaining medical care.
- Change a date of service.
- Post adjustments to generate fraudulent payments.
- Solicit, offer, or receive a kickback, bribe, or rebate in return for referring a patient to a physician, physical therapist, or pharmacy or for referring a patient to obtain any item or service that may be paid for in full or in part by Medicare or Medicaid.
- Restate the diagnosis to obtain insurance benefits or better payment.
- Apply deliberately for duplicate payment (e.g., billing Medicare twice, billing Medicare and the beneficiary for the same service, or billing Medicare and another insurer in an attempt to get paid twice).
- Unbundle or explode charge (e.g., billing a multichannel laboratory test as if individual tests were performed).
- Collusion between a physician and an employee of a third-party payer when the claim is assigned (if the physician deliberately overbilled for services, overpayments could be generated with little awareness on the part of the Medicare beneficiary).
- Bills based on gang visits (e.g., a physician visits nursing home and bills for 20 visits without furnishing any specific service to, or on behalf of, individual patients).
- Knowingly bill for the same item or service more than once or when another party bills the federal health care program for an item or service also billed by the physician.

KEY POINTS

This is a brief chapter review or summary of the key issues presented. To further enhance your knowledge of the technical subject matter, review the key terms and key abbreviations for this chapter by locating the meanings in the glossary at the end of this book that appear in a section before the index.

1. The Health Insurance Portability and Accountability Act (HIPAA) has affected confidentiality and disclosure of protected health information (PHI), completion and electronic transmission of insurance claims, fraud and abuse in claims submission, and implementation of compliance and practice standards.
2. While employed by a medical practice, the insurance billing specialist's duty is to have complete knowledge and understanding of HIPAA mandates, carry out policies and procedures that comply with federal regulations, and keep up to date with these statutes. This will assist both the physician and the patients.
3. The National Health Information Infrastructure (NHII) is an initiative set forth to improve patient safety and the quality of health care, as well as to better inform individuals regarding their own health information and to help them understand health care costs.
4. *e-Health information management (eHIM)* is a phrase that describes any and all transactions in which health care information is accessed, processed, stored, and transferred using electronic technologies.
5. The primary purpose of HIPAA *Title I: Insurance Reform* is to provide continuous insurance coverage for workers and their insured dependents when they change or lose jobs. *Title II: Administrative Simplification* focuses on the health care practice setting and aims to reduce administrative costs and burdens.
6. Serious civil and criminal penalties such as fines and imprisonment apply for HIPAA noncompliance.
7. Protected health information (PHI) refers to data that identify an individual and describe his or her health status, age, sex, ethnicity, or other demographic characteristics, whether or not that information is stored or transmitted electronically.
8. Under HIPAA, PHI may not be used or disclosed without permission of the patient or someone authorized to act on behalf of the patient, unless the use or disclosure is specifically required or permitted by the regulation (e.g., treatment, payment, or health care operations [TPO]). The two types of disclosure required by HIPAA Privacy Rule are to the individual who is the subject of the PHI and to the Secretary or DHHS to investigate compliance with the rule.
9. When comparing privileged and nonprivileged information, privileged information is related to the treatment and progress of the patient. The patient must sign an authorization to release this information or selected facts from the medical record. Nonprivileged information consists of ordinary facts unrelated to treatment of the patient, including the patient's name, city of residence, and dates of admission or discharge.
10. Under HIPAA, a Notice of Privacy Practices (NPP) document must be given to the patient at the first visit or at enrollment explaining the individual's rights and the physician's legal duties in regard to PHI. Use and disclosure of PHI is permissible for TPO because the NPP describes how PHI is used for

these purposes. Thus a consent form is not required. The health care provider is required to obtain a signed authorization form to use or disclose health information for situations beyond the TPO. This is a protection for the practice. Psychotherapy notes are handled separately under HIPAA. Such notes have additional protection, specifically that an authorization for any use of disclosure of psychotherapy notes must be obtained.

11. *Disclosure* means the release, transfer, provision of access to, or divulging in any other manner of information outside the entity holding the information. *Use* means the sharing, employment, application, utilization, examination, or analysis of IIHI within an organization that holds such information. When a patient's billing record is accessed to review the claim submission history, the individual's health information is in "use."
12. The three major categories of security safeguards include administrative, technical, and physical measures that will reasonably protect PHI from any use or disclosure that is in violation of HIPAA.
13. The difference between *fraud* and *abuse* is that fraud can occur when deception is used in a claim submission to obtain payment from the payer. Individuals who knowingly, willfully, and intentionally submit false information to benefit themselves or others commit *fraud*. *Abuse* means incidents or practices by physicians, not usually considered fraudulent, that are inconsistent with accepted sound medical business or fiscal practices.

You must strongly consider the lessons learned from the privacy, transaction, and security rules in conjunction with OIG compliance recommendations. The most important points are to read your organization's P&P manual and to ask questions about the many aspects of HIPAA or the general operations of your organization. Always use your ethical and "best practice" approach to be an informed and effective employee.

APPENDIX

B

OSHA/Bloodborne Pathogens

OSHA BLOODBORNE PATHOGENS STANDARD

PURPOSE OF THE STANDARD

The federal government established OSHA (Occupational Safety and Health Administration) to assist employers in providing a safe and healthy working environment for their employees. To provide a safe working environment for health care workers, OSHA developed a comprehensive set of regulations known as the *OSHA Occupational Exposure to Bloodborne Pathogens Standard.*

These regulations went into effect in 1992 and are designed to reduce the risk to employees of exposure to infectious diseases.

The OSHA Bloodborne Pathogens Standard must be followed by any employee with occupational exposure to pathogens, regardless of the place of employment. Employees with occupational exposure include physicians, nurses, medical assistants, dentists, dental hygienists, medical laboratory personnel, and emergency medical technicians. Employees who may have less obvious occupational exposure are correctional and law enforcement officers, firefighters, hospital laundry workers, morticians, and custodians.

Failure by employers to comply with the OSHA standard could result in a citation carrying a maximum penalty of $7000 for each violation and a maximum penalty of $70,000 for repeat violations.

NEEDLESTICK SAFETY AND PREVENTION ACT

Since the adoption of the OSHA Bloodborne Pathogens Standard, needlestick injuries among health care workers have continued to be a problem because of their high frequency of occurrence and the severity of the health effects associated with exposure to bloodborne pathogens. To address this problem, Congress passed the Needlestick Safety and Prevention Act (NSPA). The NSPA directed OSHA to revise the Bloodborne Pathogens Standard to incorporate stronger measures to reduce needlesticks and other sharps injuries among health care workers. In response to this mandate, the primary measure instituted by OSHA was to establish detailed requirements that employers identify and make use of safer medical devices. This revised OSHA Bloodborne Pathogens Standard went into effect in 2001 and is described in detail in this chapter.

OSHA TERMINOLOGY

The following definitions help clarify terms relating to the OSHA Bloodborne Pathogens Standard.

Occupational Exposure. Occupational exposure is reasonably anticipated skin, eye, mucous membrane, or parenteral contact with blood or other potentially infectious materials that may result from the performance of an employee's duties.

Parenteral. *Parenteral* refers to the piercing of the skin barrier or mucous membranes, such as through needlesticks, human bites, cuts, and abrasions.

Blood. *Blood* means human blood, human blood components, and products made from blood. Blood components include plasma, serum, platelets, and serosanguineous fluid (e.g., exudates from wounds). An example of a blood product is a medication derived from blood, such as immune globulins.

Bloodborne Pathogens. Bloodborne pathogens are pathogenic microorganisms in human blood that can cause disease in humans. Bloodborne pathogens include, but are not limited to, hepatitis B virus (HBV), hepatitis C virus (HCV), and human immunodeficiency virus (HIV).

Other Potentially Infectious Materials. Other potentially infectious materials (OPIM) include:

- Semen and vaginal secretions
- Cerebrospinal, synovial, pleural, pericardial, peritoneal, and amniotic fluids
- Any body fluid that is visibly contaminated with blood
- Any body fluid that has not been identified

- Saliva in dental procedures
- Any unfixed human tissue
- Any tissue culture, cells, or fluid known to be HIV infected

Contaminated. *Contaminated* is defined as the presence or reasonably anticipated presence of blood or other potentially infected materials on an item or surface.

Decontamination. Decontamination is the use of physical or chemical means to remove, inactivate, or destroy pathogens on a surface or item to the point where they are no longer capable of transmitting infectious particles, and the surface or item is rendered safe for handling, use, or disposal.

Nonintact Skin. Nonintact skin is skin that has a break in the surface. It includes, but is not limited to, skin with dermatitis, abrasions, cuts, burns, hangnails, chapping, and acne.

Exposure Incident. *Exposure incident* is defined as a specific eye, nose, mouth, other mucous membrane, nonintact skin, or parenteral contact with blood or other potentially infectious materials that results from an employee's duties.

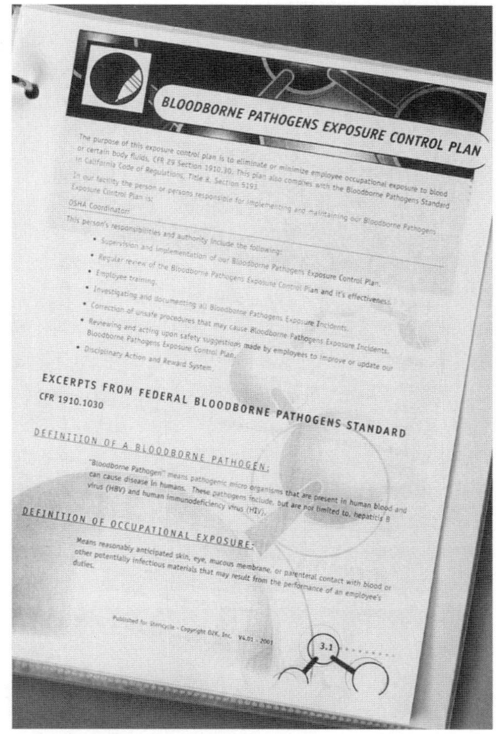

FIGURE B-1 Example of an exposure control plan.

COMPONENTS OF THE OSHA STANDARD

The OSHA Bloodborne Pathogens Standard is presented on the following pages as it pertains to the medical office and includes the following categories:

- Exposure control plan
- Safer medical devices
- Labeling requirements
- Communication of hazards to employees
- Record-keeping

Exposure Control Plan

The OSHA standard requires that the medical office develop an exposure control plan (ECP) (Figure B-1). The ECP is a written document stipulating the protective measures that must be followed in that medical office to eliminate or minimize employee exposure to bloodborne pathogens and other potentially infectious material. The ECP must be made available for review by all medical office staff. The ECP must include the following elements:

1. **An exposure determination.** The purpose of this section of the ECP is to identify employees who must receive training, protective equipment, hepatitis vaccination, and other protections required by the Bloodborne Pathogens Standard. The exposure determination must include (1) a list of all job classifications in which *all* employees are likely to have occupational exposure, such as physicians, medical assistants, and laboratory technicians, and (2) a list of job classifications in which only *some* employees have occupational exposure, such as custodians. For the second classification of jobs, the determination must include a list of tasks in which occupational exposure may occur, such as emptying the trash.
2. **The method of compliance.** The method of compliance section of the ECP must document the specific health and safety control measures that are taken in the medical office to eliminate or minimize the risk of occupational exposure. These measures are extremely important in reducing the risk of infectious diseases and are discussed in more detail later in this section (see Control Measures).
3. **Postexposure evaluation and follow-up procedures.** The postexposure evaluation and follow-up must specify the procedures to follow in the event of an exposure incident in the medical office, including the method of documenting and investigating an exposure incident and the postexposure evaluation, medical treatment, and follow-up that would be made available to the employee. (Refer to the *OSHA Postexposure Evaluation and Follow-Up Procedures* box.)

OSHA requires employers to review and update their ECP at least annually to ensure that the plan remains current with the latest information on eliminating or reducing exposure to bloodborne pathogens. The ECP also must be updated whenever necessary to reflect new or modified tasks and procedures that affect occupational exposure.

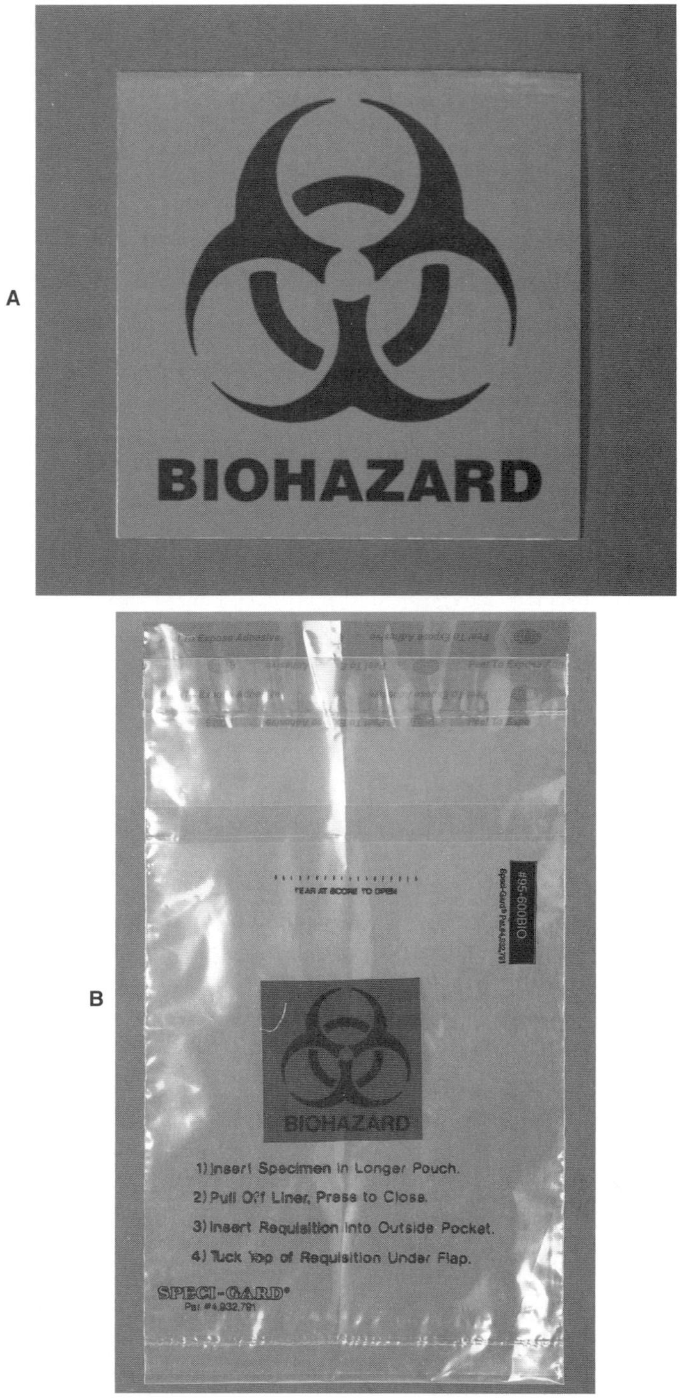

FIGURE B-2 **A**, Biohazard warning label. **B**, Biohazard bag used to hold and transport blood or other potentially infectious materials.

Labeling Requirements

The OSHA Bloodborne Pathogens Standard requires that containers and appliances containing biohazardous materials be labeled with a *biohazard warning label*. The biohazard warning label must be fluorescent orange or orange-red and contain the biohazard symbol and the word "BIOHAZARD" in a contrasting color (Figure B-2A).

A warning label must be attached to the following: (1) containers of regulated waste; (2) refrigerators and freezers used to store blood and other potentially infectious materials; and (3) containers and bags used to store, transport, or ship blood or other potentially infectious materials (Figure B-2B). Red bags or red containers may be substituted for biohazard warning labels. The labeling requirement is designed to alert employees to possible exposure, particularly in situations where the nature of the material or contents is not readily identifiable as blood or other potentially infectious materials.

OSHA POSTEXPOSURE EVALUATION AND FOLLOW-UP PROCEDURES

An exposure incident is a specific eye, nose, mouth, other mucous membrane, nonintact skin, or parenteral contact with blood or other potentially infectious materials that results from an employee's duties. In the event of an exposure incident to bloodborne pathogens or other potentially infectious materials, OSHA requires the following steps to be performed:

1. Perform initial first aid measures immediately (e.g., wash a needlestick injury thoroughly with soap and water).
2. Document the route of exposure and the conditions and circumstances of the exposure incident. This includes such information as the engineering controls, work practice controls, and personal protective equipment being used at the time of the incident.
3. Identify and document the source individual (unless the employer can establish that identification is not feasible or is prohibited by state or local law). A source individual is any person, living or dead, whose blood or OPIM may be a source of occupational exposure to the health care worker.
4. Obtain consent to test the source individual's blood. Test it as soon as possible to determine HBV, HCV, and HIV infectivity. The following guidelines apply to this requirement:
   - If consent is not obtained, the employer must document that legally required consent cannot be obtained.
   - If the source individual's consent is not required by law, the source individual's blood (if available) must be tested and the results documented.
   - If the source individual is already known to be infected with HBV, HCV, or HIV, testing does not need to be repeated.
5. Provide the exposed employee with the source individual's test results. Inform the employee of applicable laws and regulations concerning disclosure of the identity and infectious status of the source individual.
6. Obtain consent to test the employee's blood. Collect and test the blood of the employee as soon as possible for HBV, HCV, and HIV serologic status. If the employee does not give consent for HIV serologic testing, the baseline blood sample must be preserved for at least 90 days. If the employee elects to have the baseline sample tested during the 90-day waiting period, such testing must be done as soon as feasible.
7. When medically indicated, provide the employee with appropriate postexposure prophylaxis as recommended by the U.S. Public Health Service.

Communicating Hazards to Employees

According to the OSHA standard, employers must ensure that all medical office employees with risk of occupational exposure participate in a training program. The program must present the ECP for the medical office, focusing on the measures that employees are to take for their safety. Training must be provided at the time an employee is initially assigned to tasks in which occupational exposure may occur and at least annually thereafter.

The employer must maintain records of the training sessions, which must include presentation dates, content of the sessions, names and qualifications of the trainers, and names and job titles of employees who attended. These records must be maintained for 3 years from the date of the training session.

Record-Keeping

The OSHA Bloodborne Pathogens Standard requires that the following records be maintained:

1. **OSHA medical record.** The OSHA standard requires that the employer maintain an accurate OSHA record of every medical office employee at risk for occupational exposure. These records must be kept confidential except for review by OSHA officials and as required by law. The record must include the following: employee's name; social security number; hepatitis B vaccination status, including dates of vaccination; results of any postexposure examinations, medical testing, and follow-up procedures; and a written evaluation of any exposure incident along with a copy of the exposure incident report. The employer is required to maintain records for the duration of employment plus 30 years.
2. **Sharps injury log.** Employers with more than 10 employees at risk for occupational exposure are required to maintain a log of injuries from contaminated sharps. The log must be maintained in a way that protects the confidentiality of injured employees (e.g., removal of personal identification). The purpose of the log is to help employers and employees keep track of all needlestick injuries. This tracking helps identify problem areas that need attention and ineffective devices that need to be replaced. The sharps injury log must contain the following information:
   - Type and brand of device involved in the injury
   - Location of the incident (i.e., work area)
   - Explanation of how the incident occurred

CONTROL MEASURES

Specific health and safety control measures are required by OSHA to eliminate or minimize the risk of occupational exposure in the medical office. These measures are divided into six categories: engineering controls, work practice controls, personal protective equipment, housekeeping, hepatitis B vaccination, and universal precautions.

Engineering Controls

The medical office must use engineering controls to eliminate or minimize the risk of occupational exposure. *Engineering controls* include all control measures that isolate or remove health hazards from the workplace. Engineering controls must be examined and maintained or replaced as required to ensure their effectiveness. Examples of engineering controls include the following:

- Readily accessible handwashing facilities
- Safer medical devices
- Biohazard sharps containers and biohazard bags
- Autoclaves

Safer Medical Devices

Safer medical devices are one example of an engineering control. A *safer medical device* is a device that, based on reasonable judgment, would make an exposure incident involving a contaminated sharp less likely. *Reasonable judgment* refers to the judgment of the health care worker who would be using the device.

Safer medical devices include sharps with engineered sharps injury protection and needleless systems. A *sharp with engineered sharps injury protection (SESIP)* is a nonneedle sharp or a needle device with a built-in safety feature used for procedures that involve the risk of a sharps injury. Examples of SESIPs include safety engineered syringes and phlebotomy devices (Figure B-3).

A *needleless system* is a device that does not use a needle for (1) the administration of medication or other fluids, (2) the collection or withdrawal of body fluids after initial access to a vein or artery is established, or (3) any other procedure involving the potential for occupational exposure to bloodborne pathogens as a result of percutaneous injuries from contaminated sharps. An example of a needleless system is a jet injection syringe, which uses compressed air to administer an injection rather than a needle.

Employers are required to evaluate and implement commercially available safer medical devices and other engineering controls that eliminate occupational exposure to the lowest extent feasible. Input from employees involved in direct patient care must be taken into consideration in making this determination. This helps to ensure that the individuals who are using the devices have the opportunity for input. As part of the annual review of the exposure control plan, the following information must be documented: (1) safer medical devices that reflect changes in technology are being evaluated

A

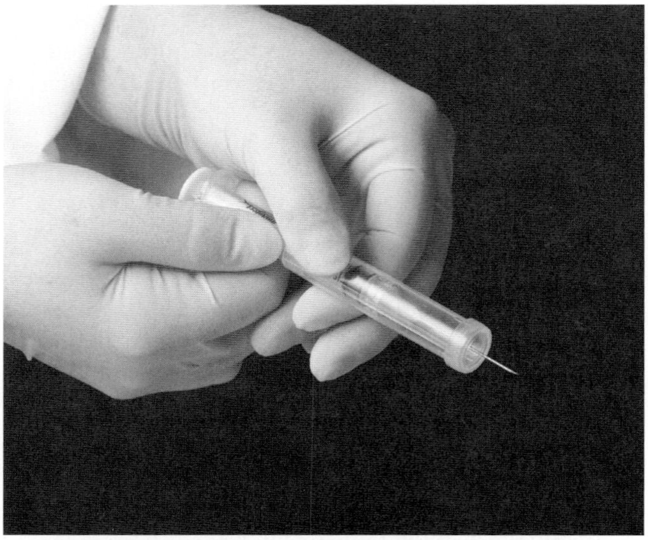

B

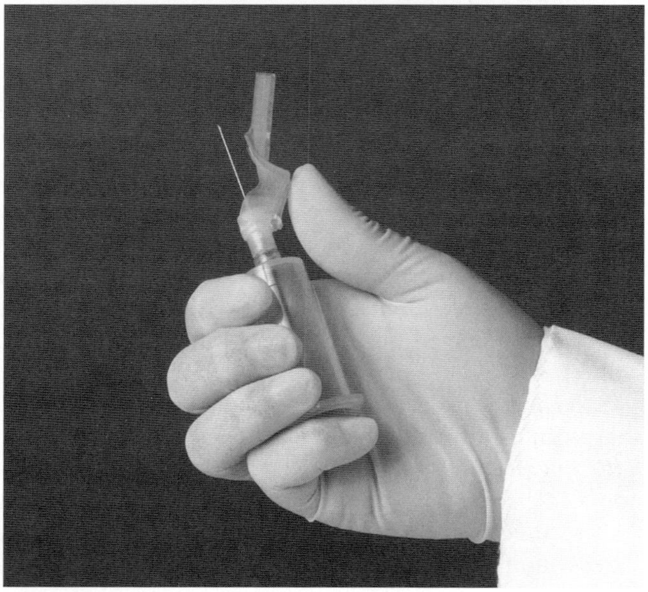

FIGURE B-3 A, Safety engineered syringe. **B,** Safety engineered phlebotomy device.

and implemented in the workplace, and (2) input was obtained from employees in selecting safer medical devices.

Work Practice Controls

Work practice controls reduce the likelihood of exposure by altering the manner in which the technique is performed. It is important to consistently adhere to these safety rules, which include the following:

1. Perform all procedures involving blood or other potentially infectious material in a manner to minimize splashing, spraying, spattering, and generation of droplets of these substances.
2. Observe warning labels on biohazard containers and appliances. Bags or containers that bear a biohazard warning label or are color-coded red indicate that they hold blood or other potentially infectious materials. Refrigerators, freezers, and other appliances that contain hazardous materials also must bear a biohazard warning label.

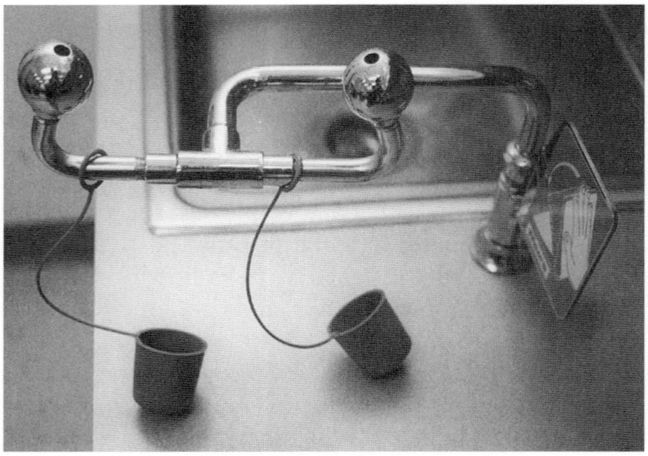

FIGURE B-4 Eye washing unit.

3. Bandage cuts and other lesions on the hands before gloving.
4. Sanitize the hands after removing gloves, regardless of whether or not the gloves are visibly contaminated.
5. If your hands or other skin surfaces come in contact with blood or other potentially infectious material, thoroughly wash the area as soon as possible with soap and water.
6. If your mucous membranes (e.g., eyes, mouth, nose) come in contact with blood or other potentially infectious material, flush them with water as soon as possible (figure B-4).
7. Do not break or shear contaminated needles.
8. Do not remove, recap, or bend a contaminated needle except in unusual circumstances when no other alternative is possible or when it is required by a specific medical procedure. Such actions must be performed by a method other than the traditional two-handed procedure. Needle removal can be accomplished with a one-handed technique using a sharps container with a well-designed unwinder. Recapping must be performed through the use of a one-handed technique; using a two-handed technique is strictly prohibited. The one-handed recapping technique involves holding the syringe in the dominant hand and picking up the needle with the cap using a scooping motion. The cap is secured onto the needle by pushing it against a hard surface. (*Note:* Sterile needles may be recapped, such as after the withdrawal of medication from a vial or ampule.)
9. Immediately after use, place contaminated sharps in a puncture-resistant, leakproof container that is appropriately labeled or color-coded. *Contaminated sharps* are contaminated objects that can penetrate

the skin, including (but not limited to) needles, lancets, scalpels, broken glass, and capillary tubes.

10. Do not eat, drink, smoke, apply cosmetics or lip balm, or handle contact lenses in areas where you may be exposed to blood or other potentially infectious materials.
11. Do not store food or drink in refrigerators, freezers, or cabinets or on shelves or countertops where blood or other potentially infectious materials are present.
12. Place blood specimens or other potentially infectious materials in containers that prevent leakage during collection, handling, processing, storage, transport, or shipping. Ensure the containers are closed before being stored, transported, or shipped and are labeled or color-coded for easy identification.
13. Before any equipment that might be contaminated is serviced or shipped for repair or cleaning, such as a centrifuge, it must be inspected for blood or other potentially infectious material. If such material is present, the equipment must be decontaminated. If it cannot be decontaminated, it must be appropriately labeled to indicate clearly the contamination site, to enable those coming into contact with the equipment to take appropriate precautions.
14. If you are exposed to blood or other potentially infectious materials, perform first aid measures immediately (e.g., wash a needlestick injury thoroughly with soap and water). After taking these measures, report the incident to your physician-employer as soon as possible so that postexposure procedures can be instituted. (See the box entitled *OSHA Postexposure Evaluation and Follow-Up Procedures.*) The most obvious exposure incident is a needlestick, but any eye, mouth, or other mucous membrane, nonintact skin, or parenteral contact with blood or other potentially infectious materials constitutes an exposure incident and should be reported.

Personal Protective Equipment

The OSHA standard specifies that personal protective equipment must be used in the medical office whenever occupational exposure remains after instituting engineering and work practice controls. *Personal protective equipment* is clothing or equipment that protects an individual from contact with blood or other potentially infectious materials; examples include gloves, chin-length face shields, masks, protective eyewear, laboratory coats, and gowns. The type of protective equipment appropriate for a given task depends on the degree of exposure that is anticipated, as outlined here:

1. Wear gloves when it is reasonably anticipated that your hands will have contact with blood and other potentially infectious materials, mucous membranes, or nonintact skin; when performing vascular access procedures; and when handling or touching contaminated surfaces or items. Gloves cannot prevent a needlestick or other sharps injury, but they can prevent a pathogen from entering the body through a break in the skin, such as a cut, abrasion, burn, or rash.
2. Wear chin-length face shields or masks in combination with eye-protection devices whenever splashes, spray, spatter, or droplets of blood or other potentially infectious materials may be generated, posing a hazard through contact with the eyes, nose, or mouth (e.g., removing a stopper from a tube of blood, transferring serum from whole blood) (Figure B-5).
3. Wear appropriate protective clothing, such as gowns, aprons, and laboratory coats, when gross contamination can reasonably be anticipated during performance of a task or procedure (e.g., laboratory testing procedure). The type of protective clothing depends on the task and degree of exposure anticipated.

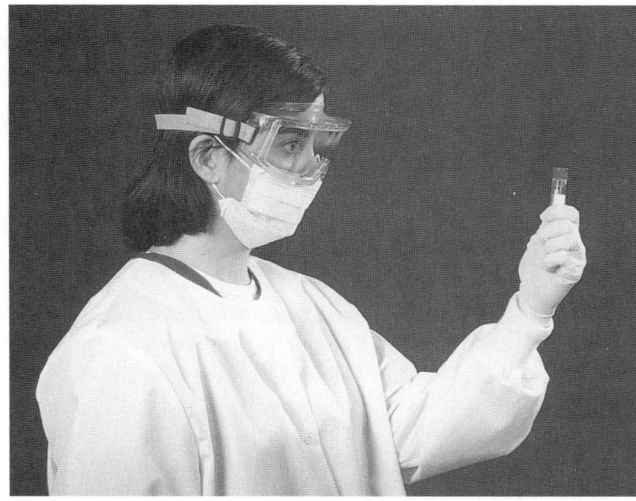

FIGURE B-5 Jennifer wears a combination mask and eye-protection device and a laboratory coat to protect against splashes, spray, spatter, and droplets of blood.

Personal Protective Equipment Guidelines. Certain guidelines must be followed when using protective equipment:

1. Protective equipment must not allow blood or other potentially infectious material to pass through or reach the skin, underlying garments (e.g., scrubs, street clothes, undergarments), eyes, mouth, or other mucous membranes under normal conditions of use and for the duration of time the protective equipment is used.
2. The employer must provide appropriate personal protective equipment at no cost to you. The employer is responsible for ensuring the equipment is available in appropriate sizes, is readily accessible, and is used correctly. In addition, the employer must ensure that

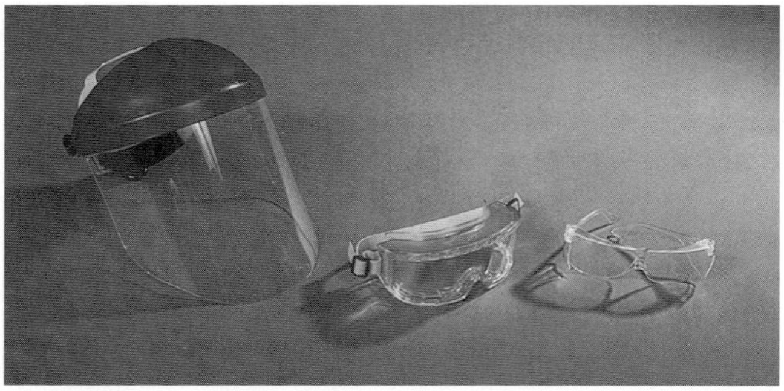

FIGURE B-6 Examples of Eye-protection Devices. *Left,* Face shield; *center,* goggles; *right,* glasses with solid side shields.

the equipment is cleaned, laundered, repaired, replaced, or disposed of as necessary to ensure its effectiveness.

3. Alternatives must be provided for employees who are allergic to the gloves normally provided. Examples of alternatives include hypoallergenic gloves and powderless gloves.
4. If gloves become contaminated, torn, or punctured, replace them as soon as practical.
5. All eye-protection devices must have solid side shields; chin-length face shields, goggles, and glasses with solid side shields are acceptable (Figure B-6); standard prescription eyeglasses are unacceptable as eye protection.
6. If a garment is penetrated by blood or other potentially infectious materials, it must be removed as soon as possible and placed in an appropriately designated container for washing.
7. All personal protective equipment must be removed before leaving the medical office.
8. When protective equipment is removed, it must be placed in an appropriately designated area or container for storage, washing, decontamination, or disposal.
9. Utility gloves may be decontaminated and reused unless they are cracked, peeling, torn, or punctured or no longer provide barrier protection.
10. If you believe using protective equipment would prevent proper delivery of health care or would pose an increased hazard to your safety or that of a coworker, in extenuating circumstances you may temporarily and briefly decline its use. After such an incident, the circumstances must be investigated to determine whether the situation could be prevented in the future.

Housekeeping

The OSHA standard requires that specific housekeeping procedures be followed to ensure that the work site is maintained in a clean and sanitary condition. The medical office must develop and implement a written schedule for cleaning and decontaminating each area

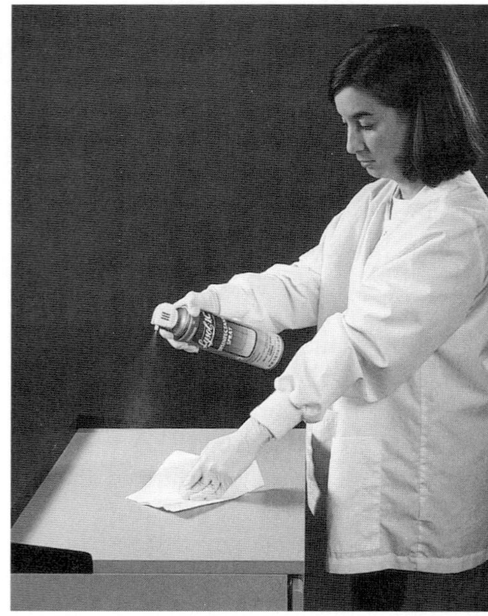

FIGURE B-7 Clean and decontaminate work surfaces with an appropriate disinfectant after completing procedures involving blood and other potentially infectious materials.

where exposure occurs. The cleaning and decontamination method must be specified for each task and should be based on the type of surface to be cleaned, the type of soil present, and the tasks or procedures being performed in that area. Housekeeping procedures include the following:

1. Clean and decontaminate equipment and work surfaces after completing procedures that involve blood or other potentially infectious materials. Cleaning is accomplished using a detergent soap, and decontamination is performed using an appropriate disinfectant (Figure B-7).
2. Clean and decontaminate all equipment and work surfaces as soon as possible after exposure to blood or other potentially infectious material. For the decontamination of blood spills, OSHA recommends the use of a 10% solution of sodium hypochlorite (household bleach) in water (1 part bleach to 10 parts water).
3. Inspect and decontaminate all reusable receptacles, such as bins, pails, and cans, on a regular basis. If contamination is visible, the item must be cleaned and decontaminated as soon as possible.
4. Do not pick up broken, contaminated glassware with the hands, even if gloves are worn. Use mechanical means, such as a brush and dustpan, tongs, and forceps (Figure B-8).
5. Protective coverings, such as plastic wrap and aluminum foil, may be used to cover work surfaces or equipment, but they must be removed or replaced if contamination occurs.
6. Handle contaminated laundry as little as possible and with appropriate personal protective equipment.

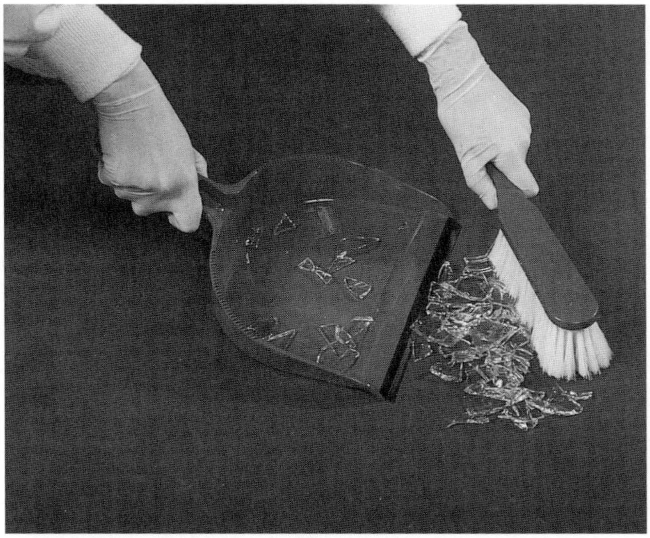

FIGURE B-8 Use mechanical means to pick up broken contaminated glass.

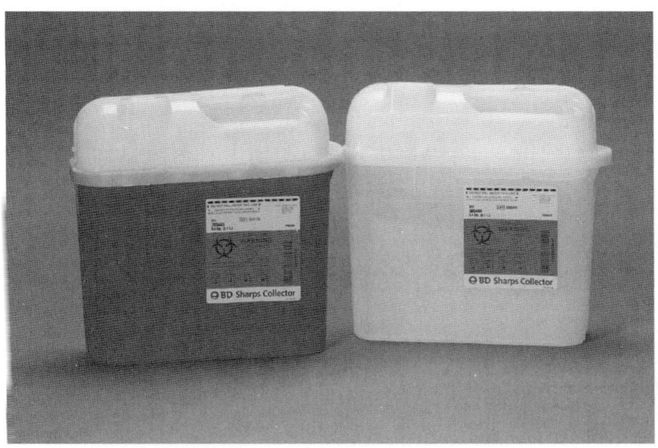

FIGURE B-9 Biohazard sharps containers.

Place all contaminated laundry in leakproof bags that are properly labeled or color-coded. Contaminated laundry must not be sorted or rinsed at the medical office.

7 If the outside of a biohazard container becomes contaminated, it must be placed in a second suitable container.

8. Biohazard sharps containers (Figure B-9) must be closable, puncture-resistant, and leakproof. They must bear a biohazard warning label and be color-coded red to ensure identification of the contents as hazardous. To ensure effectiveness, the following guidelines must be observed:
   - Locate the sharps container as close as possible to the area of use to avoid the hazard of transporting a contaminated needle through the workplace.
   - Maintain sharps containers in an upright position to keep liquid and sharps inside.
   - Do not reach into the sharps container with your hand.
   - Replace sharps containers on a regular basis, and do not allow them to overfill. (It is recommended that sharps containers be replaced when they are three-quarters full.)

HIGHLIGHT ON OSHA BLOODBORNE PATHOGENS STANDARD

General Information

The exposure control plan must be made available to OSHA on request.

OSHA inspectors are responsible for determining whether the medical office meets the Bloodborne Pathogens Standard. This is accomplished through a careful review of the exposure control plan, interviews with the medical office employer and employees, and observation of work activities.

Feces, nasal secretions, saliva, sputum, sweat, tears, urine, and vomitus are not considered by OSHA to be potentially infectious material unless they contain blood.

Control Measures

Employees must be trained in the proper use of the following: engineering controls (including safer medical devices), work practice controls, and personal protective equipment.

General work clothes, such as scrubs, uniforms, pants, shirts, and blouses, are not intended to function as protection against a hazard and are not considered personal protective equipment.

Employees are not permitted to launder contaminated clothing at home; it is the employer's responsibility to have contaminated clothing laundered.

If an employee is allergic to the standard latex gloves, the employer must provide a suitable alternative, such as hypoallergenic gloves.

Needlestick Injuries

The CDC estimates that every year 600,000 to 800,000 health care workers in the United States experience needlestick and other sharps injuries, and 1000 of these individuals contract serious infections as a result of these injuries. The CDC estimates that 62% to 88% of sharps injuries can be prevented by the use of safer medical devices.

A wide variety of commercially available safer medical devices have been developed to reduce the risk of needlestick and other sharps injuries.

Safer medical devices that eliminate exposure to the lowest extent feasible must be evaluated and implemented in the health care setting. The lack of injuries on the sharps injury log does *not* exempt the employer from this provision.

Hepatitis B Vaccination

The OSHA standard requires physicians to offer the hepatitis B vaccination series free of charge to all medical office personnel who have occupational exposure. The vaccination must be offered within 10 working days of initial assignment to a position with occupational exposure, unless the following factors exist: (1) The individual has previously received the hepatitis B vaccination series, (2) antibody testing has revealed that the indi-

HEPATITIS B VACCINE REFUSAL

I understand that due to my occupational exposure to blood or other potentially infectious materials, I may be at risk of acquiring hepatitis B virus (HBV) infection. I have been given the opportunity to be vaccinated with hepatitis B vaccine at no charge to myself. However, I decline hepatitis B vaccination at this time. I understand that by declining this vaccine I continue to be at risk of acquiring hepatitis B, a serious disease. If in the future I continue to have occupational exposure to blood or to other potentially infectious materials and I want to be vaccinated with hepatitis B vaccine, I can receive the vaccination series at no charge to me.

____
Employee Name (printed)

______________________________ _______________
Employee Signature Date

______________________________ _______________
Witness Signature Date

FIGURE B-10 Hepatitis B vaccine waiver form. This form must be signed by an employee with occupational exposure who declines hepatitis B vaccination.

vidual is immune to hepatitis B, or (3) the vaccine is contraindicated for medical reasons.

Medical office personnel who decline vaccination must sign a hepatitis B waiver form documenting refusal. This form must be filed in the employee's OSHA record (Figure B-10). Employees who decline vaccination may request the vaccination later, which the employer must then provide according to the aforementioned criteria.

Universal Precautions

Before the release of the OSHA standard, the CDC issued recommendations for health care workers known as the Universal Precautions. According to the concept of Universal Precautions, all human blood and certain human body fluids are treated as though known to be infectious for HIV, HBV, HCV, and other bloodborne pathogens. The OSHA standard states that the Universal Precautions must be observed; these precautions form the heart of the OSHA standard itself.

REGULATED MEDICAL WASTE

Medical waste is generated in the medical office through the diagnosis, treatment, and immunization of patients. Some of this waste poses a threat to health and safety and is known as **regulated medical waste (RMW)**. The OSHA Bloodborne Pathogens Standard defines RMW as follows:

- Any liquid or semiliquid blood or OPIM
- Items contaminated with blood or OPIM that would release these substances in a liquid or semiliquid state if compressed
- Items that are caked with dried blood or OPIM and are capable of releasing these materials during handling
- Contaminated sharps
- Pathologic and microbiologic wastes that contain blood or OPIM

HIGHLIGHT ON HEPATITIS B VACCINE

The hepatitis B vaccine became available in 1982 and is 95% effective in providing immunity.

The hepatitis B vaccine is well tolerated by most patients. The most common side effect is soreness at the injection site, including induration, erythema, and swelling. Occasionally, a low-grade fever, headache, and dizziness occur.

Current data show that the vaccine-induced antibodies may decline over time, but the immune system memory that programs the body to produce these antibodies remains intact indefinitely. Because of this, an individual with declining antibodies is still protected against hepatitis B. At present, the CDC does not recommend a booster dose once an individual has received the initial (three-dose) vaccine series.

The hepatitis B vaccine is recommended for all infants, children, and adolescents who are 18 years old or younger. It also is recommended for adults older than 18 years who are at increased risk for developing hepatitis B. This population includes employees with occupational exposure (e.g., health care workers), hemodialysis patients, hemophiliacs, individuals with multiple sex partners, homosexually active men, injection drug users, and household and sexual contacts of individuals with chronic hepatitis B.

The number of individuals contracting hepatitis B has decreased sharply since the development of the hepatitis B vaccine. As more people become immune to hepatitis B through the immunization of infants, the goal of eliminating hepatitis B in the United States may be realized.

Regulated medical waste must be discarded properly so as not to become a source of transfer of disease. According to the OSHA definition, a dressing saturated with blood is considered RMW and must be discarded in a biohazard bag. A bandage with a spot of blood on it is not considered RMW and can be discarded in a regular waste container.

Handling Regulated Medical Waste

Regulated medical waste must be handled carefully to prevent an exposure incident. The OSHA Bloodborne Pathogens Standard outlines specific actions to take when handling regulated medical waste, as follows:

1. Separate regulated waste from the general refuse at its point of origin. Disposable items containing regulated medical waste should be placed directly into biohazard containers and not mixed with the regular trash.
2. Ensure that biohazard containers are closable, leakproof, and suitably constructed to contain the contents during handling, storage, and transport. These containers include biohazard bags and sharps containers.
3. To prevent spillage or protrusion of the contents, close the lid of a sharps container before removing it from an examining room. Never open, empty, or clean a contaminated sharps container. If there is a chance of leakage from the sharps container, it should be placed in a second container that is closable, leakproof, and appropriately labeled or color-coded.
4. Securely close biohazard bags before removing them from an examining room. To provide additional protection, some medical offices double-bag by placing the primary bag inside a second biohazard bag.
5. Transport full biohazard containers to a secured area away from the general public, using personal protective equipment (e.g., gloves).

Disposal of Regulated Medical Waste

Each state is responsible for developing policies for disposal of regulated medical waste. To avoid noncompliance, it is important to know and understand the specific regulated waste policies and guidelines set forth in his or her state.

Most medical offices use a commercial medical waste service to dispose of regulated medical waste. The service is responsible for picking up and transporting the medical waste to a treatment facility for incineration to destroy pathogens and render it harmless. The waste can then be safely disposed of in a sanitary landfill. Regulated waste treatment facilities must be licensed and hold permits issued by the Environmental Protection Agency (EPA), allowing them to dispose of regulated medical waste.

A series of steps must be followed for preparing and storing regulated medical waste for pickup by the service. Although these steps may vary slightly from state to state, general measures required by most states include the following:

1. Place biohazard bags and sharps containers into a receptacle provided by the medical waste service. The receptacle is usually a cardboard box. The box should be securely sealed with packing tape, and a biohazard warning label must appear on two opposite sides of the box.
2. Store the biohazard boxes in a locked room inside the facility or in a locked collection container outside for pickup by the medical waste service. This step is aimed at preventing unauthorized access to items such as needles and syringes. The regulated waste storage area should be labeled with one of the following:
   - "Authorized Personnel Only" sign
   - International biohazard symbol
3. Many states require that a tracking record be completed when the waste is picked up by the medical waste service. The form includes such information as the type and quantity of waste (weighed in pounds) and where it is being sent. The form must be signed by a representative of the medical waste service and the medical office. After the waste has been destroyed at the regulated waste treatment facility, a record documenting its disposal is mailed to the medical office.

VENIPUNCTURE SAFETY PRECAUTIONS

The OSHA Bloodborne Pathogens Standard presented earlier must be carefully followed during the venipuncture procedure to avoid exposure to bloodborne pathogens. The following OSHA requirements apply specifically to the venipuncture procedure and to separation of serum or plasma from whole blood (see later):

1. Wear gloves when it is reasonably anticipated that you will have hand contact with blood.
2. Wear a face shield or mask in combination with an eye protection device whenever splashes, spray, splatter, or droplets of blood may be generated.
3. Perform all procedures involving blood in a manner so as to minimize splashing, spraying, splattering, and generating droplets of blood.
4. Bandage cuts and other lesions on the hands before gloving.
5. Sanitize hands as soon as possible after removing gloves.
6. If your hands or other skin surfaces come in contact with blood, wash the area as soon as possible with soap and water.
7. If your mucous membranes (e.g., eyes, nose, mouth) come in contact with blood, flush them with water as soon as possible.
8. Do not bend, break, or shear contaminated venipuncture needles.

9. Do not recap a contaminated venipuncture needle.
10. Locate the sharps container as close as possible to the area of use. Immediately after use, place the contaminated venipuncture needle (and plastic holder) in the biohazard sharps container.
11. Place blood specimens in containers that prevent leakage during collection, handling, processing, storage, transport, and shipping.
12. If you are exposed to blood, report the incident immediately to your physician-employer.

MICROBIOLOGIC SPECIMEN COLLECTION

If the physician suspects that a particular disease is caused by a pathogen, he or she may want to obtain a specimen for microbiologic examination. This examination identifies the pathogen causing the disease and aids in the diagnosis. If a urinary tract infection is suspected, a urine specimen is obtained for bacterial examination. In this instance, a clean-catch midstream collection is required to obtain a specimen that excludes the normal flora of the urethra and urinary meatus.

A **specimen** is a small sample or part taken from the body to represent the whole. One might be responsible for collecting specimens from certain areas of the body, such as the throat, nose, and wound. One might also be responsible for assisting the physician in the collection of specimens from other areas, such as the cervix, vagina, urethra, and rectum. In most instances, a sterile swab is used to collect the specimen. A *swab* is a small piece of cotton wrapped around the end of a slender wooden or plastic stick. It is passed across a body surface or opening to obtain a specimen for microbiologic analysis.

To prevent inaccurate test results, good techniques of medical and surgical asepsis must be practiced when a specimen is obtained. One must be careful not to contaminate the specimen with *extraneous microorganisms.* These are undesirable microorganisms that can enter the specimen in various ways; they grow and multiply and possibly obscure and prevent identification of pathogens that might be present. To prevent extraneous microorganisms (i.e., normal flora) from contaminating the specimen, all supplies used to obtain the specimen (e.g., swabs and specimen containers) must be sterile. In addition, the specimen should not contain microorganisms from areas surrounding the collection site. When obtaining a throat specimen, the swab should not be allowed to touch the inside of the mouth.

The OSHA Bloodborne Pathogens Standard presented in this chapter should be carefully followed when performing microbiologic procedures. Specifically, one must wear gloves when it is reasonably anticipated that hand contact might occur with blood or other potentially infectious materials. Eating, drinking, smoking, and applying makeup are strictly forbidden when one is working with microorganisms because pathogens can be transmitted through hand-to-mouth contact. In addition, labels for specimen containers should not be licked, and any break in the skin, such as a cut or scratch, must be covered with a bandage. If some of the material in the specimen is accidentally touched, the area of contact should be washed immediately and thoroughly with soap and water. If the specimen comes in contact with the worktable, the table should be cleaned immediately with soap and water followed by a suitable disinfectant, such as phenol. The worktable also should be cleaned with a disinfectant at the end of each day.

After collection, the specimen must be placed in its proper container with the lid securely fastened. The container must be clearly labeled with the patient's name, the date, the source of the specimen, the worker's initials, and any other required information.

Handling and Transporting Microbiologic Specimens

After the microbiologic specimen has been collected, care should be taken in handling and transporting it. Delay in processing the specimen may cause the death of pathogens or the overgrowth of the specimen by microorganisms that are part of the normal flora usually collected along with the pathogen from the specimen site. If the specimen is to be analyzed in the medical office, it should be examined under the microscope or cultured immediately. Otherwise, it should be preserved (if possible) with the method used by the medical office.

Specimens transported to an outside medical laboratory by a courier service are usually placed in a transport medium. The transport medium prevents drying of the specimen and preserves it in its original state until it reaches its destination. Transport media are discussed in more detail in the section on "Collection and Transport Systems."

Outside laboratories provide the medical office with specific instructions on the care and handling of specimens being transported to them. These specimens must be accompanied by a laboratory request that designates the physician's name and address; the patient's name, age, and gender; the date and time of collection; the type of microbiologic examination requested; the source of the specimen (e.g., throat, wound, urine); and the physician's clinical diagnosis. There is usually a space on the form to indicate whether the patient is receiving antibiotic therapy. Antibiotics may suppress the growth of bacteria, a factor that could produce false-negative results.

OSHA SAFETY PRECAUTIONS

To avoid exposure to bloodborne pathogens and other potentially infectious materials, the OSHA Bloodborne

Pathogens Standard presented earlier should be followed when performing first aid. The following guidelines help reduce or eliminate the risk of infection:

1. Make sure that your first aid kit contains personal protective equipment, such as gloves, a face shield and mask, and a pocket mask.
2. Wear gloves when it is reasonably anticipated that your hand will come into contact with the following: blood and other potentially infectious materials, mucous membranes, nonintact skin, and contaminated articles or surfaces.
3. Perform all first aid procedures involving blood or other potentially infectious materials in a manner that minimizes splashing, spraying, spattering, and generation of droplets of these substances.
4. Wear protective clothing and gloves to cover cuts or other lesions of the skin.
5. Sanitize your hands as soon as possible after removing gloves.
6. Avoid touching objects that may be contaminated with blood or other potentially infectious materials.
7. If your hands or other skin surfaces come in contact with blood or other potentially infectious materials, wash the area as soon as possible with soap and water.
8. If your mucous membranes (in eyes, nose, and mouth) come in contact with blood or other potentially infectious materials, flush them with water as soon as possible.
9. Avoid eating, drinking, and touching your mouth, eyes, and nose while providing emergency care or before you sanitize your hands.
10. If you are exposed to blood or other potentially infectious materials, report the incident as soon as possible to your physician so that postexposure procedures can be instituted.

LABORATORY HAZARDS

Chemical Hazards

The clinical laboratory is home to chemicals that are fl ammable, **caustic**, poisonous, **carcinogenic**, and/or **teratogenic**. Exposureto these dangers can be through inhalation, direct absorptionthrough the skin, ingestion, entry through a mucous membrane,or entry through a break in the skin. OSHA is involved in regulating the standards directed at minimizing occupational exposure to hazardous chemicals in laboratories. The OSHA hazard communication standard (known as the employee "right to know" rule) became law in 1991 and ensures that laboratory workers are fully aware of the hazards associated with their workplace. The law necessitates the development of a comprehensive plan to implement safe practice throughout the laboratory insofar as chemicals are concerned. This chemical hygiene plan must outline the specific work practices and procedures that are needed to protect workers from any health hazards that may arise from working with in-stock chemicals. Information and training must be provided to all workers. There must be a Material Safety Data Sheet (MSDS) on file for all chemicals in use in the laboratory. OSHA requires the manufacturer of the chemical to make the sheets available, usually as a package insert.

Each MSDS contains the basic information about the specific chemical or product. This includes the trade name, chemical name and synonyms, chemical family, manufacturer's name and address, emergency telephone number, hazardous ingredients, physical data, fire and explosion data, and health hazard and protection information (Figure B-11).

Following principles of proper handling will reduce your risks of harmful effects. Harmful exposure can be reduced by using proper devices for pipetting; never pipet by mouth. If a chemical produces toxic or fl ammable vapors, work under a fume hood that exhausts air to the outside. In case of accidental exposure to the skin, rinse the affected area under running water for at least 5 minutes. Remove any clothing that is contaminated. If chemicals are splashed in the eyes, fl ush the eyes with water from an eyewash station for a minimum of 15 minutes. Prompt medical attention must be given to victims of chemical exposure.

Chemicals should be tightly sealed and properly labeled. A hazard identification system was developed by the National Fire Protection Association that provides, at a glance, information on the potential health, fl ammability, and chemical reactivity hazards of materials. This identification system consists of four small, colored, diamond-shaped symbols grouped into a larger diamond shape. The top diamond is red and indicates fl ammability hazard. The diamond on the left is blue and indicates hazards to health. The bottom diamond is white and provides special hazard information including radioactivity, special biohazards, and other dangerous situations. Finally, the diamond on the right is yellow and indicates reactivity or stability hazard. The system indicates the severity of the hazard by using numbers imprinted in the diamonds from 0 to 4, with 4 being extremely hazardous to 0 being no hazard (Figure B-12).

MATERIAL SAFETY DATA SHEET

MSDS NO. 396
PAGE 1

SECTION 1 IDENTIFICATION

MANUFACTURER'S NAME: Corelis Corporation
ADDRESS: P.O. Box 93
Camden, NJ 08106

EMERGENCY TELEPHONE NUMBER: 1 (800) 733-8690

TELEPHONE NUMBER FOR INFORMATION: 1 (800) 331-0766

ISSUED: 10/99

IDENTITY: 2% Aqueous Glutaraldehyde Solution

PREPARED BY: Regulatory Affairs

PRODUCT CODE: 3345

TRADE NAME: Aldecyde

SYNONYMS: None

CHEMICAL FAMILY: Aldehydes

MOLECULAR FORMULA: $OHCC_3H_6CHO$ (Active)

RTECS #: MA 2450000 (Active)

MOLECULAR WEIGHT: 100

HAZARD RATING – HEALTH: 3 (Serious Hazard) FLAMMABILITY: 0 REACTIVITY:0 SPECIFIC: NONE

SECTION 2 HAZARDOUS INGREDIENTS/IDENTITY INFORMATION

COMPONENTS (SPECIFIC CHEMICAL IDENTITY)	CAS #	%	OSHA PEL	ACGIH TLV	OSHA 1910.1200
Glutaraldehyde (active)	111-30-8	2	0.2ppm, C	0.2ppm, C	n/a
Inert buffer salts	n/a		None	None	Nonhazardous
Water	7732-18-5	98	None	None	Nonhazardous

SECTION 3 PHYSICAL/CHEMICAL CHARACTERISTICS

APPEARANCE AND ODOR: 2 components: colorless fluid and liquid salts; turns green when activated. Sharp odor masked with peppermint fragrance.

BOILING POINT: 212°F

SPECIFIC GRAVITY (H_2O=1): 1.003 g/cc

VAPOR PRESSURE (mm Hg): same as water

MELTING POINT: n/a

VAPOR DENSITY (AIR=1): same as water

EVAPORATION RATE (H_2O=1): 0.98

SOLUBILITY IN WATER: complete

pH: 8

FREEZING POINT: same as water

ODOR THRESHOLD: .04 ppm, detectable. (ACGIH)

SECTION 4 FIRE AND EXPLOSION HAZARD DATA

FLASH POINT (METHOD USED): None FLAMMABLE LIMITS – LEL: nd UEL: nd

EXTINGUISHING MEDIA: If water is evaporated, material can burn. Use carbon dioxide or dry chemical for small fires. Use foam (alcohol, polymer or ordinary) or water fog for large fires.

SPECIAL FIRE FIGHTING PROCEDURES: Self-contained breathing apparatus and protective clothing should be available to fireman.

UNUSUAL FIRE AND EXPLOSION HAZARDS: None

TOXIC GASES PRODUCED: None

SECTION 5 REACTIVITY DATA

STABILITY: 212°F

CONDITIONS TO AVOID: None

INCOMPATIBILITY (MATERIALS TO AVOID): None

HAZARDOUS DECOMPOSITION OR BYPRODUCTS: None

HAZARDOUS POLYMERIZATION: Will not occur

FIGURE B-11 Material safety data sheet (MSDS). *(From Bonewit-West K: Clinical procedures for medical assistants, ed 6, Philadelphia, 2004. Saunders.)*

MATERIAL SAFETY DATA SHEET **MSDS NO. 396**
PAGE 2

SECTION 6 HEALTH HAZARD DATA

ROUTE(S) OF ENTRY – INHALATION: yes SKIN: yes INGESTION: yes EYE: yes

SIGNS AND SYMPTOMS OF EXPOSURE:

EYES: Contact with eyes causes damage.

SKIN: Can cause skin sensitization. Avoid skin contact.

INHALATION: Vapors may be irritating and cause headache, chest discomfort, symptoms of bronchitis.

INGESTION: May cause nausea, vomiting and general systemic illness.

EMERGENCY AND FIRST AID PROCEDURE:

EYES: Flush thoroughly with water. Get medical attention.

SKIN: Flush thoroughly with water. If irritation persists, get medical attention.

INHALATION: Remove to fresh air. If symptoms persist, get medical attention.

INGESTION: Do not induce vomiting. Drink copious amount of milk. Get medical attention.

HEALTH HAZARDS (ACUTE AND CHRONIC):
Acute: As listed above under Signs and Symptoms of Exposure
Chronic: None known from currently available information.

MEDICAL CONDITIONS GENERALLY AGGRAVATED BY EXPOSURE: None known from currently available information.

LISTED AS CARCINOGEN BY – NTP: yes IARC MONOGRAPHS: no OSHA: no

TOXICITY:		
	ORAL LD50 (Rat)	Toxicity Rating 1: 500-5000 mg/kg.
	OCULAR (Rabbit)	Toxicity Rating 2: Irritating or moderately persisting more than seven days with.
	DERMAL LD50 (Rabbit)	None by dermal route.
	INHALATION LC50 (Rabbit)	Irritating but non-toxic at highest concentration achieved (2.89 ppm).

SECTION 7 PRECAUTIONS FOR SAFE HANDLING AND USE

STEPS TO BE TAKE IN CASE MATERIAL IS RELEASED OR SPILLED: For LARGE spills, use ammonium carbonate to "neutralize" glutaraldehyde odor. Collect liquid and discard it. For SMALL spills, wipe with sponge or mop down area with an equal mixture of household ammonia and water. Flush with large quantities of water.

WASTE DISPOSAL METHOD: Triple rinse empty container with water and dispose in an incinerator or landfill approved for pesticide containers. Discard solution with large quantities of water.

EPA HAZARDOUS WASTE NUMBER: n/a

PRECAUTIONS TO BE TAKEN IN HANDLING AND STORING: Use normal storage and handling requirements.

SECTION 8 TRANSPORTATION DATA AND ADDITIONAL INFORMATION

DOMESTIC (D.O.T.): Aldehydes, N.O.S.

PROPER SHIPPING NAME: Glutaraldehyde

HAZARD CLASS: None

LABELS: None Needed

REPORTABLE QUANTITY: None

INTERNATIONAL (I.M.O.): Aldehydes, N.O.S.

PROPER SHIPPING NAME: Glutaraldehyde

HAZARD CLASS: None

LABELS: None Needed

UN/NA: 1989

FIGURE B-11, cont'd Material safety data sheet (MSDS). *(From Bonewit-West K: Clinical procedures for medical assistants, ed 6, Philadelphia, 2004, Saunders.)*
Continued

MATERIAL SAFETY DATA SHEET — **MSDS NO. 396** PAGE 3

SECTION 9 CONTROL MEASURES

VENTILATION:
ROUTINE: Product should be used in a covered container. Use with standard room ventilation (air conditioning); natural draft.
EMERGENCY: Enhanced ventilation

RESPIRATORY PROTECTION:
ROUTINE: None required
EMERGENCY: Organic vapor cartridge, canister mask

EYE PROTECTION:
ROUTINE: Safety glasses recommended
EMERGENCY: Safety glasses

SKIN PROTECTION:
ROUTINE: Impervious gloves
EMERGENCY: Impervious gloves; Protective clothing; Rubber boots

WORK/HYGIENIC PRACTICES: Avoid contamination of food

SECTION 10 SPECIAL REQUIREMENTS

None

KEY:
n/a = Not Applicable
nd = Not Determined
C = Ceiling
PEL = Permissible Exposure Level
RTECS = Registry of Toxic Effects of Chemical Substances
* = Trademark

FIGURE B-11, cont'd Material safety data sheet (MSDS). *(From Bonewit-West K: Clinical procedures for medical assistants, ed 6, Philadelphia, 2004, Saunders.)*

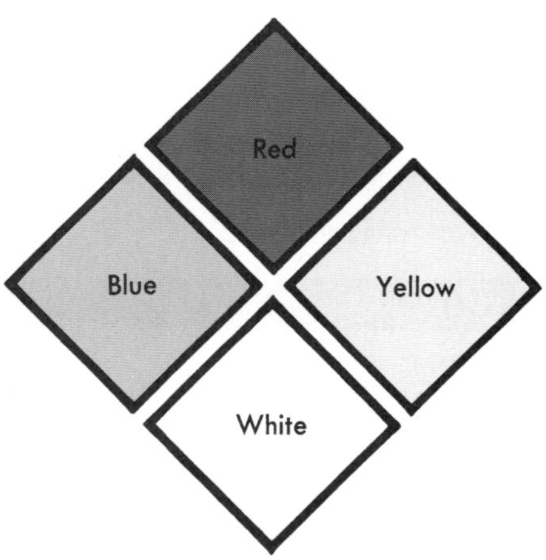

FIGURE B-12 Identification system of the National Fire Protection Association.

APPENDIX C

Acknowledgments

CCi
CORINTHIAN COLLEGES, INC.

RECEIPT OF HANDBOOK

Date: ____________________

To: All Allied Health Students

Subject: Acknowledgment

I have received a copy of the Student Handbook.

______________________________ ______________________________

Print Name Here Date

____

Signature

CCi
CORINTHIAN
COLLEGES, INC.

STUDENT VERIFICATION OF HIPAA TRAINING CURRICULUM CONTENT

Student Name

____

Last First Middle Initial

Date of Birth: ____________________ Social Security Number: ____________________

Profession for Which Student Is Training: ____________________

This form certifies that the above named participant has successfully completed the required HIPAA (Health Insurance Portability and Accountability Act) training. Additionally, the student has passed a HIPAA exam based on this material, with a score of 75% or higher. This test has been placed in the student's permanent academic file.

Date of HIPAA Training: ____________________

I certify that the above individual has been presented with the HIPAA handout. The student has read the handout and agrees to comply with all requirements.

Instructor Name: ____________________

Title: ____________________

CCi
CORINTHIAN
COLLEGES, INC.

School/Program: ____________________

Date of Verification: ____________________

CCi
CORINTHIAN
COLLEGES, INC.

OSHA PROTECTIVE PRACTICES

Date: ____________________

To: All Allied Health Students

Subject: OSHA Blood / Airborne Pathogens Protective Practices

The attached handout is required reading for all Allied Health students. If any student does not understand the material, he/she should ask the instructor for clarification.

The instructors have presented this material as well as shown the film.

I have received the OSHA Blood / Airborne Pathogens handout. I have read the handout and will comply with all requirements.

______________________________ ______________________________

Print Name Here Date

____

Signature